Molecular Diseases
4

Prof. Dr. Sami AL-Mudhaffar

1

Contents

Chapter one

Techniques used in Medicine

It is used in the separation and diagnosis of many chemical compounds, biological, etc. There are many types of chromatography including adsorption and ion exchange retail and gel filtration and other technical methods for the purpose of use paper and thin layer and gas chromatography.

Chromatography include multiple ways that all based on the separation of compounds based on the difference in migration through the passage in the center of force, as well as the tendency to face hard "Stationary phase" for central transgeneration and face the hard nature solid or gaseous, or liquid depends on the tendency of various materials to hard to face multiple methods such as adsorption "Adsorption" ion exchange "Ion exchange" may include all kinds of chromatography of these methods.

Based on the tendency of the ions or molecules to materials other than for mobile and non- soluble, which owns the distinct shipments, or molecules that carry one or more of the positive charge exchange with the positive charge associated with the Ionia face, the mobile Resins "Resins" with a negative charge is called this ion exchange process with the positive charge "Cation exchange" and reverse ion exchange is called a negative charge. Examples of the reciprocals of the ion non- animated "Immobile Ion Exchange" that are used in chemical research.

Polystyrene where will attend the multi-way styrene polymerization contributory "Copolymerization" with composite "Divinyl benzene", which adds to the styrene chains cross- shaped multi- written and added then aggregates the active ions altering the chemical composition of the original units that can be prepared for example, styrene resin that contains strong acid groups such as SO_3H hold process of "Styrene-Divinyl Benzene sulfonation". In the same way can be prepared that contains the totals as strong as NR^{3+}, or weak acid groups such as the COOH groups or grass- roots groups such as NH^{3+} and types of preparation depends on the ion concentration reciprocals composite "Divinyl benzene" the amount of strings cross referred to the number listed after the name of the resin, such as "8X" Dowex 50, which contains 8% of the "Divinyl benzene".

The type of chromatography by gel filtration on the difference in the movement of compounds during the gels with regular pores partially used for the purpose of the way in a column filled with from one type of granulated gel filtration.

The pores is able to expel particles with, partial weights more than 10000 if we, for example at the top of the column a small scale solution of dissolved protein and molecular weight of 70,000 with ammonium sulfate the following happens:

• Protein molecules expelled from the pores of granulated gel filtration.

- The migration of protein size start "void volum" outside the granules column.
- Interference ions NH^{+4} and SO^{-4} small pores of the gel granules nomination so there is the amount of liquid required for the expulsion of these molecules outside the pores.

The granules are gel filtration where proteins are separated by major united ammonium by successive periods of time and be dependent on the size of the separation- free liquid, gel filtration is very important ways often used to separate proteins from salts "Desalting". Electrophoresis is applied techniques migration electric technology application. It is accurate in the middle of an insulator as a result the electric field moves in a minute steady pace, and can then measured the balance between the electric power Eq, and the light of that we get the equation.

The gel gromotography is the primary means of separation and purification of various enzymes and proteins, as well as the fragmentation of nucleic acids and proteins in the treatment, especially when quantitative diagnosis of some human diseases, as well as by the method of the exchange of tritium to test the protein structure or the structure of DNA and a study of the link between proteins and small molecules. The thin layer chromatography is mainly used for amino acids, polysaccharides and simple sugars, fat and various steroids and other small molecules. The ion exchange chromatography applications, including chromatography cellulose DNA, to purify proteins associated with DNA to separate in general the Bio-compounds according to molecular weights. The affinity chromatography is used to purify the enzymes and antibodies and transport proteins, membrane proteins and the chips and sugary proteins and the separation of animal cells in particular.

Immunological methods

5

The developed immunologic tests, which are used to estimate small quantities of antigenic non- radioactive compounds in a mixture of large numbers and quantities of miscellaneous materials testing immune- ray equivalent to or greater than the sensitivity tests of natural chromatography. That the purpose of radio-immunoassay test is to assess the basic particles:

- Those that were not labeled by radioactivity within the body by proper specific activity or without adequate labeling of other compounds.
- Those do not know the identity, it could interact jointly and thus to compete with the antigen known.

There are many substances that are measured in the test radioimmunoassay, including the hormones and pharmaceutical agents, vitamins, and factors assigned and materials in the blood and viral antigens (viral) nucleic acids and nucleotides. In some cases, there is no acceptable method for the preparation of labeled antigen, which is permitted by measuring these materials using immuno-radio metric method, which can be measured by an unknown amount of antigen directly, through its combination with specie labeled. Examples of immunological methods that used in the biological tests of:

- Diagnosis and weakening the various types of bacteria by agglutination.
- Diagnosis of (viruses) by inhibition of virus generated by agglutination of red blood cells especially the antibody present in the serum.
- Diagnosis of gonadotrophin in the urine of pregnant women by testing the inhibition test and complements.
- Measurement of making DNA in phage infected by complement fixation.
- Diagnosis of relations between proteins by specific reaction.
- Diagnosis of tumors.
- Testing materials of clinical importance in children.

Immunoassay

The development in many areas of clinical medicine by "Yallow & Berson", which developed a radio- immunoassay technique "RIA" for the purpose of measuring the concentrations of very low- lying materials and the offer of "displacement" antigen, which is marked by radiation from the body own by adding increasing concentrations of antigen, the record is marked by radiation and this applies well in the science of hormones, as the hormone levels in the bloodstream always be very low, making it difficult to measure ways of life and conventional chemical. There are many hormones that can be measured easily and quickly test by radiation immuno assay including, prolactin, which was found to be associated with spinal tumor glandular "anterior pituitary gland tumor" and more permanent with symptoms by menstrual "Menstrual disturbance". In fact, the measurement become a part essential to the tests of modern futility "infertility".

Measurement by radio- immunoassay and other methods of link

There are three methods of test for the purpose of measuring the materials of life:

- Biological assays.
- Binding assays.
- Physical chemical assays.

There are also two types of tests in cases of binding namely:

- Test the link "Ligand".
- Tests of Binder.

The test of linking section are all kinds of bands that can be used, namely:

- Cell receptors.
- Circulating binding protein.
- Antibody.

The types of acquisitions "Tracers" used are included:

7

- Particle.
- Fluorescent.
- Enzyme.
- Isotope.

Applications of the main principles of radio- immunoassay test

Radio-immunoassay test depends on the competition between the antigen, which is labeled and non-labeled sites on the anti body component complexes ratio on the amount of antigen without radioactivity.

Using these antibodies tagged for the diagnosis and distribution of antigens by the optical microscope or electron microscope in tissue sections and sandwich technique used widely. The unlabeled antibody is 88

placed on the section washed with labeled antibody increases and the layer enzyme linked or marked by "fluorescence" against immune "Immunoglobuin" and can therefore be signaling antigen under examination.

This technique in applied research (Bio and medical research) Examples using antibodies "antisera ordinary polyclonal" on the "Topographical mapping" of the various types of cells in tissues such as "islets of Langerhans".

The immuno tissue chemistry containing various anti blood serum describes beta cells of containing insulin, located in the central mass of the island "islet" cells while the A cell that secrete glucagon in the peripheral side linking them to the cells D secreting "somatostatin". An examples on these the use of monoclonal antibody in the clinical diagnosis of tissue "histopathological" of the disease when the test of the "Lymph nodes biopsy" where it help in the classification of a certain type of lymphoma "lymphoid tumor" (e.g. Hodgkin's disease and various types of lymphoma "Lymphoma").

These antigens are characterized by being glycoprotein's present on the cells, especially white blood cells in humans and is then called human white blood cells, "Human leukocyte antigen" (HLAs). Carrying this antigen genes of the immune response status, where they control antigens were present in different tissues in the body, in addition to genes, there are mismatch humoral immune response "Humoral" and cellular "Cellular".

Immunodeficiency resulting from the lack of a genetic condition in the inability to create an immune cell, or one of its outputs and symptoms of the disease- causing immune deficiency commensurate with the degree of destitution and accompany him.

One of the examples on the case the disease resulting from this deficiency (AIDS), "Acquired immunodeficiency syndrome" (AIDS) or acquired immune deficiency syndrome and was attributable to a virus of the type of regression "retrovirus" with a tendency to lymphatic cells "T" in humans, called "Human T cell lymphocyte".

This virus has several methods to spread such as blood and mucus and the interface is accompanied by injury to the virus to many diseases, so called on the situation of the disease and syndrome of one disease. The assumption is based on the perception of geometric depends on logic that a collapse of the immune system caused by AIDS, produced by relationship engineering between HIV (human immunodeficiency) in the body of the infected and the immune system where it is can do the following:
- Cloning of the virus rapidly that destroy large number of cells of the system as there are two types of tests in cases of a binding.
- Faces a viral reproduction for many years through every defensive response to prevent the virus from reproducing.

9

- An imbalance in the latter for the benefit of the virus "HIV" event leading to AIDS.
- It can show new geometric forms of the virus as a result of mutations that be able avoid the defense forces of the body in some way, and confuse the immune system, which enable many patients to stay healthy for many years, finally collapse due to the boom continued, speaking of the virus.

Diagnostic Imaging

In medical diagnosis it is adopted mainly on the knowledge of diagnostic imaging technology spectrum, including the use of X-rays and gamma rays from, which is characterized by being electromagnetic radiation ionizing radiation, then began to think about using the term of this non- ionizing radiation infrared or microwave radiation and technical NMR magnet. The examples of spectral techniques used in diagnostic imaging:

- X- rays
- Gamma- ray
- Ultrasound
- Infrared
- Anti electric tissue
- Visual mechanisms

X-ray

The oldest techniques that is used in diagnosis and therefore will not focus on the importance of being where they were getting on the first pictorial representation of various tissues obtain after the development that is built on a limited computer assistance.

Gamma rays

The purpose of gamma-ray is the imaging profile then it was developed as computer- assisted also in the eighties which was called "ECT" and was then developed using imaging "Postiron emission tomography (PET)" where the radiation of tissue is carried out by position (positively charged) and thus can get a picture to clarify the life processes of the tissues that carry electrons and draw.

Ultrasonography

The speed of these waves are characterized by being less of electromagnetic waves, which provides an opportunity to measure the fetus as well as during the stages of development in the womb, added to that the fact that this technique is based on the fact that the X-ray is not ionized therefore it is not a preferred use in diagnostic imaging

Nuclear magnetic resonance imaging

Despite this technology it is old, but it was then developed for the purpose of medical diagnostic imaging has gone from the seventies, where the nuclei of atoms is measured by the disposal of certain substances found in different body tissues. The criterion for the disposal of these seizures depends on the radio pulses that are similar to the frequency in the field of outer-core magnet and thus to obtain a diagnostic can be used.

In the medical applications for the purification of nuclear magnetic resonance imaging to obtain imagery of infarction that occurs in some parts of the brain and important developments in this area the integration of multiple techniques and access to advanced apparatus for nuclear resonance imaging, including the "TMR" and "MRI".

It is important experiments that experiments are used the magnet resonance imaging of kidney transplantation, which was filmed nearby parts of the kidney and then infected the interactions that take place within the body after transplantation and efficiency of the cultivated parts. As well as imaging of tumors within the liver and liver imaging at the time of myocardial fibrosis or within, as possible, filming parts of the stomach and colon and to identify tumors. It was also to obtain information about stroke and is believed to imagery obtained of cancerous tumors of the brain were more pronounced than the use of X-ray.

It can be measured by any inflation occurs as a result of heart disease, and can also study the problems of the heart due to the presence of any obstruction or infarction in one of the blood vessels and could also portray the evolution of stroke, heart attack and its impact on the heart.

A nuclear magnetic resonance imaging "MRI"

This device is used which was created as a result of the development in the technology of magnetic resonance spectrum by the registration of spectra of life processes taking place within the animal body where the magnet- making with full slot by placing the human within the magnet and thus these devices provide a complete picture of the part which is conceived, and the advantage of the fact that this device magnetic field is not harmful, and the microwave radiation used is not harmful too.

It is possible through this device to study the effects of ongoing parts of the human body while taking a particular medicine can also be follow-up of the various core elements and sequentially, as well as to study the changes occurring stereoisomers of chemicals inside the cell as a result with other molecules.

Labeling with radioactivity

Require a lot of chemical analysis revealed small amounts of material with amount of concentrations $10^{-4} - 10^{-6}$ molari therefore it requires the development of other ways to respond to the concentration of low- lying, such as the development of experimental   methods by radioactive to solve many of the other problems that might face them. Some of these methods that could be used by dual- labeling for follow-up of two similar materials formed at various times by pulse method for follow-up fugitive substance at a time after the configuration without interference of other material. An example is the use of radioactive materials in the chemistry of life:

- Choose a material that resides on small concentrations, which are difficult to measure by direct chemical methods.
- Distinguishing similar molecules in different chemical sites.
- Analysis of mixtures that are very complex, which can not be done by various conventional chemical methods. Including:
- Enzyme interactions (DNA polymerase).
- Measurement of molecular weight of the DNA by labeling the final group.
- Diagnosis particle by settling with the anti body. Protein purification, which does not have a chemical test.
- Diagnosis of active centers of enzymes.

The isotopic properties will make the labeled compound more easily identifiable. For example, the radioiodine – labeled thyroxine molecules can be identified and quantified easily by virtue of their radioactivity.

The use of isotopes, both stable and radioactive, has proved great body of information in the medical scince. Stable isotopes are non radioactive and are suitable for use as tracers in humans. Especially infants children and pregnant women, stable isotopes

13

have also been used in the quantative analysis of various substances in recent years.

Isotopes in clinical chemistry:

The isotopic properties will make the labeled compound more easily identifiable. For example, the radiodine-lablled thyroxine molecules can be identified and quantified easily by virtue of their radioactivity.

The use of isotopes, both stable and radioactive, has provided great body of information in the medical science. Stable isotopes are non radioactive and are suitable for use as tracers in humans, especially infants children and pregnant women, stable isotopes have also been used in the quantitative analysis of various substances in recent years.

Radioactivity measurments depends on the ability of radionuclides to produce ionized or excited atoms within the detector. Two basic types of radiation detectors are in common use : gas ionization and scintillation. Radioisotopes allow the detection of minute quantities and differentiate physically between substances.

The use of radioactive isotopes in biochemistry and clinical chemistry has provided us with a wealth of information about biological processes, that offers such as adiverse range of applications, using enzyme assays, biochemical pathways of synthesis and degradation, analysis of biomolecules, measurements of antibodies, binding and transport studies. The use of radionuclide in nuclear medicine began when Frederick proescher published the paper entitled the use of radium for therapy of various diseases. Early experimental and diagnostic applications were performed with naturally occurring radionuclides, then the radioisotope with physical short half lives have become increasingly popular for imaging applications.

The first commercially available radioisotope generator was the 134Ie-132I, several other generators (such as ^{99}Mo-^{99m}Tc, ^{68}Ga, ^{113}Sn-^{113}In, ^{87}Y-^{87M}Sr---etc,) subsequently evolved (6-9). These generators must meet certain physical basic criteria to be useful. It should be simple and converient to operate, its radiation must be adequately shielded_____ yield adaughter product of high purity in terms of both radioaetivity and stable contaminants during every elution throughout the life of the generator, the product should be in achemical form suitable for use with aminimum of additional chemical or physical manipulation, lastly the radioactive yield of the daughter product during each elution should be high.

Labeled compounds either be used in biochemical research or for routine medical diagnosis were carried out in vivo for medical diagnosis such as those labeled with gamma emitting isotopes to permit detection external to the patient, but those

15

labeled with beta-emitting isotopes such as: C, H, S, and P were principally used in biochemical research.

There are various methods which were used for preparing labeled compounds such as of the following:

(1) isotope exchange reactions, in which one or more atoms in the molecule, exchange with atoms of the same element and of different mass, these atoms may be radioactive or stable isotopes, according to the follwing:

$$AX^*+BX-BX^*+AX$$

The comound BX under certain reaction conditions will exchange its X atoms (s) with the compound AX* where X* atom (s) is an isotopic form of the element X, awide range of compounds labeled with different stable or radioactive isotopes are prepared by exchange methods, which have the advantage that they can normally be carried out on a small chemical scale, an example is the preparation of urea- C, .

$$CO(NH_2)_2+14CO_2-CO(NH_2)_2+CO$$

(2) chemical synthesis: involves the construction of complex molecules from simple isotopically labeled intermediates, yields are usually expere___ as a percentage radiochemical yield:

$$\%radiochemical\ yield = \frac{Total\ radionactivity\ in\ product \times 100}{Total\ radionactivity\ in\ substrate}$$

For example, the preparation of earboxyl-labelled fatty acids
by reation with the corresponding Grignard reagent or acetic
C (16-19)4C and amino acid-1°C, steroids-14°anhydride-14

(3) biochemical methods : these include different
procedures such as enzymatic synthesis which is very
similar to chemical synthesis in that such a conversion
usually occurs without any change in the specificity of
the labeling or the molar specific activity (16). Total
biosynthetic methods are normally of value only when
microorganisms are employed, but the production of
uniformly labeled carbohydrates by photosynthesis in
detached leaves is an exception to this .

(4) Recoil labeling this method depend on the ability of
recoil atom produced in a nuclear reaction to form a
stable bond with an organic (or an inorganic)
compound. For example, if an organic compound is
mixed with a lithium carbonate or chloride and
irradiated in anuclear reactor at fixed neutron flux,
tritium compounds are produced by the recoiling
"tritond" from the nuclear reaction $6Li (n, \ ) 3H$.

One pure radioisotope or in labeled compounds is technetium-
^{99m}Tc, which have a short half-life, about six hours, with a
predominate single photon gama emissiom having an energy of
140 kev. ^{99m}Tc-labelled compounds are diagnostic imaging

agents used in the field of nuclear medicine to visualize tissue anatomical structures and metabolic disorders. After intravenous administration ^{99m}Tc or its labeled compound localized in specific target organ or tissue, can then be imaged using stable instrument.

Radioactivity measurements depends on the ability of radionuclides to produce ionized or excited atoms within the detector. Two basic types of radiation detectors are in common use: gas ionization ans scintillation. Radioisotopes allow the detection of minute quantities and differenate physically between substances.

The use of radioactive isotopes in biochemistry and clinical chemistry has proved us with a wealth of information about biological processes, that offers such as adiverse range of applications, using enzyme assays, biochemical pathways of synthesis and degradation, analysis of biomolecules, measurement of antibodies, binding and transport studies.

The use of radionuclide in nuclear medicine began when Frederick proescher published the paper entitled the use of radium for therapy of various diseases. Early experimental and diagnostic applications were performed with naturally occurring radionuclides, then the radioisotope with physical short half loves have become increasingly popular for imaging applications.

The first commercially available radioisotope generator was the ^{132}Tc-^{132}I, (5) several other generators (such as Mo-^{99m}Tc, ^{68}GE-68Ga, ^{113}Sn-^{113}In, ^{87}Y-^{87}mSr....etc) subsequently evolved. These generators must meet certain physical basic criteria to be useful.
It should. It should be simple and convenient to operate, radiation must be adequately shielded------- yield adaughter product of high purity in terms of both radioactivity stable contaminants during every clution throughout the life of the generator, the product should be in a chemical form suitable for use with amininmum of additional chemical or physical manipulation, lastly the radioactive yield of the daughter product during each elution should be high.

Labeled compounds either be used in biochemical research --- routine medical diagnosis were carried out in vivo for medical diagnosis such as those labeled with gamma emitting isotopes to permit detection external to the patient, but those labeled with beta-emitting isotopes such as: ^{14}C, ^{3}H, ^{35}S and ^{32}P were principally used in biochemical research.
There are various methods which were used for preparing labeled compounds such as of the followings:

1- isotope exchange reactions, in which one or more atoms in the molecule, exchange with atoms of the same element and of different mass, these atoms may be radioactive or stable isotopes, according to the following:

$$AX^* + BX \rightarrow BX^* + AX$$

The compound BX under certain reaction conditions will exchange its X atom (s) with the compound AX* where X* atom (s) is an isotopic form of the element X. awide range of compounds labeled with different stable or radioactive isotopes are prepared by exchange methods, which have the advantage that they can normally be carred out on a small chemical scale.

An example is the preparation of urea C,

$$CO(NH_2)_2 + {}^{14}CO_2 \rightarrow {}^{14}CO(NH_2)_2 + CO$$

2- chemical synthesis in volves the construction of complex moleculry from simple isotopically labeled intermediates, yields are usually expre   as a percentage radiochemical yield: For example, the preparation of carboxyl-labelled fatty acids by reaction with the corresponding grignard reagent or acetic anhydride- ${}^{14}C$, steroids ${}^{14}C$ and amino acids-${}^{14}C$.

3- biochemical methods: these include different procedures such as enzymatic synthesis which isvery similar to chemical synthesis in that such aconversion usually occurs without any change in the specificity of the labeling or the molar specific activity. Total biosynthetic methods are normally of value only when microorganisms are employed, but the production of uniformly labeled carbohydrates by photosynthesis in detached leaves is an exception to this.

4- recoil labeling (19, 20): this method depend on the ability of recoil atom produced in a nuclear reaction to form a stable bond with an organic (or an inorganic) compound. For example, if an organic compound is mixed with a lithium carbonate or chloride and irradiated in anuclear reactor at fixed neutron flux, tritium compounds are produced by the recoiling "tritons" from the nuclear reaction $^6Li(n, \alpha)^3H$

One of the most radioisotopes used in clinical application in both cases as pure radioisotope or in labeled compounds is technetium-99m, which have a short half-life about six hours, with a predominate single photon gama emission having an energy of 140 kev. ^{99m}Tc-labelled compounds are diagnostic imaging agents used in the field of unclear medicine to visualize tissue anatomical structures and metabolic disorders. After interavenous administration ^{99m}Tc or it labeled compounds localized in specific target organ or tissue, can then be imaged using stable instrument.

.

^{99m}TC-APPLICATION IN NUCLEAR MEDICINE

The following are some applications of ^{99m}Tc and its labelled compounds in unclear nedicine.

thyroid imaging:

The trappng of ^{99m}Tc as sodium pertechnate by thyroid is useful for assessing both function and its anatomy of the gland, although thyroid gland requires iodide ion for the production of thyroxine and triodothyronine the iodide ions are transported across the memberans of the epithelial cells in the thyroid follicles by means of an active transport process, but the radius of iodide is comparable to that of pertechnetate and each of the ions has asingle negative charge then hey have asimilar charge densities, so that $^{99m}TcO4$ is taken up readily by thyroid cells, evenm though iodine has several gamma-energies, so $^{99m}TcO4$ is preferred.

. Brain imaging:

Its is limited to the detection of ruptures of tumours and vascular lesions that impair the function of the blood brain barrier which is normally impermeable to he highly water-soluble $^{99m}TcO_4$. The rate at which substances penetrate brain tissue through the blood-brain barier is inversely related to their size and directly related to their lipid solubility, therefore attempts have been made to design small Tc-complexes with hydrophobic ligands such as bis-aminoethanethiol, propylene amine oxime. Each of these agents readily croses the blood brain barier but subsequently clears the brain tissue in a matter of minutes due to the lack of affinity for any particular recptor sites to these agents.

. kidney imaging:

Nearly all ^{99m}Tc –labelled compound will be excreted by the kidneys and eliminated in the urine, becaue of the kidneys are the principle organ responsible for the exceretion of water-oluble substances from the body the functional unit of the kidney is called the nephron, it is composed of afiltering apparatus referred to as the glomerulus, which is encapsulated in a structure called the bowman's capsule, following the glomerulus is a multisegmented tubule system which reabsorbs nutrients and secrets unwanted substances. Dynamic imaging of the glomerular filleration process is normally carried out with tc-DTPA (T-diethyl enetriamine penta acetic), the tc DTPA) readily passes through the glomerular filtration apparatus.

liver maging

The use of 99mtrc-labelled compound in hepatobiliay imaging was introduced in 1972 with the use of tc-penicillamine and then awide variety of 99m tc-complexes have been designed for this purpose (64). In designing any labeled compound to image bepatobilary function, one must attempt to minimize excretion by the kidneys and maximize extraction by the liver. The physical properties determining the favored excretory pathway of an agent are its size, charge, protein binding and functional group hydrophobicity, the more lipophilic species tend to be excreted by the liver and the hydrophilic species by the kidneys .

Two general types of ligands have been combined witb technetium to form hepatobiliary imagng agents, these include the iminodiacetic acid complexes, and the pyridoxylideneaminate complexes. The latter are composed of Schiff basses to which various hydrophobic amino acids are attached, these complexes are believed to have 99mtc in the Illoxidation state, best owing a (-1) charge on the complexes. This means that the uptake in hepatocytes is determined primarily by the anionic active transport process and by the way the complexes fit into the carrier proteins of that system.

heart imaging:

^{99m}TC -complexes may become a major competitor of 201TI. ^{99}IC is preferred because o its shorter half-life, six hours compared to 72 hours for the 201TI, lower cost, and greater availability. Although group I cations (K_{+1}, CS_{+1} and R_{b+}) accumulate in normal myocardium through the action of the Na+/K+ ATPase system, so radioactive isotopes of these cations can be used for heart imaging. Awide variety of other cations including TI, also accumulate in normal heart tissue, however, not through this enzyme system. Instead they are beleived to bind to relatively nonselective recpetors which appear to recobnize a variety of positively charged speciese. This has been the basis for the development of an entire group of potential technetium based heart-imaging agents .

Many authors have puplished th use of ^{99m}TC -labelled compounds in heart imaging agents. Because the 201TI and ^{99m}Tc isonitriles complexes will only reveal an absence of uptake in damaged heart tissue, localization of myocardial infarctions with these agents is difficult so ^{99m}Tc-complexes which accumulates specifically in the infarction tissue is necessary to quantity heart damage.

A number of 99mTc bone imaging agents have been found to localize in infaracted myocardium, most notably 99mtc-pyrophosphate was localized in damaged tissue producing a hot-spot rather than a cold-spot image of the infarct, it is agued that the localization is the result of irreversible deposition of calcium in the mitochondria due to the combination of cell membrane damage plus residual coronary blod flow to the damaged area.

bone imaging:

Many radionuclides have been used in the investigation of bone metabolism both in animals and in human, include, phosphorous ^{32}P, calcium, ^{40}Ca, strontium, ^{87m}Sr, and barium, ^{137m}Ba.. The production of ^{99m}Tc-labelled phosphorous complexes has led to adistinct improvement in bone scintigraphy largely due to the lower energy of the gamma-ray and the greator radioactivity administered as compared to the previously used radionuclides,

25

several abnormal patterns of bone scintigrams with ^{99m}Tc-labelled phosphorous complexes have been reported in patients with metabolic bone diseases.

The properties of an ideal bone imaging agent may differ according to the clinical application:

1- to delineate benign or malignant focal lesions, which is the most frequent indication a high ratio of lesion-to-normal bone uptake, at the same time there must be sufficient activity in normal bone for accurate localization of lesions, balanced against low background activity in soft tissues such as the muscles and major viscera (liver, spleen, kidneys and lungs).

This is achieved by rapid clearance of plasma activity without diffusion into the red blood cells, which in turn requires a high renal extraction efficiency. Fortunately, MDP do not undergo gastrointestinal or biliary exeretion so that gastrointestinal activity dos not obscure the lumbar spine or pelvis.

2- To as a vascular necrosis, both normal uptake and the bone-to-soft tissue ratio must be high. For quantitation of skeletal activity at 24 hours in patients with generalized bone disease, Fogelman prefers ethane -1-hydroxy-1, 1-diphosphonate (EHDP) because of its lower overlap between normal and abnormal bone uptake than with other diphosphonates.

COMPETITIVE – BINDING STUDIES

In the last 1960's it has become possible to quantify great variety of organic substances by means of competitive protein-binding techniques using radionuclide labelled substat. These have offered so many advantages over the others and have become so widespread in their applications. These studies are based on the non-covalet reverable binding of ligand to aspecific binding protein, according to the following general reaction:

Ligand + binding protein → binding protein –ligand……..(1)

Examples of specific binding protein are antibodies coricosteroed binding globuline (CBG), estrogen receptors, thyroglobulin (TBG) and others. These proteins are characterized by their ability to bind ligands (varied antigens, cortisol, corticosterone, estrogen, vitamin B12….etc) with high specificity and affinity. The competitive-binding assay can be imaged as the addition of increasing amount of unlabelled ligand to reaction mixtures containing known constant amounts of labelled ligand which compelte for the binding site of specific inding protein.

$$Ab + L \rightarrow Ab{:}L \dots\dots\dots\dots 2$$

$$L^* + Ab \rightarrow Ab{:} L \dots\dots\dots\dots 3$$

$$L^* = \text{labelled ligand}$$

$$Ab = \text{antibody}$$

If the conditions are selected correctly, then over a certain dose range of non radioactive will be bound to the binding protein and does response curve in term of non radioactive added and either bound to the binding protein or existing free unbound solution may be dr wn. Common types of markers used to labell ligands include radioisotopes, enzymes, and fluorphores. These can be used both homogenous and hetergenous competitive binding assays. The sensitivity of binding reaction assay is function of the affinity of the binding protein for its ligand. The specificity of binding protein for its ligand is measured by its ability to bind only the ligand and not other substances. Avarious assay techniques using the same basic principles of competive binding assays include:

1- radioimmuno assay, which have the ligand and constant amount of radioactively labelled ligand compete for alimited number of antibody binding sites. Redioimmuno assay is applicable to the measurement of both low-molecular weight and high molecular weight ligands.

2- Enzyme-linked immunosorbent assay (ELISA):
Are heterogenous nonisotopie assays that usually have an antibody immobilized onto a solid support and the ligand labelled with the enzyme.

3- Homogneous enzyme immuno assay: the binding of antibody to the enzyme-labelled ligand changes the enzymatic activity of the labell so that antibody – bound enzyme can be distinguished from unbound labelled ligand.

4- Substrate – labelled flurescance immno assay:

This assay is based on a lebel that is a flurogenic enzyme substrate. When the label is hydrolyzed by aspecific enzyme (β-galactosidase) it yields afluorescent product.

5- Florescence polarization immunoassay : is based on the amount of polarized fluorescent light detected when the fluorophore label is excited with polarized light.

6- Apoenzyme reactivation immunoassay system (ARIS):

Has bee applied to dry reagent strip tests for analysis of therapeutic drugs such as thophylline,phenytouin.

·

Protein engineering

It is the technique that allows the installation of structural proteins desired in order to build a clone- mediated DNA "Cloned DNA". There is no relationship between the latter and engineering of proteins used, including the building of protein functionally, chemically and physically.

The DNA could be modified by two ways using:

- Mutagenic in private venues.
- Switch sections of the nucleotides.

The protein engineering include modify the structure with protein mediated by genetic engineering and most protein engineering is carried out currently in the field of enzymes, either to speed up its response to the incentive or to become more receptive to acid and heat.

Example: "Cloning" the cDNA for the receptor of "acetyl choline receptor" facilitated the technology which is called site directed mutagensis for getting sequences skilled "Deletions" or substituting some of the amino acids in an additional unit "subunits" of the receptor and then it can test these changes on the functional aspect, and are also defined as follows:

There are many examples of this type of modification for production of complex of organic compound that have catalytic activity have of it chemically synthesized for example the myoglobin of which associated with oxygen, but it docs not have catalytic activity. This Bio-molecule with three complexes of ruthenium "ruthenium" carrier of the electron through the surface of the histidines components generate a complex that has the ability to reduce oxygen and the oxidation of the natural ascorbate.

The construction of DNA contributed significantly to the development to the stage of protein engineering to construct proteins that do not exist in nature. The technique has evolved to the point can modifies the gene by an engineering to change the protein in a predictable and have to improve some functional characteristics such as:

- No. transformation "turnover number".
- Static Km of substrate specific.
- Thermostability.
- temperature optimum.
- Stability and activity in non-aqueous solvents.
- Privacy of interaction and substrate "Specificity".
- Requirements of co- factors.
- Protease resistance.
- Allosteric regulation.
- Molecular weight and composition of the structural unit "Sub- unit structure".

And for engineering the protein molecule, it is clearly necessary to ensure a series of rules relating to major synthetic building blocks of proteins that recipe as desired. After seeing the structural composition of protein crystals, it is then possible to diagnose those areas in which it occurs possible modifications to improve the catalytic molecule, protein, and this is done to modify the sequence of amino acids in the protein.

Major modifications protein

The use of site-directed mutagenesis determined then what is aimed to, because the change in one base in the gene result in a change in the sequence of amino acids in the protein, which in turn improve the protein in question. Large modifications in proteins by removing the "delete" section mediated by enzymes or by the unequivocal chemical structure of part of the gene. In this way, the production of spare "klenow fragment" "DNA polymerase" free of analytical activity, also can add sequence of amino acids through docking to improve the stability of proteins made in E. coli and finally can collect or part of a fusion gene or the whole of all or part of the other, thereby generating new proteins.

Determination the general features of the installation of the structural protein. Protein engineering based on the availability of information on the district and synthetic building blocks that are obtained from the methods of X-ray diffraction and nuclear magnetic resonance two- way "Two dimensional nuclear magnetic resonance NMR" and the latter is the alternative method in the future. Many researchers expect success in engineering of proteins "Protein Engineering", especially after the great progress which has been in embryonic technique, where each protein is produced by genetic conditions of its own machine of the cell consisting of enzymes when they become three characters of the genetic material and arranged in advance and checked that then wrap as a specimen to be specific proteins effectively.

When you know the rules that allow the protein to form belts wrapped can then change the genetic information of proteins and identified so that it works in another way as soon as a large and powerful grants stability, and thus can benefit economically from the proteins of the broad areas of application by micro- organisms and can be more clear: for example, improved production of proteins (new physical properties and functional).

Important notes that are related to protein engineering is to clarify the potential relationship of proteins, where the protein for example, a specimen 15- amino acid. There are 103×3 possible sequence of these acids is larger than the number of atoms that make up technical enzymes immobolized on board, the development of these enzymes are restricted or limited to a solid surface to be in constant contact with the foundation to which the article in the mobile phase "mobile phase". It is clear from this that there is a possibility to use the many pathways that retains its effectiveness.

Enzyme Technology

The biotechnology is considered as one of the technical life in science and engineering. It was one of the enzymatic technology trends that have grown with the technology of life, despite being preceded by technical life, keeping in mind that enzymes from an engineering standpoint is special case of the factors that have qualities such as privacy.

Bio- systems are used in critical periods in history to get the desired chemical conversions such as transformations of like milk to cheese and fermenting of liquids that contain sugar to alcohol, but such research trends have changed during the evolution of Biotechnology with the fact that these processes such as cheese, bread and alcohol industry still very important.

The history of enzymatic techniques started with the developments that have emerged a number of chemical transformations using the tissue of life, which include, for example hydrogen peroxide decomposition and degradation of starch to sugar and digestion of proteins.

Immobilized enzyme technology

At present, there are important industrial applications of immobilized enzyme technology represented by the following enzymes:

- Glucose isomerase.
- Aminoacylase.
- Penicillin acylase.

Lactase. Technical features of immobilized enzymes"

- Prevent the entry of the immobilized enzyme in the mobile phase.
- The product is characterized by being cleansed of the enzyme and does not accumulate.
- Using the enzyme for long.

The globe, despite the lack of clear understanding of the rules that govern protein engineering, but the equipment contribute to give some

suggestions on how to achieve a stereo structure of the protein. In this area one can not expect for example bacterial cell to produce human that differs in form of human protein.

The latter has been "Immobilized" on the particles of silica. It is used to convert the lactose in whey to glucose and galactose.

Applications to include of immobilized in the future as follows:

- Use enzyme "Cholinesterase" for the purpose of pesticide detection "Pesticides" and watching the inhibition of this enzyme either by the method of electrical "Calorimetrically electrochemical" or by the color method.
- Other enzymes that may be used in the same method in order to detect toxic chemicals, the enzyme "Carbonic anhydrase" is very

33

sensitive to low concentrations of chlorinated hydrocarbons from low-lying "Chlorinated hydrocarbon" and "Hexokinase" to "Chlordane".

- Immobilized diisopropyl phosphor fluoridate extracted from the nerve cells.

General aspects of enzymes immobilization

This process is intended as we mention it to determine kinetics of enzymes, as yell as cells that characterized by (desorption) on the surface such as fibers gels, etc., also can be used as phenomenon shooting accordingly.

Advantages of the immobilization process are the followings:

- Finding the status of enzymes similar to those found within cells and tissues.
- Prolonging the period of use and has repeatedly given to the survival of catalytic activity and stability.
- Use appropriate concentrations and may be high for the purpose of increasing the speed of the reaction, given the focus to fit with the speed in specific circumstances of the reaction.
- Contributing of the immobilization process to facilitate the purification process of related to products of reaction.
- The use of multiple systems from the fermentation (continuous and open).
- Reducing energy consumption and cost.

The immobilization methods are numerous, including:

- Chemical methods: they are similar to affinity chromatography such as use the covalent and casual.
- Physical methods: such as packaging inside a capsule adsorption and shooting.

As for choosing the appropriate method to be immobilized it is determined according to the specific bases represented by measurement of activity and stability. So it must be taken into account the business side which means less expense. And choose the easiest method because they are all tough and stay away from hazardous substances to human health, and the technical side is important in the selection process since there is a special mechanical pressure during the operation.

The immobilization cells vary from cell since it is being more of enzymatic system builders with the installation of diverse chemical content, therefore, requires that the appropriate modalities, simple and stay away from these that require to use extreme circumstances. It also requires that to taken into account the number of cells to be immobilized so the method must be convenient and linking cells are good and avoid the use of hazardous materials. The characters of the immobilized cells are numerous advantages including the use of small amounts of carbon and energy sources and re-use of cells, so it is possible separate the growth phase from production phase, where it is possible control the fermentation. Immobilization depends on the type of cells, microbial cell reduce the size of the manufacturing process and thus reduce the cost of the production process. The Eukaryotic cells which are characterized as specialized capable of limited division of which are specific plant or animal cells and preferred to be immobilized, particularly those that are separated as any single and are generally used for the purpose of the immobilization of adsorbed on the hollow fiber.

Human Genome Project

The initiative of (HGP) came the first time in 1988 and aimed at finding the sites of some 100000 human gene in DNA and the (HGP) expresses 24 pairs of the human of chromosomes, is turning into information content when it follow the sequence of rules need to be resolved based on computer science, mathematics, statistics and experimental sciences.

The computer science often provided in contributions in programs and solutions that are characterized by the skills that led to the invention of language access code information described the performs a particular order and provides methods to describe complex biological processes by the number of code rather than their natural language with hundreds of pages. Then the researchers and observers said that the twentieth century be the century of biology and analytical power resulting from the HGP that will explain drastically all life and medical research as it was:

- Research on the nature of genomes and the nature of the composition and organization of various scientific institutions.

- Acceleration in the implementation of the project, which was planned to complete within 15 years of technical progress, but then shortened   the   time   to   ten   years .The search of the genome to find the type of information or material contained in the communication as well as identifying the sequence about three billion chemical bases.

- Study the nature of the information stored in the computer and the evolution of elaborate by efficient techniques of and sequence evolution in the tools that contribute to the analysis of information.

- Study the effects to be set in the community and to what extent this

can be achieved, and the type of response.

In spite of all reported studies and research conducted by methods and techniques in various vital information as well as numerous writings and published in this area, there are still many other fields and various study and research. Some of these fields has not been touched so far in the country, especially the human genome projects, and areas to attract the attention of researchers, but it's mostly a few problems, mostly dealing with partial or subsidiary.

Bio-engineering

There are a number of scientific developments resulted from the diving in the world of molecules to push medicine forward through the discovery of technical of recombinant DNA (engineering life) and this new knowledge has led to the understanding of the causes of the disease that has eluded science until now, and thus to find new treatments to them. Engineering of life had an impact on medicine borders these have become easier with the forgotten youth of this important scientific field.

The reality is that James Watson and Francis Crick did not reach a structural installation with a double helix molecule of DNA. And then it was identified the gene (genes), which manages the production of individual proteins, and then we obtained the tools of partial strong, and in the early seventies researchers began snapped genes of the DNA. One of the species and planting it in DNA another kind for the manufacture of new molecules and in a few years researchers were able to transfer these genes and to produce objects that are within during the eighties and became a human gene transfer to many microscopic organisms and bacteria turning them into factories for medically useful proteins.

After it has been cloned of human genes in the micro-organisms for a number of hormones, including growth hormones and insulin in human as well as bacteria many of the genes responsible for human proteins with diagnostic value was produced at the level of marketing. It is noteworthy that human insulin is derived from living with diabetes, and also for the development of techniques for the production of antibodies "monoclonal antibodies".

Many applications, there is a steady increase in the use of enzymes in the diagnosis and treatment as well as in planting (farming) tissues and cells, "Tissue and cell transplantation" and that the development of engineering of life is still in the young stage, but there have major impacts on medicine and industry is synergy between electronic systems, electrical and life- component electrons so-called life "Bioelectronics" and electrochemistry of life "Bioelectrochemistry". Then there have been the following design of a number of devices depending on what is stated in the above examples include "Glucose monitors" for the purposes of medical sensors and nerve gases for medical purposes and sensors nerve gases "Nerve gas sensors" to military uses.

Based on sensors that have been most developed in the present time to reveal the exact products enzymatic activity mediated by the traditional pole "Conventional" where is the install (restricted) "Immobilization" new approaches that lead to devices with more sensitivity that depends on the movement of electrons between the direct-polarization and the redox centers protein "Protein redox centers" In brief the enzymes, which is based on the sensor depend on the medical sensor "Glucose sensor" and other sensors that measure chemicals in blood such as immune sensors include the electronic life "Bioelectronic immunosensors", which was commercially manufactured during the current decade, are measured in a large number of materials in the fluid of life, causing a revolution in the diagnosis, in addition to the incremental progress that has been happening as a result the development of a wide range of models "Sensors", which depends on the synergy between micro-organisms substantiated grants stability, "Immobilized and Stabilized". Finally, various data indicate that the microbiology of life through the engineering involved in the medical field in the production:

- Antibiotics.
- Vitamins.
- Nucleotides.
- Hormones.
- Enzymes.
- Vaccines.
- Antibodies.

The progress that accompanied the engineering of life has affected in particular the daily practice of doctors, because of the speed that accompanied the evolution of knowledge and techniques in the laboratory and hence to the industrial production and then patient care. The expression of human insulin gene in bacteria E. coli, for example, has been studied in 1979 and that this insulin, with the original engineering-

life of "Recombinant DNA" has been tested by volunteers with non-diabetes "non- diabetic" in 1950 and clinical trials that have been in patients with diabetes began in 1981.

The attention of most doctors on the applications of modern life engineering in medicine, which tend to be very important in areas which have helped to revolutionize the diagnosis, treatment and understanding of many diseases, and examples of this therapeutically important protein, which was manufactured by engineered mediated microbiologist, microbiology, applications of single origin "Monoclonal antibodies", enzymes and others that arise out of uniform origin from lymphoid cells, where used in:

- Treatment of cancer.
- Diagnosis of many diseases.

Pharmaceutical industry, pharmaceutical companies have been choosing some clinically significant produced cheaply, such as insulin, which was previously mentioned, and which treats patients with diabetes and extensive use of interferon for the treatment of many diseases, including cancer.

The Bio-engineering worked towards a second method by increasing the secretion of microbiology by called anti- life penicillin produced in fungi, and the third trend in the medical field that is the development of drugs already in the nature and turn them into centers of drugs more effectively.

Containing anti-bacterial drugs that have contributed to engineering life and developed vaccines, hormones, vitamins and antibiotics and life for the purpose of producing these materials from micro-organisms after it was restricted to human and animal cells.

Hormones are the most advanced in terms of the accuracy of the technique used and the large economic returns through the engineering of life and led to great successes through the production of materials likes of the hormones which are stimulated, and stimulating the flesh wounds and the growth of the affected nerves that affect the sense of pain. The success of engineering in the provision of life-hormones of the study and treatment has become a boom due to technical difficulties in extraction, which vaccine and growth hormones as well as the instigator of the secretion of pituitary adreno "ACTH" used to treat infections and diseases is used to treat wounds, burns, and stunting and release thyroid hormones pituitary as well as insulin used to treat diabetes, where possible transmission of their genes to bacteria.

Production of hormones is mediated by microbiology research center in the fields of engineering life in general and genetic engineering in particular, where microbiologists used to convert steroids and the production of hormones from the human body can not produce in sufficient quantities. Then it was grown in importance after the custom of cortisone and its derivatives and their effective role in the treatment of arthritis, which draw many medical companies of steroids from plants, animals and chemical methods of trying to turn them into other steroid prescriptions.

The methods of microbiology steroids is turning quickly but with less degree, there is in the addition of specialized microorganisms capable converting steroids quickly. There is also the addition of specialized microorganisms is added hydroxyl group of any carbon atom present in the steroid.

There are also some working to add hydrogen to steroids or withdrawal of hydrogen or oxidation or separate pools of chemical side effects. Using growth hormone that is released from the pituitary gland for the treatment of dwarfism find the hormone extracted from the animals be in a non-pure from, but according the production of this hormone is preferred to be extracted from microbiology such as the production from the bacteria E. coli after treatment genetically.

The plant hormones have been possible to produce from fungi, especially those produced from rice, as it is known that plant hormones industry is still expensive despite their limitations. In addition, there are a large number of proteins found in the blood such as the factors that contribute to coagulation missing by patients with hemorrhage as well as the albumin found in serum. These materials have been contributed to the development of production by engineering life in medicine (drugs).

The pharmaceutical industry, which includes anti-bacterial drugs, vitamins, vaccines and hormones of the biggest industries that relied on engineering techniques of life for the purpose of producing these materials from microbiology.

Medical applications of Bio-engineering

There are many faces, can be addressed when studying the medical applications of bio- engineering after the gene was designed, including:

Production of therapeutic: include hormones, such as somatostatin insulin, interferon and anti- biotic, where it was initially isolate the hormone somatostain for regulating secretion of growth hormone from the pituitary gland in the traditional way that requires half a million sheep brains to produce 5-10 mg of this material.

Treatment of many of the genetic diseases: the treatment of many genetic diseases is possible to treat many genetic diseases due to loss of protein production remedying these proteins from bacteria, and the examples of this case the planting and production of large amounts of genes to produce hemoglobin, which decreases in "Thalassemia" through the introduction of genes responsible for hemoglobin the patient's bone marrow, and then returned the cells to the patient.

Diagnosis of a number of diseases before birth: the fetus diagnosed in the prenatal stage, through the identifying the defects in a specific gene that causes the disease, such as some "Gamma- Globuinemia" and the disease lest Nhin as well as Tay- Sachs "Tay- Sachs".

There has been progress in some areas of medical engineering technology due to the recombinant DNA such as "cloning" the human insulin gene as well as growth hormone and its expression in bacteria that has been marketing of human insulin derived from microbiology and used for the treatment of patients with diabetes in addition to:

-       Production of interferon by a large clone human genes in microorganisms.
-       The development of production techniques and monoclonal antibodies and their uses.
-       The increase in the use of enzymes for the diagnosis and treatment in instilling the cells and tissues "tissue and cell transplantation".
-       Treatment of many diseases of genetic mediation by protein that being lost, which can be mediated by production of bacteria.
-       Diagnosis of diseases before birth by identifying the defect in a gene or several genes.

Turning to the relationship between engineering, medicine, is taken into account the following things:
• Mutant cells and the cells unmodified organisms and their products such as antibiotic cellular life and plants, as well as other life transitions "Bioconversions".
• Modified cells "Modified cells" and their products to ensure that objects Monoclonal "Monoclonal antibodies" of the following uses:
-       Immunological Studies.
-       Immunohistochemistry.
-       Tissue typing for trans- plantation.

- Diagnosis and monitoring of malignancy.
- Preparation of medicinal products with a "Prepartion of medically important products".
- Recombinant DNA technology and its use for the production of insulin, interferon and growth hormone and vaccines "Vaccines" and enzymes.
- The application of Bio-engineering techniques of molecular

Genetics and techniques diagnosis recombinant DNA in the diagnosis and (pathological) human disease:
- Patriarchal diagnosis of genetic diseases.
- Effects of genetic diseases on the specie disease.
- Features of the future.

It is believed to that Bio- engineering represented by "Clinical biotechnology" has begun in the application management and industrial production of penicillin in 1940 that the success of the full insulin has created a growing demand for medicine (drugs).

The production of penicillin by fermentation and used in the treatment of diseases using the Bio-engineering problems that has been accompanied by the emergence of side effects and put some Bio-engineering solutions, and the problem of production has been developed through genetic improvement producing strains and control the components of the center other conditions contribute to the process of fermentation.

Bio-engineering and cancer

Bio- engineering has succeeded results in the field of cancer better than other diseases, as shown in the eighties that the main thing vs. cancer is a change in the genes (genes) from an engineering standpoint.

It was clear from the following entries in the relationship between the Bio- engineering and cancer.

Through analysis of a group of viruses called regressive "Retroviruses", which cause cancer in animals, as a number of these viruses carrying cancer-causing genes or tumor genes "Oncogenes". It appears that the retroviruses that cause cancer have been captured from the normal gene, cell; or one animal that is made part of their own genetic material. The retroviral infection of new cells in the later planted with genetic material, leading to the transformation of healthy cells into cancerous cells.

The researchers show that DNA extracted from human tumors can shift the cancer cells to cancer cells in test tubes. Or that a specific gene in a human cell that can transform sound cell into the tumor cell and a tumor-causing gene for bladder cancer in humans.

.

The gene tumor is often due to the mutant or increase in production and there is general consensus about the fact that any of the original tumor gene mutations may be some inherited mutations.

The studies of funmor contribute to inherited breast or ovarian caner, the physician may be able to use that gene to assess the patient's condition and prospects and to provide more effective treatment for patients who have multiple copies of inherited suspicious. Harold Varmus and Michael Bishop has concluded that "Lancogen" the legacies of the genes responsible for causing cancer.

Bio-Engineering and AIDS

To understand the relationship between Bio- engineering and the AIDS requires a study of the topic in two cases:

How should the immune system to destroy virus: the defense forces resulting from the immune system to attack multi- directional and of different media for the virus (a specific target) to:

- Phagocyte and other cells relevant to specific viral antibodies are chewing.

- These cells installed in the grooves on proteins known as antigens of human white blood cells.

- Construction immune complexes on the surface of cells identified by a type of white blood cells (T-help) "Helper T".

- The recipients are on the T- cells help identify the peptide superficial "epitopr", associated with divide, and secrete small proteins that stimulate and activate T-cells and the toxic or lethal trait.

- The killer T cells directly attack infected cells and fragmentation of viral particles and peptides associated with molecules of antigens of human white blood cells, when identified by toxic T cells by antigenic recipients on the surface of infected cells and destroy them by producing more of them.

- The B- cells recognize the antigen norepinephrine viral surfaces as a prelude to their destruction.

- Immune response and the virus "HIV" contribute the immune steps in defense against the virus "HIV", where they are:

▪ Invasion of the virus of T- lymphocytes and cells assistance, followed by cloning and increase the virus and help decrease the number of cells, death, and loss of infected T cells.

▪ Launch of viral particles from the cell membrane of T cells after being wounded by the T cells and B- toxic responses to be dispatched a strong defense which resulted in killing infected cells, viruses, and thus is determined by the breeding assistance and reference cells to a normal level.

▪ A high level of virus gradually with the decline in the number of cells to help patients and reflects the so- called phase of AIDS when the number of cells less than 150 assistance cell in the blood followed by a rise in the level of virus with the decline of the immune system.

Monoclonal antibodies

The areas of application for the production of these antibodies where the potential for many therapeutic and diagnostic enormous, including:

• Treatment of patients with leukemia and production of specific antibody alien objects on the cancerous blood cells, leading to the union of antibodies with and removed from the bloodstream.

• Accepting the objects of a transplanted organ which are used Monoclonal antibodies or clone in the development of the body accept a transplanted organ such as the kidney.

• Birth control through private industry specific antibody to proteins found in human sperm.

• Determining the sex of the fetus through a special antibody to sperm of own unwanted sex.

• Models are highly sensitive and privacy are being used as opposites, and a single origin and widely high sensitivity and privacy in early screening for malignant tumors by using specific proteins associated antigen and the presence of tumor presence.

• Determining the levels of hormones in the body and used Monoclonal antibodies to determine the levels of hormones in the body and determine the effectiveness of the glands.

• Search for the presence of some drugs in the body tissue and blood used Monoclonal antibodies in the search for the presence of some drugs in the body tissue and blood to prevent the occurrence of cases of poisoning or addiction.

• Diagnosis of crimes using Monoclonal antibodies in the search also in the diagnosis of crimes. The food industry also used Monoclonal antibodies in the field of food industries, especially in the diagnosis and determination of the purity of food, processed meat, and free of

•

unwanted substances and preventing fraud in this area.

Of the significant developments that have taken place for Immunology and molecular biology and biochemistry and the discovery of antibodies and the creation of a single origin "The Monoclonal antibodies" is characterized by privacy "Specificity" and sustainability of production,

"Immortality" huge quantities "Large ruantities" and high purity "High Purity" for periods of a very long time.

However, these antibodies Monoclonal antibodies created by the multiple origin (clone) the molecular composition and effectiveness. Studies have shown that the use and applications of antibodies only be successful to detect very small quantities of tumor functions that can be used in early diagnosis of many tumors and by diagnosing the effectiveness of these antibodies could be argued that a large proportion of blood diseases can be categorized.

The advantage of imaging the immune flashlight as we have mentioned that the blue single antibodies prepared in the body of a patient associated antigen, surface of cancer cells without other cells and sputtering when labeling these antibodies with radioactive isotope, it can locate the radioactive iodine, for example by gamma cameras and thus can be located and the size of cancerous tumors, including colon, ovarian and skin cancer.

The unilateral clone in addressing some of the tumors where it can be linked to medicine as well as radioactive materials to these antibodies, such as chronic leukemia and thyroid cancer lymphoma and colon cancer has been found that these antibodies injected intravenously is grappling with the tumor cells and selectively and is disposed of, where became can direct these drugs directly to tumors by linking them to the catalytic antibodies to these tumors. Used monoclonal antibodies to treat cancer when there is a high toxic concentrations in the tumor. It could also be linked Monoclonal antibodies radioactive isotope and alive in the body of a cancer patient at which time the radioactive material to the site of the tumor and therefore within the cancer cells and it crashed. There are many researches addressing the use of monoclonal antibodies in the early diagnosis of the body rejecting the case of the tissues and the transplanted organs as well as a lot of studies on the use of these antibodies in the treatment of the case of rejection.

47

Some applications objects Monoclonal

Improving the sensitivity of the current immune for tests or tests new Histocompatibility

Fibronnectin

Blood groups Antigens

Sperm antigen

Interleukins IL

Interferons

Progesterone gastrin

Blood   clotting   factors Estrogen

Human growth hormone

Monoclonal antibodies has clear impact and important role in clinical medicine before developing the "hybridoma technology", which provides heterogeneous objects "Homogenous antibodies". The research carried out by each of the "Kohler & Milstein" in the early seventies, created a method used for the manufacture of the anti body homogenized with a quantity of non- specific proliferation applied at large.

The researchers "Kohler" and Mlesstin have participated in the production of monoclonal antibodies, which is derived from specific tissue culture which is called hybridoma, where the latter's has the ability to produce one type of antibodies but does not produce more. This is done by crossbreeding or mating types of cells, the first is produce the antibody and the second for the growth of cancer cells have the ability to reproduce. And then treated with hybrid that has to be the formation of antibodies, where antibodies are produced for this body alone, and perhaps it carries the qualities of cancer, the production of antibodies is very large quantities. It is possible in the light of the use of a composition for the manufacture of an unknown antigen monoclonal each part, and then used these antibodies to probe the chemical composition of the real knowledge of the unknown substance.

Monoclonal antibody can be used for treating patients with cancer of the blood through the manufacture of these antibodies is specific to the alien objects on the cancerous blood cells united for the purpose of removal from the blood stream, and used these antibodies for early detection of the presence of tumor cells through the tests that require purity too high to measure the presence of proteins associated with its existence of these tumors and their locations in particular antigen-mediated tumor.

These antibodies are used in determining the levels of hormones in the body and to determine the endocrine events are also used in the search for the presence of certain drugs in the blood and tissues because of the poisoning have also been introduced in the diagnosis of bacteria in the development of the transfer of the body of a transplanted organ, in particular   kidney

Preparation of medically important products

The use of monoclonal antibodies the purpose of purification and preparation of medical materials which is represented by the task done by the "Secher, Burks" and that covalently bound to anti- body unilateral origin against assigned to drive in "Sepharose" and therefore can refine 5000 times.

There are a number of the production of insulin- led company "Eli Lilly & Co", which used the Bio- engineering, including recombinant DNA technique as a base for the manufacture of human insulin. The production process has been carried out by "Lilly" in cooperation with "Genentech Inc." According to the following steps:

• Determination the sequence of DNA From the known sequence of amino acids m insulin.

- Chemical structure of genes for the series "A" and Series "B" of insulin, contains each and every one of them in the codon methionine at the end "O".
- Each gene enter in 2 mentioned in the beta- 2 gene "B-galactosidase" of the plasmids, which are the same within the" E. coil".
- Because of the fact that the bacteria had grown in the medium that contains the galactose and not glucose that urges enzyme B- galatosidase and then with a series of insulin "A" or "B" linked with methionine.
- After the breakdown of bacteria, treated with cyanogens bromide "CNBr", that breakdown the proteins at the site where the
- methionin is present.
- Purification of the two strings "A& B" and then returned to their union with the natural production of insulin, the two strings.

The bacteria do not carry enzymes that change the pro insulin to insulin through manufacture the lofty strings "A, B" in the bacteria followed by purification separate chains bilateral, ties with the sulfide.

It is noteworthy that human insulin that is produced by E. coli was tested by healthy human volunteers and with diabetes (and there were no adverse that there is capacity similar to purified pork or with decrease the blood glucose when injected under the skin or injected inside the vein.

The trials have been carried out on human and compared with animal insulin producer from the pancreas of pork produced then was shown similar effects. This was in the hospital, "Guys" in London and Osaka in Japan.

The department of food and drugs in the United States the U.S. approved marketing of insulin produced by the micro- organism, which called the "Humalin", also got the same thing by Britain in the same year 1982.

Growth hormones

These hormones are used in the treatment of growth disorders in children, dwarfism some cases of infertility in women and because of the high cost of treatment using these hormones and the difficulty of obtaining and the need for a large number of the pituitary gland the high cost of the hormone and the likelihood of infection with viruses and expected such as uses future growth of the tissues, and the flesh wounds after surgical operations the flesh of fractures and the assist once in the treatment o burns, sores and the used in the study of malignant diseases.

Researchers have made efforts to extract it and its production in bacteria by bioengineering after the successful transfer of genes responsible for hormone production from human cells to bacteria which was done in 1979.

The length of human growth hormone, 191 amino acid with a molecular weight of 2200 excreted by the pituitary gland, secreted of from the front gland of the longitudinal growth of the structure which means the isolation from the pituitary gland.

The pharmaceutical kebi have cooperated with the company "Genetech" for the production of growth hormone from E. coli using Bio-engineering of life recombinant DNA techniques.

The technical difficulties have been overcome in the collection of pituitary glands as well as the cost that accompany and other problems, including lack of access to one type of the hormone, but a mixture composed of several different forms in the installation of structural and molecular weight than did patients with antibodies inhibiting their production.

Interferon

The interferon is extracted from the cells infected by virus and studies have shown that these cells, the immune system stimulates the production of this hormone during the infection by virus.

Then overlap with the later injuries to the work therefore it is called "Interferon" used to treat the casualties.

The cost of purification of interferon is very high and extracted from white blood cells, and the other efforts made to develop the production method for human interferon non-blood through tissue culture (artificially), and then methods developed to produce interferon from

51

bacteria, it is done successfully in 1980 and it became clear that there several species produce a number of genes.

Interferon has been isolated in 1957 and considered at that time the first line of defense against attack by viruses, used to treat many viruses diseases and including:

- Cold.
- Hepatitis.
- Cancer Diseases.

Because of the interferon ability to prevent abnormal complications of the cells studies have shown that the immune system of these cells motivated during virus infection leading to secrete very active material is to overlap with the later injuries to the work.

The interferon's a family of proteins, discovered as a result of infection which flows into the cells by viruses "Virally infected ceils" are characterized by the following characteristics:

- Antiviral in other cells.
- Inhibition of "Cellular proliferation" "anti cancer drug".
- Internalization of the immune system "Modulation of the immune system".

It is possible to re-classify the life can be interferon's to the following types:

- α- alpha- interferon leucocyte "α leucocyte interferon".
- β- beta, interferon cell Fiber "fibroblast interferon".
- Gama of lymphocytes, immune interferon "immune interferon", "Lymphocytes T".

Leucocyte interferon reduces the spread of a vesicular composition "vesical formation" and responds to fear of infection of the liver "Hepatits B" as well as in various malignancies "malignancies" such as breast cancer spread "metastatic breast cancer" and non- Hodgkin's lymphoma "Non- Hodgkin's lymphoma" and osteoma flesh "Osteosarcoma" and malignant melanoma "Malignant melanoma".

Research has shown that there are about 20 types of interferon, which produces a number of genes mediated for the purpose of genes engineering more effective against viruses or against tumors.

Production of interferon's

- Using 50000 liters of human blood, produced from 0.1 g of pure interferon for the treatment of acute viral diseases.
- A culture producing cells and white blood cells of some healthy donors and encouraging the virus "Sandi Virus" for 24 hours and then isolated interferon-mediated by centrifuge in the Central Laboratory of Public Health in Helsinki, France and the United States.
- DNA recombinant technology.

Protein map "Proteome"

The term "Proteome" which appeared in 1994 to the total pool of proteins present in each cell type the amount of a hundred trillion in each individual and the total proteins produced by cells of the body during different life stages.

After discovering the human genome, which includes (full content of genes (genes) in the amount of the 34 thousands people only, and not one hundred thousand. I think scientists for a long time) and also all the genes inherent in the cells of the body at the present time highlights the important question, what the protein content of these cells.

The type of each protein has to be known as a result of these cells and what function each protein and then what order of these proteins. Asking this question came after attrition rationale the concept of the genome and its consumption and is not enough to know as responsible for stimulating cells to produce the kinds of protein, but only requires the knowledge of the situation in its entirety in routine cases of disease and natural and in accordance with these questions and answers on the back of proteome.

Proteome contains information more complicated and the secrets of the genome is more dangerous than those found in the genome and extensive knowledge and synthetic for more than a million different types of proteins. The concept of proteome is known later human proteome is doing now by scientists and they hope that these will be the beginning of the main achievements under this project, despite the severe difficulties faced by these scientists, in excess of those related to the human genome.

The analysis (cell proteome), reached some of the researchers in 2000 to
build automated device called the molecular scanner "Molecular Scanner", which is carried out by measuring by mass spectrometer, from which tens of thousands of known proteins in a single day, and at the speed of more than ten times what was known before.

These researchers also managed to build a million boosted the analysis of protein per day to build bigger infrastructure database proteomics mankind. The draft of human proteome or other whereupon many of the laboratories and big budgets and international companies, different research directions, the analysis of three-dimensional protein structure and interactions between proteins, which performed many of the key characteristics of the human proteome would pay off represented by the following:

- Specification of fungus or yeast proteome with a single- cell, the first that has been done in the world of proteome.
- This project change from how to design drugs in the near future.
- The appearance of the so-called science and technology human proteome, which will focus on the conversion of most of the drugs manufactured by genetic engineering and biotechnology.

Advanced sciences and technologies

That the era of advanced technologies "High Technologies" or high-technology "Super Technologies" in which we lived the last three decades of the twentieth century, the era in which we do not know how many decades it will take, representing a number of scientific areas and new technology comes on top of these technologies, laser and fiber-optic and space technology, new materials, pharmaceuticals, chemicals, minute nanotechnology, and finally biotechnology and genetic engineering.

The forthcoming technical applications that are difficult to know the extent of today and its impact on humanity can be viewed as the era of advanced technologies as the following day when mankind as a whole interconnected network giant relies on a wide range of communications satellites such as radio waves and X-ray laser, so that every part of the ground contact one of the satellites in the moment and will be available electricity in remote areas with farms, genetically engineered to convert sunlight into carbon and then to the crude stream, and can then run all the equipment and facilities, communications equipment, including satellite and the Internet.

The future applications of these technologies will be radical changes in the forms of life activities and practices relevant to the interests of individuals, groups and the process of coordination between these advanced technologies is a strategic way to bring about a surge in operations research and industrial beginnings began to appear, for example, a draft genome and bioinformatics. We will try in this article and subsequent articles offer examples of advanced technologies

Nanotechnology, the technology that deals nanometer scale (metric unit of measurement), which is manipulating atoms for the manufacture of automatic equipment and information does not extend far a handful of atoms, and then anything can be made by micro- physics is quite different. The first part of the term to reflect the unit of measure (nano= 190^9 meters) the term nanotechnology in Engines of Creation written in 1986 and said the possibility of seeing the future of the armies of machinery hidden carry oxygen and nutrients and waste, and manufacture of atomic- sized machines called complexes pads that hold individual atoms. It was found that the control of the maize one and move freely and easily from attributes of nanotechnology.

This technique showed high density in the form of recent innovations in many of the global scientific publications. Including the mutations responsible for many genetic diseases and therefore provide in the future and relevance of information is indicated task to determine the organism is an information system for the manufacture of proteins and other compounds in spite of the inability to resolve the issue of structural triangular shape of proteins, despite the existence of mathematical models serve the purpose.

A fruitful field of nanotechnology research in many parts of the world and in government labs, commercial and academic, have emerged, according to the products on this technique such as sewing pants of fiber and manufacture of precision tennis balls retain flexibility. In the near future, computers will appear smaller tubes made of carbon atom chips represent the atomic scale wires and high strength to build elevator to space, and plants that will manufacture computers minute integrated directly with the human brain to increase intelligence.

It is clear from the examples mentioned that nanotechnology is a technology that will change very little minutes every aspect of human life and giving people the ability to control the material, and this technique is the most important applications of medical treatment of human beings through the introduction of precision instruments within the cells to repair infected objects from within or for the diagnosis of patients as well as some developments on the mechanisms of control cells. The first medical use of this technology has been developed a device implanted in the body that may manufacture.

The energy comes from bio-fuels in the cell and the purpose of this engine is to integrate machines in living systems fully, and use some of the scholars of this technology to produce nano-bombs to kill cancer cells. A team of other customers of this technology to produce nano-bombs to kill cancer cells. A team of scientists of any other industry, the crew of siliceous teeth not larger than the size of the cell that can swallow the red blood cells and re-launched into the bloodstream, either antibiotics nano-particles "Nano biotics", which new types of antibiotics contribute to solving the problem of resistance of some types of bacteria to drugs, as well as the modified bacteria organisms, are converging nano- tube micro- rings 2.5 nm diameter amino acids and small hole walls of bacteria are infectious.

Researchers believe that the future of medicine is moving towards nanotechnology that will change medicine, as future devices that will work within the human body to diagnose many diseases and treatment. Russian scientists in the field of quantitative light and laser physics to reach a new discovery has been called the needles agency, a new type of X- ray beam, or special characteristics, as containing the elements of nano- any electronic material on subatomic particles that do not exceed the measurements of nanometer dimensions .

It has also developed the first computer chip companies auction that could contribute to increase the power of computers and a reduction, while reducing the amount of energy consumed by the chip is composed of cylindrical molecules of carbon atoms in diameter than a billion to a part of the linker carbon (smaller than a hair a hundred thousand times).

Femto means the number 15 and the chemistry of femto, to understand the reasons that lead to some chemical reactions without the other, one of the achievements made at the end of the twentieth century and the efforts of the world that have emerged Ahmed Zewail, who won the Nobel Prize in Chemistry in 1999 and showing the possibility of seeing how to move the atoms within molecules during chemical reactions using laser technology and the rapid use of a new standard of time is Alfmto seconds (10^{15} seconds). Zewail has been used pulses of laser beam of a partial vacuum in the middle of materials to study the chemistry of high- speed stages of the transition, working within the Alfmto seconds be managed after the suddenness of molecules in the interim period and then became a pioneer of so- called Alfmto chemistry using laser technology (laser Alfmto) camera and a very fast, sophisticated and very accurate to portray the ongoing chemical reaction between the molecules in three- dimensional image Alfmto time in its three dimensions, not one dimension only.

Finally, what scientist do is to identify cases of transition of chemical reactions as broken links and new links up, and the development of new chemistry carried the name Alfmto result of invention, or a new laser called laser Alfmto or laser technology and through rapid as we were filmed for the moment the chemical reaction within the atoms in the process of only one part of a billion a second, and therefore this technology and its owner, Dr. Zewail laser secrets complex world characterized by inventing something new the properties of new energy and knowledge of the movement of particles from birth or docking to know what was happening in record time is a million billionth of a second the proportion of this period to the second equivalent of one per second span of time to 22 million years ago.

To reach Dr. Ahmed Zewail of the use of laser microscopy to clarify the picture may have been the most difficult times in less than two and thanks to the time factor has been developed to see things, whether internal or external speed and one millionth of a billionth of a second.

The features of Applied Chemistry Alfmto side is represented as medical, industrial and agricultural in nature and changes in the human body, such as treatment of diseases such as cancer, diabetes, a cell can be imaged in the human body, and according to that disease can be determined in the light of the nature of these cells.

Bioinformatics

The modern scientist characterized by the advantages and new versions is in the lab trying to understand the practical environment in which he lives and solve puzzles and formulates symbolic formats for a network of information and communication for the purpose of creating and responding to inquiries, questions of science resulting from a novel link between health and genetics. The question that presents itself is to us after the introduction on the topic of bioinformatics. The term is relatively new view and bio-informatics is also new. As is the case for many of the terms introduced in modern science, scientists have so far failed to agree on a single definition of the term. It may therefore suffice here to say that the (computing life) is the process whereby the relationships between technologies, biotechnology and computer technology, for the purpose of exchanging information and experiences and the related transfer of ideas and information for the purpose of understanding of life and death of organisms and also represents the integration of mathematics, statistics, computing and life sciences for the purpose of organizing (computing life) and analysis and interpretation.

In spite of informatics is modern science that he knew very complex rooted in and accountable to the most important multi-disciplinary mathematics and computer science as well as many explanations of the science or medical studies resulting from the human genome (genetic content) for different organism as well the use of electronic informatics to understand Genetic Network Models and the development of three-dimensional views of the complex molecules of the computer.

The basis of bioinformatics has taken different forms and the use of methods and tools for a variety of information consistent with the idea of the basic units of DNA. The gene, but at the same time vary according to the sequence of these units themselves and the simplicity or complexity.

The conditions and circumstances that prevailed in the incidence of different diseases and conditions associated with this aspect of the major change is largely in the increasing trend towards the modernization of information about human biology, including chromosomal abnormalities and related diseases for example, inherent "Down" is characterized by the fact that cell individual contains a third copy of chromosome 21, and is determine by microscopic examination, but tremendous progress has been possible to monitor changes in the DNA including the mutations responsible for many genetic diseases.

The important thing anyway is that recent data are heavily dependent on modern technologies that are designed to connect researchers, these operations become aware of the basics of bioinformatics associated with sophisticated and effective, hence the importance and seriousness of these means which undoubtedly provide the benefit greatly from this knowledge and its applications in health and genetics.

The inter-relationship between computer scientists and molecular biologists can computer world help to provide interpretation of the rules and the necessary to encrypt the DNA and therefore provide in the future and relevance of information indicated the task to determine the organism. Moreover, there is a possibility for the development of computer using DNA and the use of mathematical symbols rules when you're adding a certain amount of DNA that can store all the information in the computer world. The idea of computer life which appeared in the 1995 adaptation of DNA affords. For information processing finally, the biology is no longer limited to specialists, but it entered the computer science and scientists, who began learning these sciences and participate in the research teams of specialists to develop computer- life, as it can be envisaged that biology has become a note in terms of information called bioinformatics and the size of the smallest components of the computer-life billions of times the size of silicon chip is that characterized by very huge storage capacity and speed of processing to resolve some complex issues.

From the standpoint of the computer, the DNA and its installation of structural system is an intelligent and sober for the storage and dissemination of information and computer scientists had been accustomed to dealing with a binary digital expression of the alphabet, numbers and symbols, and diagnosed a direct letter of the alphabet of letter DNA. In order to encrypt messages, and all three relay in DNA is an information system for the manufacture of proteins and other compounds in spite of the inability to resolve the issue of structural triangular shape of proteins, despite the existence of mathematical models that serve the purpose.

Due to the fact that the storage of information in sophisticated computers to evoke a dramatically different senses, as a researcher actually lives inside a computer, a view of human life, all stored images of modern technology and not necessarily be tapped and developed. As several researchers in countries that have contributed to the success of the development of this human means and comparisons, as were studied in the genetic makeup of living non- human colon fruit flies.

The inter-relationship between scientists and molecular biologists can offer a update knowledge, interpretation of the rules and necessary to encrypt the DNA and therefore provide in the future and relevance of information is indicated task to determine the organism. Moreover, there is a possibility to develop the use of DNA and the use of mathematical symbols rules when adding a certain amount of DNA that appeared in the 1995 adaptation of DNA afford to address the NMC and finally, biology is no longer limited to specialists, but it came to the attention and scientists are beginning to learn this science and to participate in the research teams, of specialists to develop life, as it can be envisaged that biology is located in the heart of a paradigm shift led by scientists and biology became the so- called informational note.

Vital components and the size of vital billions of tunes smaller than the size of silicon chip and is characterized by very huge storage capacity and speed of processing to resolve some complex issues. From the standpoint of DNA and installation of structural system is an intelligent and sober for the storage and dissemination of information that scientists have accustomed to dealing with binary digital expression of the alphabet, numbers and symbols, and diagnosed a direct letter of the alphabet in the four DNA.

In order to encrypt messages, and all three relay in DNA is an information system for the manufacture of proteins and other compounds in spite of the inability to resolve the issue of structural triangular shape of proteins, despite the existence of mathematical models serve the purpose due to the fact that the storage of information in the accounts of sophisticated evoke a dramatically different senses, where a researcher is already in the arithmetic of human life, finds its stock, all images of modern technology and not necessarily be tapped and developed, as several researchers in countries that have contributed to the success of the Human Genome Project, the development of this means and comparisons, as were studied in the genetic makeup of living non-human colon fruit flies.

Research on the nature of genomes and the nature of the composition and organization of various scientific institutions. Acceleration in the implementation of the project, which was planned to complete within 15 years of technical progress, but shortened the time to ten years

Search the content of the genome to know what kind of information or material contained in the communication and diagnosis of all the genes strictly speaking, the number 100000 in the amount of DNA human as well as identifying sequences around three billion chemical bases. Study the nature of information storage in the computer and the evolution of elaborate techniques of efficient and sequence evolution that contribute to the analysis of information.

Study the effects to be set in the community and to what extent this can be achieved, and the type of response. In spite of all reported studies and research conducted by methods and techniques in various vital information as well as numerous writings in this area, there are still many other fields, and a variety of study and research. Some of these fields has not been touched so far in the country, especially the human genome projects, areas and areas to attract the attention of researchers, but it's mostly a few problems, mostly dealing with partial or subsidiary.

Diagnostic

Securing the different types of health services, preventive, curative and rehabilitation of the basic necessities of the individual and society is part of the economic and social development, the Ministry of Health before the embargo the country and the terms of reference of modern medical equipment and refurbished medical equipment, such that the health services in the country in all its aspects to the stage of qualitative and quantitative development admittedly many of the specialized agencies and international experts. That the imposition of the embargo has negatively impacted on the level of health services and spare the necessary medical supplies such as vaccines, medicines and laboratory solutions. In spite of that medicines and medical supplies but not prohibited under UN resolutions, but that the need for medicines and medical supplies that have increased due to the deteriorating state of health, environmental and food, which led to the emergence of many diseases, and chronic diseases and malnutrition. For example, Iraq was clean and free of cholera; the disease returned and appeared again significantly in 1991.

The scarcity of essential drugs and lack of availability of the required quantities led to the deterioration of the situation of citizens suffering from chronic diseases such as sugar and heart disease, hypertension, epilepsy, kidney failure and cancer diseases.

The laboratory tests were not no better than drugs, because the lack of laboratory materials and equipment used to conduct those tests and lack of maintenance and sustaining them available because of the acute shortage of spare parts and failing to be delivered to Iraq as well as the lack of diagnostic kits necessary to conduct examinations and laboratory1 tests, all that reflected negatively on the number of tests performed annually following table shows the percentage decline in the monthly Madal to prepare laboratory tests compared to 1989.

Impediments to the implementation of the diagnostic kits (negatives)

- The lack of some raw materials necessary for the completion of diagnostic kits, including:
  -       Chemicals.
  -       Other essentials.
  -       Hardware.
- Difficulties in meeting the needs of the researcher:
  -       Chemicals.
  -       Services in the local market.
- Continuing attempts to obtain materials and devices from other outlets outside the country led to:
  -       The survival of the need for quite a few of the resources vernacular.
- The cost of scientific resources, stationery and print the necessary reports to parents of high.
  -       The difficulty in obtaining journals and literature of modern world.
- The area of examination and evaluation
  -       Assigning one for the purpose of examination and evaluation.
  -       Not possible to give a certificate of inspection for some diagnostic kits for the following reasons the amount of material sent for testing are limited, instabilities of some materials, lack of some modern techniques and equipment.
  -       Unable to implement a number of these numbers.
- A steady increase in prices of materials and equipment and the cost of sustaining an impact on services:
  -       Estimates of the prices offered by the researchers.
  -       A number of research and is now paragraph of materials and devices is the amount greater than what they have as much time of signing the contract.

• Lack of standard materials and solutions for a number of diagnostic as reference material for the purpose of comparison scanned materials and productive and the lack of number of standard delay in conducting the tests or they can not be implemented .

Chapter Two

Development of biotechnology in medicine /the Iraqi perspective

Biotechnology

The concepts of traditional genetics known for thousands of years and then evolved into the development of Mendel's laws, famous, and then changed, according to the progress of various technologies and discoveries.

The increased in gene progress in terms of chemicals, then was reached as to how the work of the gene at the molecular level with the adoption of methods of biochemistry, rather than traditional methods in the interpretation of genetics, which paved the way to the evolution of the concept of genetic engineering.

The high and low living organism from units can only be seen with a microscope, a cell, which contains the kernel and the last, which includes chromatin materials that turn into chromosomes (chromosomes). Studies show that both the egg and sperm contain half the number of chromosomes (chromosomes) and therefore half the number of genes in human egg contains, 23 chromosomes. Chromosomes chemically composed of proteins and the "DNA". Studies have indicated that the gene is made up of sections from the chemical DNA. The latter consists of chemically according to the double helix model of Watson and Kirk.

That has been proven that DNA is the genetic material according to the following:
• The amount of DNA constant in all cells of the individual, regardless of the quality of tissue that make up the member.
• The DNA ability to configure a mirror image of himself during the division.
• The DNA characterized to contain all the genetic information in the order of succession of base nitrogen.

Genetic engineering

Genetic engineering is intertwined with the vitality and technology based on several basic sciences such as cell science, genetics, biochemistry, physics, and others.

The content of genetic engineering the human ability to control the mechanisms of gene transfer from one cell to another and how to express them within the cell for the future.

To understand the genetic engineering practice to be done the following:

- Isolation of DNA of the object which is meant the transfer of its genetic material.
- Cut the DNA to the sections that each end section to a particular gene.
- Identify the gene required between these parties.
- Ensure the presence of a carrier "vector" suitable for gene transferred in order to carry the gene of the object to the donor organism.

Discoveries that paved the way to genetic engineering:

- Carrier "vector".
- Types of bacteria contain a small chromosome called "Plasmid".
- Restriction enzymes DNA, you cut it off at specific sites.
- Ligases close the gap left by the restriction enzyme.
- Select a succession bases in the DNA Sequencing.
- Synthesis of pieces of DNA "Oligonucleotide synthesis" for the purpose of identifying genes within the cell for the purpose of diagnosis of many genetic diseases and led to begin the implementation of the Human Genoma Project.
- Using "Probe" in the processes determining the existence of gene and diagnosis and genetic makeup of the individual.

The genetic engineering since its birth in the seventies of this century a lot of fear, it is double-edged sword usable for good or evil and see the use in the prevention of disease or treatment, whether genetic surgery that change the genes with other as well as another gene in the filing of another object to obtain large quantities of secretion this gene for use as a drug for some diseases. After the success of the possibility of transferring genes from one cell to another, there were some concerns, including the following:

- The possibility of introducing genes that are synthesized toxic material within the cells of bacteria and make them so harmful effect.

- The introduction of parts of DNA Tumor Virus in another virus bacteria.

- Disable the genetic diversity, where the plants or animals that were subject to genetic engineering are usually homogeneous, making it vulnerable to bacterial and viral diseases and others.

Scientists played down such fears, the development of standards and controls to reduce the risk of manipulation of genes and these terms:

The issue of genetic engineering, genetic since its birth in the seventies of the last century a lot of fear, they double- edged sword usable for good or evil and see the use in the prevention of disease or treatment, whether surgery, genetic change since intra gene in the cells of the patient and the gene in the filing of another object for large quantities of secretion of this gene for use as a medicine for certain diseases while preventing the use of genetic engineering on sex cells "Germ Cells" for the legitimacy of the dangers.

And taking into account that it also may not be used in genetic engineering purposes, evil and aggressive, or to overcome the genetic barrier between the different races of creatures in order to create objects out of shape, mixed curiosity.

It is not permissible use of genetic engineering policy to alter the genetic structure in so- called improvement of the human race and any attempt to tamper with the genetic character or human intervention suited to individual responsibility is legally.

The prospects and risks of genetic engineering (genetic) after the success of the possibility of transferring genes from one cell to another, there were some concerns, including the following:

- The possibility of introducing genes are synthesized toxic substances within the cells of bacteria and make them so harmful effect.
- The introduction of parts of DNA tumor virus in another virus in bacteria, with the spread of these viruses and bacteria spread of the - disease.
- Loss or interruption of genetic diversity, as the plants or animals that were subject to genetic engineering are usually homogeneous, making it vulnerable to bacterial and viral diseases and others.
- It is known that human intestine contains different types of bacteria the bacteria can thus be dealt with genetic engineering techniques to live in the human intestine and increase the chances of the spread of diseases and epidemics.

However, the scientists played down such fears, the development of standards and controls to reduce the risk of manipulation of genes, some of these precautions: Controls for the design of laboratories and security measures to prevent the spread or leakage of bacteria and viruses treatment.

Although the benefits of biotechnology in many areas such as medicine, agriculture, industry and conservation of the environment there is increasing data show that diversity of thought began to intervene in the subjects continued to reduce the time from the jurisdiction of social thought and reason. The evaluation process of biotechnology has not yet started, does not believe that the limited studies on the impact of bad to launch microorganisms genetically engineered has no real value. These studies resulting from the overlap of politics in science and nothing to do with the problems faced by our communities

Genetically Modified organisms (GMO)

Biotechnology, which contains the processes of nucleic acid technology and molecular biology to separate the specific gene from one organism and transferred to a particular object of another district called gene transfer technology, "Transgenic" or may be called the genetic change or genetic modification "Gene modification" and called on the living modified organisms has been applied this technique recently on agricultural crops in the recent developments in genetics, which is also hot topics in it. A number of genetic modifications on some common food organisms, the addition of a specific gene or several genes, for example when carrying out genetic modification of wheat plant is usually a small percentage due to the fact that this plant has about 80.000 genes.

The process of genetic modification is possible in practice so as not to become genetically modified plant to another object or to plant malicious, but maintains the general attributes of the amendment with relative injury. According to some voices of opposition to the process of genetic modification, that could cause damage to humans and the environment, including poisoning or allergies.

The number of countries including the United States of America, Canada and China that will produce genetically modified crops, including soybeans, corn, flax, beets, potatoes in different proportions. From a technical point of view alone, there are a number of benefits of genetic modification of crops to convert to regular crops resistant to pesticides and weed, disease and insects and reduce pesticide use and increase productivity and improve the nutritional value of crops, and make it more a shift of the circumstances, including salinity, drought and an increase in the quality of the crops for use in food as well as in withstand the transport and storage and make crops resistant to pesticides, insects or insect resistance or both groups.

The genetic modification was still in use in plant breeding has a significant impact in providing food for humans and methods that have been used traditionally to improve the crops, but they are not specific or accurate results of modern genetic modification in which the change is unknown in most cases, things such as crops and breeding plant breeding and mutations.

Iraq occupies a very diversified geographic and climate zone and assumes a great deal of importance. However, its wealth is under U.N. resolutions. Its health and agricultural problems are diverse.

For almost twenty years (1970-1990), its Biotechnological activities have sought to bear on various problems on Agriculture and Medicine. In recent years (1990s), these activities have turned in a very limited way, to use some of new developments in Basic Biotechnology such as Molecular Biology and Genetic Engineering.

Various Centers and Departments are involved in the National Biotechnology research systems in Iraq. The Biological and Agricultural research Centers also integrate such activities into their research program.

Presently, these centers established different types of programs (long term, short term) in Agriculture and Medicine, for generation, development and transfer of Biotechnology. Major components of these programs; include development of technology transfer facilities and establishment of international collaboration in the field of Biotechnology.

Medical Biotechnology in Iraq, as a whole, demands strong collaboration in order to reduce the present gap between Iraq and the developed countries. Whereas, Agricultural Biotechnology seeks to increase food crop resistance to insects and diseases, utilize a wide varieties of techniques, including Biological control and various forms of Biotechnology, such as tissue cultures, molecular genetics and genetic engineering.

This part of the analyses of the major activities of Biotechnology in health, Agriculture and Basic Science in Iraq offers general background information on the development of Biotechnology. Then examines the current of Biotechnology research and potential, and suggests an outline of the strategies for the future of Biotechnology in Iraq.

Iraq, which has already entered the biotechnology era, whether on purpose or by chance, will in any case inevitably suffer the consequences of the widespread use of such techniques in industrialized countries. Therefore, the question is no longer whether such a move is desirable. but more how can best be put into use.

Currently people of Iraq are suffering from poor quality of life because of U.N. sanctions, which resulted in:

- Food shortage and malnutrition.
- Unsafe drinking water.
- Improper sanitation system.
- Poor health care.

This is why Iraq needs to have at least a basic level of skills to make it possible to define and implement policies in Biotechnology and the other technologies. Biotechnology alone will not feed Iraqis or give them better health, but it would be irresponsible not to see it as one of the available tools. A certain number of social, cultural or institutional conditions also have to be satisfied before technical success can be converted into economic and social progress.

This part analyses the major activities of biotechnology in Iraq; then examines the prospects of strengthening biotechnology in conjunction with conventional technologies; and finally it outlines the strategies for the promotion of biotechnology in Iraq.

Historical Aspects of Biotechnology in Iraq

Biotechnological activities were known to ancient Iraqis in Samaria and Babylon. For instance, fermentation processes and perfume extraction were very well-known to them.

It has been reported that the first experiment in scientific research was performed in the palace of one of the kings of Babylon. The experiment was carried out by two palace ladies who prepared perfumes by distillation from plants (steam distillation).

Cheese making is believed to have started in Mesopotamia at approximately 8000 years ago.

In the early 1970s scientific infrastructure construction began and several research activities were planned and set up.

Most of these biotechnological activities were limited to traditional methods to serve their needs; i.e. industrial fermentation, soil microbiology and bioconversion of waste products.

The government showed its interest in providing support to biotechnology by offering to host the first Arab Conference on Genetic Engineering in 1984. As   a consequence of the meeting, the council of Scientific Research established "Genetic Engineering Center", which became responsible for all research and development in this field; then in the agreement that Iraq established an affiliation of the International Center of Genetic Engineering (ICGEB) with the Scientific Research Council, as the principle Liaison Institute.

Since then during early 1990s research in agricultural biotechnology dealing with production of Biocides and Biofertilizer and Tissue Culture Technique were carried out by (IPA) Center.

The Ministry of Higher Education in the middle of 1990s, established a new centers for Genetic Engineering, involved in research on biotechnology. The main research objective on biotechnology of these centers involved the application of basic genetic engineering particularly in the following fields:

- **Molecular biology**: for enzyme production, industrial and clinical diagnosis.
- **Cell biology**: for animal cytogenesis (chromosome and gene mapping).
- **Microbial genetics**: for the production of useful microbial compounds through genetically improved strains.

Iraq through a new council of biotechnology at the University of Al-Nahrain (previously Saddam University) is monitoring international development in biotechnology in order to apply some of these techniques. As a result, this council has developed plans for biotechnology and genetic engineering in the sectors of health, agriculture and basic biotechnology. The major components of this plan are:

- Generation, transfer and development of biotechnology.
- Development of trained personnel.
- Strengthening of research and technology transfer facilities.
- Establishment of international and regional collaboration in the field of biotechnology.

Approaches of biotechnology in Iraq

Most biotechnological activities, which are applied in Iraq, are limited to traditional methods and serve their needs through:
- Fermentation
- Antibiotic industry
- Single cell protein
- Plant biotechnology
- Tissue culture
- Soil fertility, through biological activities
- Increasing food production through plant cell-culture
- Bioconversion of waste for food and feed ingredients

Fermentation

Iraq in early 1970s established traditional fermentation industries, bakers yeast production, ethanol, acetic acid, acetone, butanol and citric acid production. In 1970, a factory for making bakers yeast from sugar-beet molasses was established with plans for the production of compressed yeast.

This industry was faced by many problems, especially in dried yeast production:

- There are abundant sources of raw materials for fermentation in Iraq. Large quantities of hydrocarbons, and carbohydrate by-products (molasses) and lignocelluloses waste are found.
- Fermentation of food crops like dates, which enjoy comparatively large market sizes, does not receive sufficient attention. Local research on bioreactors is therefore needed to support the development of new processes and improve the performance of food industry in Iraq. Bioreactors also play a key role in the production of enzymes used in the beverage, detergent and leather industries.

Antibiotics industry

The antibiotics industry in Iraq started in 1970 for the production of penicillin and tetracycline. On the other hand, tetracycline production continued until 1980. This industry was discontinued for economical and technical reasons as a result of sanctions. The involvements of research and development programs have positive effect for restarting bio-industry and production of different types of antibiotics.

As the pharmaceutical industry in Iraq is directed to satisfy the local market by satisfying the market needs, it is therefore necessary to develop appropriate biotechnologies against various diseases that are endemic.

Single-Cell protein

A research and development program for single-cell protein (SCP) production at pilot plant level started in Iraq in 1982. The production of SCP from methanol using local and imported strains of Candida Utilis was investigated. The research plan included an economic feasibility study and the assessment of technological and nutritional aspects of SCP under local conditions. Then, another pilot plant was established to utilize date syrup for the production of bakers yeast and SCP.

The most important achievements of this program were the establishment of pilot research facilities, training of personnel, the nutritional assessment of available commercial SCP products and the isolation of several methanol- utilizing bacterial cultures.

Plant biotechnology

Plant biotechnology applications in Iraq include soil fertility (nitrogen fixation) using yeast strains in a mixed culture and cell conversion. Scientists have carried out research on nitrogen fixation by grain legumes. The main objective of this research was to increase the yields of grain legumes while decreasing the input of inorganic nitrogenous fertilizers

Tissue culture

- In view of the importance of the date-palms in Iraq, a tissue culture laboratory was established in 1979 at the Agriculture and Water Resources Research Center in Baghdad. Another laboratory was initiated at the Genetic Research and Biotechnology Scientific Research Center for the improvement of plant production. Tissue culture laboratories were also established at the Universities of Basra and Musol and also at the Ministry of Agriculture. The latter worked in collaboration with FAQ through regional center for date-palms in the near east and North Africa. The major objective was the commercial propagation of plants by in vitro techniques.

- Then in 1982, the vegetative micro propagation through tissue culture was carried out as a promising technique. However, future research is needed to early following and lack of uniformity of the closed plant.
- Date palm propagation by tissue culture was also implemented at research institutes and universities in Baghdad and Basra. Other species such as lettuce and potatoes were propagated by tissue culture at the department of Biology of Mosul University.

Other activities

- Research at the Faculty of Agriculture and Biology in the Nuclear Research Center was concentrated on the study of a sexual embryogenesis techniques and the induction of mutations by mutagenic agents.
- Agricultural and forest residues in Iraq are considered renewable resources that can be utilized by bio-technological means for the production of food, fertilizers and fuels.

The situation of Biotechnology in Iraq, since the imposition of sanctions

As a result of sanctions, many fields in public health system are affected sector by sector including critical areas such as: food security and nutrition, water resources, women's health, children health, national health emergencies, hospital care, humanitarians' donations and international cooperation. Scientific fields are also affected such as Oncology, Cardiology, Nephrology, Endocrinology, Ophthalmology, Diagnostic Testing and Protection of Blood Supply and Scientific Information and medical education, pharmaceutical and biotechnology inputs.

In agriculture, the U.N. sanctions ban the importing of fertilizers. Shortages in production of crops led to the deterioration in the Iraq's populations and nutritional intake (daily caloric intake).

- Iraq is facing the following three main threats: food supply, health improvements and environmental protection. Millions of people in Iraq under poor and risky growing conditions are suffering from poverty and poor health. They go to bed hungry due to U.N. resolution and security problems.
- Food security in Iraq is unique; it is not related directly to biotechnology problems. Genetically altered seeds are not necessarily needed to feed Iraq. This view rests on two critical assumptions, which we question:

The First is that poverty is not due to a gap between food production and growth of population. **The Second** is that biotechnology is not the only or best way to increase agriculture production.

- Iraq is not able to undertake effective agricultural biotechnology research for its own urgent needs without the scientific support of developed countries. Iraq needs more investment in developing appropriate agricultural biotechnology.
- Iraq which is subtropical country is basically an agricultural country. Approximately 80% of the total area is devoted to cereal production mainly wheat, barley, rice and corn. The remaining 20% includes a wide variety of crops, date-palm, citrus, tobacco, cotton and others. In general the average production level of all the important crops in Iraq is very low compared to those in developed countries. In the last 10 years, plans have been organized by the Iraqi government with cooperation of agricultural scientists to improve both the quality and quantity of crops per capita, using proper machinery equipments, fertilizers and suitable control measures.
-

Applications of biotechnology in Iraq in the experimental stage

Animal production

• The use of biotechnology in animal production in Iraq has occurred, in the field of reproduction, animal health, feeding, nutrition, growth and production.

• In the field of reproduction, new biotechnologies such as embryo transfers, in vitro fertilization, cloning, and sex determination of embryos have been studied experimentally for different types of livestock at the faculty of Agriculture and Biology in the Nuclear Research Center.

• Animal health can be improved with new biotechnology methods at experimental stage of diagnosis, prevention and control of animal diseases.

• Biotechnology in animal nutrition concentrates on improvement of feed; enzymatic treatment, the decreasing of the anti-nutritional factors in certain plants, such as legumes, which are used as feed.

Plant production

At present, more traditional aspects of biotechnology such as the followings are used:

• Tissue culture

The application of tissue culture does not require very expensive equipment. This technology was applied in Iraq to improve local varieties of food, crops for example using traditional methods for propagating potatoes for example.

• Pest and weeds

In Iraq, most of the land is affected by many weeds causing big losses in the agricultural crops. Since 1970s several herbicides were used to control the weeds of corn, cotton and vegetable fields.

Bio-control programs used for controling pests

The plant production research center is a State Board for agricultural research. College of Agriculture, Baghdad and Mosul Universities, Agriculture and Biology Research Centers and Iraq Atomic Organization are the main research centers in Iraq, which carried out different research studies on the biology, taxonomy and control of the pests. These research centers successfully adopted control measures on the most important pests attacking crops, vegetables and by applying chemical and agricultural methods. Promising results were obtained from many plant extracts against pests, by inhibition pest life cycle.

In Iraq, most of the agricultural land subjected to grow many of weeds causing big losses to the agricultural crops, as many research workers confirmed the positive results of the weed control measures to increase the yield of the crops.

Researchers started to evaluate herbicides since 1965, and mid of seventies, herbicides were applied to control the weeds in wheat, rice, corn, cotton, potatoes and tomatoes. Increased support is needed to expand research designed to develop new herbicides that are not likely to pollute ground water and that will provide reliable control.

Several centers are involved in bio-control programs.

commercially, research centers introduced two bio-control mutant fungi. Both fungi successfully were applied to control plant parasitic nematodes and soil born fungi on vegetables and citrus. Also the center used another fungus against date-palm stern borer insects.

State Board for agricultural research successfully adopted several control measures on the most important pests attacking field crops, vegetable and fruit trees by applying chemical, biological and agricultural methods. Many insect growth regulators, bio-control agents, fungi and plant extracts were experimentally applied on small and large scale fields.

Most of the research studies of the graduate students in the department of plant protection concentrated on the biological control, and plant extracts.

At the present time, the U.N. sanctions which have been imposed on Iraq since 1990, destroyed most of biological control programs and Iraq is facing lack of well trained personnel and shortage in facilities. As a result the first generation biotechnologies used in Iraq such as insect resistance, herbicides resistance are not easy to address any more.

Health biotechnology
• Several centers are interested in carrying on research on health biotechnology. The following may be mentioned.
  - Previously Saddam Center for Cancer and Medical genetics Research (SCCMGR).
  - Institute of Biotechnology and Genetic Engineering for Graduate Students, University of Baghdad.
  - Department of Genetic Engineering, College of Science, University of Baghdad.
  - Genetic Engineering Departments in a number of Universities.
• SCCMGR is engaged in several lines of biotechnological activities in health:
  - Cloning of tetanus toxic gene into tumor cells.
  - Preparation of tumor cell lines in vitro for gene therapy technique
  - Preparation of restriction enzymes vectors for gene therapy.
  - Studies on disorders of mitochondrial DNA in muscular dystrophy.
• Several biochemists have participated in various research projects that deal with diagnosis, and monitoring of several types of tumors.

Future biotechnology
The need for the application of biotechnology to face the basic needs regarding food and health in Iraq is real. There are different approaches such as the development of plant biotechnology, biotechnology applied to livestock production and biotechnology applied to food processing.

So, the suggested components of biotechnology plan include:

- Micro propagation: through e.g. tissue culture for multiplication.
- Genomics: the molecular characterization of all species.
- Bioinformatics: the assembly of data from genomics analysis into accessible forms.
- Diagnostics: the molecular characterization and identification of pathogens.
- Molecular breeding: the identification and evaluation of desirable traits in breeding programs with the use of marker assisted selection
- Transformation: the introduction of single genes conferring potentially useful traits into crops, livestock, fish and tree species.
- Vaccine technology: use of modern immunology to develop recombination DNA vaccine for control of lethal diseases.

Plans for future biotechnology research should be formulated through several priorities:

- Food security.
- Increase and improvement of agricultural production. Breeding for higher- yielding plant varieties and improve nutritive development values. Pest and pathogen-resistant genotypes and conservation of plant genetic diversity.
- Production of pharmaceuticals for the extraction of biologically active plant substances.
- Immunology: Production of vaccines and monoclonal antibodies.
- Use and recycle of agricultural products for the production of ethanol, acetone, butanol and methanol.

Food security

The applications in agricultural biotechnology in Iraq have the promise of bringing about the much-needed requirements in agricultural production, such as carrying resistance / tolerance to a biotic stresses (drought and salinity) and to provide options for better rotation to conserve natural resources.

Iraq is neither in the process of testing genetically enhanced products in number of crops, nor in the process of testing commercial products in the market to-date. Many technological advances are not visible in the farmers fields in Iraq but in the future are expected to provide ways to improve crops in a precise and fast manner. Use of functional genomics to address complex traits, marker assisted breeding to ensure presence of key genes, improving nutritional quality and managing natural resources better by use of efficient monitoring tools, Iraq must be an active participant in this area so that specific needs of food security are achieved.

Agricultural production

Despite the importance of health and industry sectors, the suggested priorities in the plan should have great emphasis on agro biotechnologies for two reasons. **First**: research on plants for crop improvement directly relates to specific ecological conditions predominant, whereas biotechnology applications for industry and human health are more difficult in Iraq. **Second**: preliminary data indicate that most biotechnology research activities in Iraq relate to agriculture.

The following classes of agricultural biotechnology are suggested to be used in Iraq in the future:

- Gene transfer technologies, which provide transgenic plant, resistant to many pests' pathogens, herbicide resistant to stress such as temperature, drought and salinities.
- Non transgenic biotechnological approaches for improving the efficiencies and effectiveness of conventional plant breeding methods.
- Technologies for better monitoring of natural resources and environment.

Additional suggestions for the implementation of the plant are the following:

Plant biotechnology

The establishment of biological treatment plants for sanitary wastewater and utilization of the treated wastewater for landscaping and agriculture.

- The establishment of the commercial production of inoculants such as Rhizobium and developed efficient methods for recycling agricultural waste such as beet molasses and maize and rice straw. Research should be carried out on the use of bio-fertilizers to increase rice yields in Iraq.

- The use of biotechnological techniques for the development and improvement of bio-insecticide for control of plant pests.

- Increasing protein content of rice by the application of biotechnological techniques. Rice is one of top five cereals grown in Iraq with its unique capabilities desirability to grow in stress conditions it is a crop of choice for Iraqi people. Rice has received comparatively less attention for research in general.

- The creation date-palm clones resistant to disease, and the application of tissue culture to improve date-palm varieties.

- Future research is needed to overcome the difficulties related to early flowering and lack of uniformity of cloned plants.

- Production of secondary metabolites, by tissue culture, the selection of plant cell lines for stress tolerance to salinity and drought and also the production of virus- free potatoes planting material; and the micro propagation of plant.

Animal biotechnology

Biotechnological application in livestock and fish production, and the adoption of embryo culture to improve local animal breeds through embryo transfer technology, are samples on pre-implantation and embryo freezing.

Microbial biotechnology

- Microbial biotechnology for ethanol production from sugar by-products and methanol production from Agro- industrial wastes.

- Microbial genetics: elimination or degradation of pollutants transformation of cellulolytic nitrogen fixers; construction of

Saccharmyces cervical strains capable of cellulose, cellobiose or lactose consumption.

- Proper technology to convert biomass into bio-fuel and biogas to convert agricultural biomass and animal droppings into bio-fuel and manure; of the various wastes used for biomass production. Rice straw is one of the possible applications.

- Bioconversion of lignocelluloses wastes to protein- enriched fermented materials followed by the production of microbial biomass from the hydrolyzed cellulose product.

- The use of bacterial treatment for the removal of oil and chromium; and also in the nitrification-denitrification process to remove ammonia

Health biotechnology

Medical Biotechnology in Iraq, as a whole, will demand a strong collaboration in order to reduce present gap between developed countries and Iraq to achieve this aim:

• A center of bone marrow transplant should be established in one of the hospitals. This requires the availability of experts, equipment and materials.

• Iraq is facing cancer and genetic diseases hence, research projects in gene therapy should be initiated.

Pharmaceutical industry

The pharmaceutical industry in Iraq should be expanded and developed so as to meet at least the local requirements. Biotechnological techniques should be introduced.

Environment

- Applications of natural occurring organisms (e.g. yeast, fungi and plants) should be used to convert hazardous substances in soil.

- Using microorganisms' pollutants from sewage systems to clean up industrial sites.

- The use of biotechnology to avoid pollution is of increasing importance such as the use of bioreactors to treat hazardous products.

Bioinformatics

This new discipline (biology and computing), which will be the core of biology in the 21st century, should be used for measuring and monitoring thousands of genes at one time. This computer-aided bioinformatics will stimulate future developments in the pharmaceutical industries.

cooperation with International Agencies

- Cooperation with Islamic and International agencies and countries are required.
- Well trained scientists from Arab and Islamic countries, directly involved in the training and transfer of various biotechnologies are also required.
- Post-graduate short training courses sponsored by international organizations such as the United Nations Educational, Scientific and Cultural Organization (UNESCO) should be organized in the various fields of biotechnology.
- Training of medical personnel in bone marrow transplantation, to help in gene therapy especially for cases of leukemia and lymphoma.
- Broadening the biotechnology base is a must for characterization, collection and conservation of germplasm that is already in the gene bank collection around the world and providing information for collection of gene pools that are not currently available in gene bank.
- Strengthening capabilities, developing projects, visits, and training programs of mutual interest to all participating countries in the following areas of biological control:

  - Exchange of biotic agents on a case to case basis.
  - Mass production of host insects and natural enemies.
  - Biological suppression of crop pests by developing joint projects.

- Computerization of information and networking research organization in different countries.
- Training in different aspects of biological control.

Ethical issues related to biotechnology

The Islamic world needs to have sharp opinions on various current issues related to biotechnology and genetic engineering such as genomics, human cloning and genetically modified organisms.

The National Programme for the Biotechnology / proposed research projects

Bio-technologies represent the modern mosaic of knowledge, rooted in the world of genetics, biology, evolutionary biology and molecular knowledge of chemistry. Bio-technologies are unique among other technologies for being a tool for dealing with life itself. They include technical applications that use the vital systems of organisms or their components or products to modify products or vital processes for specific purposes, and therefore include many operations and have wide application in agriculture, industry and other sectors.

Despite the benefits of bio-technologies in the fields of medicine, agriculture, industry, however other biological fields increasingly intervene with many other subjects and indicate that the diversity of thought began to appear. Therefore, a significant problem surfaced when preparing the National Programme for bio-technologies. Then, there was a significant overlap between the main axes of the programme and its affiliates. It developed themes and sub- themes according to different areas of bio-technologies that can be investigated by the Iraq meaningful progress particularly in the areas of food and health and strengthening pharmaceutical industries.

Major components of the programme

- The biotechnology and food security
- The production of bio-pesticides.
- The production of bio-fertilizers.
- Tissue culture.
- The production of potato tubers and seedlings free of viral disease
- Production of broad Date Palm
- The production of Fruit assets.
- Production of secondary materials
- Education programs and improvement.
- Technical embryo implantation in cattle.
- Manufacture of food products with curative nature.
- The production of liquid sugar from Iraqi dates.
- A study of pesticide residues in food.
- Improving the nutritional values of feed.
- Single-cell protein production.
- Improving the conditions of storage of foodstuffs.

Health and medical technologies

- Gene therapy and diseases
- Markers of neoplasm
- Genetical markers
- The production of vaccines
- The production of antibiotics
- The production of hormones and enzymes
- Vaccine production

- The production of antibodies to microorganism and toxins from snake bites and insect bites
  - The production of antibodies (monoclonal antibodies)
  - Development or establishment of cancer lines in the laboratory
  - Transfer of bone marrow and cultivation of bone marrow
  - Using molecular indicators in human lymphatic cells
  - Diseases of hereditary Cancer
  - Diagnostic kits
  - Forensic-genetic fingerprint

Biotechnology and safety pharmaceuticals

- Extraction of drugs from living organisms (plants, animals and microorganisms) for use against cancer and other diseases.
  - Extracting of active substances.
- The production of pharmaceutical materials and medicines through the revival of genetically modified microorganisms.
  - Preparation of medicines from medicinal herbs.

Plant Bio-technology

- Plant tissue culture, both at the level of cell or tissue or at the level of protoplast.
  - Improving the quality attributes of different crops.
  - Production of plants of potential environmental conditions.
  - Production of plants resistant to pests and agricultural bush.
- Increased production of medical and pharmaceutical plants and medicinal herbs.
  - The genetic diversity of plant.
  - The production of fertilizers and bio- pesticides.
- Development of insecticides to control plant pests.
193
- Reproduction development of resistants to diseases and the application of tissue culture.

- The production of secondary materials using tissue culture.
- Production of plants that have the capacity to fix Nitrogen.
- The production of new crops resistant to pesticides and pests salinity.
-

Animals and microorganisms technologies

- The production of genetically modified animals characterized by the attributes of high productivity.
- Animal tissue culture.
- Improvement animal resistance to environmental conditions.
- The production of veterinary vaccines.
- Artificial insemination.
- The diagnosis of hereditary diseases and germ using the PCR (Polymerase Chain Reaction).
- The cultivation of embryos.
- Applications of biotechnology in improving livestock.
- DNA technique.
- Vaccination of livestock against diseases.
- Transmission of embryos in cattle and fish.

Microbial Bio- technologies

- The production of hormones
- Fermentation
- Producing bacterial strains of anti- cancer
- The production of bacterial strains of high productivity of enzymes
- The production of bacterial strains of high productivity of antibiotics
- The production of microorganisms strains which have desirable qualities for use in bio- pesticides and fertilizers

- Producing microorganisms strains with high productivity of industrial materials
- Ethanol production by microbial Bio-technologies from sugar and methanol production of industrial and agricultural waste
- The removal and crushing and transformation of nitrogenous cellulosic fixtures
- Bio-conversion to cellulose waste materials rich in nitrogen

Environmental Bio- technologies

- The Use of living organisms in purification of heavy metals of the environment.
- Preparation biocides to combat agricultural pests.
- Preparation of bio-fertilizer to improve agricultural product.
- Finding microorganisms to revive the disintegration of some hydrocarbons and turned into a simple compound.
- Bio-technologies in the ecological balance.
- Bio-treatment of sewage.
- The use of microbial treatment to remove oil, chromium and ammonia.
- Using natural organisms to convert hazardous substances in the oil.
- Clearing industrial sites and avoid pollution.
- Oil Pollution by breaking chemical compounds.
- Isolation of bacterial strains that have the ability to remove sulfur.
- Using Bio-Markers and Bio-controls for detecting pollution levels.

Bio-technologies of Water

- Aquaculture techniques
- Techniques of bio- actors of water
- The use of bio- sensitivity
- The use of drugs and vaccines to preserve the health of fish.
- The cultivation of fish.

Biotechnology and basic sciences

- Genetic engineering techniques
- Genetic fingerprint (D.N.A. Finger Printing)
- Production of restriction Enzymes
- Production of standard D.N.A.
- Diagnosing the production of certain genes
- Amplification of genetic materials

Genetically modified organisms

- Genetic manipulation of farm animals to produce therapeutic human proteins
- Methods of genetic manipulation of farm animals
- Genetically altering poultry for the production of therapeutic proteins
- The use of animals in the production of genetically therapeutic proteins
195
- Adverse effects on animals that may arise due to genetic manipulation
- Genetically engineered animal, models for human diseases
- Genetically modified plants
- The production of much meat with low fat
- Improving the quality of protein from milk cows
- Gene transfer techniques to provide resistance to many of the insects and plants resistance to high temperatures and drought salinity

Bio-technologies in industry
- The production of antibiotics
- The production of enzymes and drugs

- Production of energy materials such as ethanol and methanol and acetone
- The design and analysis of Bio- reactors

Transfer Bio-technologies

- Technique of PCR (Polymerase Chain Reaction)
- Technique of PCR- STP (PCR with Short Tandem Repeats)
- Other techniques

Cloning
- Cloning techniques

Genome (genetic content)
- Studying the genetic content of the bacterial isolates
- Isolating and purifying D. N. A.
- Determining the content of the Plasmid isolates
- The safety of animal products and genetically modified organisms
- Building gene maps of plants of economic importance

Studies related to bio-technologies

- The systems and regulations for genetically modified animals
- The importation of transgenic animals
- Economic feasibility of genetic modification in animals farm to produce therapeutic human proteins
- Controls systems in the use of genetically modified organisms
- Ethics and social values and bio- technologies
- Bio- informatics
- The Bio-safety and bio-technologies
- Laws regulating the use of genetically modified crops
- Medical, religious and security considerations of bio- technologies

Development of scientific incubators in Iraq

To introduce technological incubator in Iraq it is proposed to bring these ideas systematically in line with the global approach by doing the following general functions:

• Absorbing the output and achievement within the country at the level of master and doctorate degrees and transnational consulting offices of these colleges.

• Absorbing the achievements of research and development centers in different quarters in the state (achievements of pharmaceutical, veterinary, programming and packaging materials)

• Employing the achievements of some companies from the public sector- private or mixed-dealing with specific technologies of the functions of these products, including incubators, and feeding of the proposed technologies as well as industrial products.

These technological incubators cover:

• Biotechnology
• Technology of drugs, medicine, veterinary medicines, herbal medicines, medicinal agricultural materials
• Technology of new materials, packaging, canning
• Information technology
• Technology of food industries

The importance of technological incubators in Iraq

To support the private sector, these is a clear desire to encourage this sector and meet the urgent need of the Iraqi people, especially in the sector of pharmaceutical, medical, veterinary, and food industries, packaging, information technologies, means of education and industrial sector.

Elsewhere, there are efforts to link interaction of institution of higher education, scientific research and technical institutes with productions, services as well as benefit from the ideas of creativity and innovation among individuals and institutions of Iraq. The embodiment of these trends has issued new laws and established special institutions that have national initiatives to achieve the required states of the initiative "cooperation mechanism" between the colleges and universities with various ministries and increase the number of graduate students, particularly at the stage of doctorate.

This shows that the economic climate and scientific activity and legislation in Iraq encourage the development of technological incubators at the present time (to be on   a trial basis), and the objectives for that are the following:

- The first objective is to gain experience in how to achieve Iraqi "product development" or how to move from search result to the investment, or how to transform idea and innovations or developments and renovations to the scientific and technical institutions to factories or services. This experience and expertise that produces them, if successful, must be repeated in dozens of places and scientific and technical areas.

- The success of the idea of incubators leads to diversify the Iraqi economy greatly, especially when it beats the experience of being beyond generating tens of incubators in Iraq.   The success of incubators leads to achieve substantial added value in production processes and services, not only in limited profits, leaving the added value of large foreign companies, the concessionaire or have intellectual property rights.

- Generating jobs and real productive for Iraqis, especially their graduates.

- Lifting returns of laboratories, equipment of universities, research centers and industrial development during the period of its life produced by investing in the work for production and service sectors and thus improve the conditions of their investment.

- The success of the experiment, solving these problems and constraints encountered will transform the experience of adoption by large companies in Iraq. Technology incubators associated with these companies will lead to significant results in the generation of existing industries (down stream industries) as well as in creating nutritious industries of these companies by generating (upstream industries), and feeding industries.

- The technological incubators will benefit in the marketing of output of scientific and technical universities, research centers and industrial development and linked to the national economy more deeply.

There are many justifications for the introduction of such regulation of such regulation, because the economic situation and its structure include more coordination, such as the following:

• Supporting the industrial sector in charge of the proposed technology incubator, including (medicines, information, food industries).

• Supporting the private sector which deals with these technologies to invest in the industry.

• Contributing to the provision of products for purchase of Iraqi citizens within its possibilities.

• Providing services not normally available.

Starting with incubators of this kind goes back to the physical possibilities available as well as the provision of appropriate venues as well as the fact that the process is not easy for the existence of many obstacles, yet this is a new experiment in which many elements have been evolved.

The private companies of special paper, cardboard, plastic, aluminum sheets, the National Center for Mobilization and packaging at the Ministry of Industry, conservation and packaging supportive of the pharmaceutical and food industries (dates, vegetables, and fruits) can play many functions.

Moreover, technological incubator in Iraq could play a special assignment, including:

- Linking universities and research centers in the industry.
- Marketing output of scientific and technical communities.
- Transfer of technology from home and abroad to invest in production and service sectors.

Developing job opportunities for graduates.

- Serious desire to support the industrial sector and agriculture and the private sector.
- Generating companies in the feeder industries and expanding in the market and- added value and the generation of new industries.
- Increase the added value in production sector.

Specifications of technological incubator

The establishment of technological incubator in Iraq should be connected to the Ministry of Higher Education, to meet the urgent need for the existence of an institution that play a role of assistance and contribution in providing advisory services to medium and small- sized enterprises and individuals. Incubator package of facilities and support and consultative mechanisms can be provided during the period or periods of time until the relevant qualification is set to start production and actual work.

These incubators specialize in general successes of the features and services including:

- Medicines and Medical herbs.
- Medical and veterinary supplies.
- Informatics area, computer software and the Internet.
- Packaging, preservation, packaging (materials technology)

The private sector will participate in the sectors of pharmaceutical, food industries and information technology sector and other feeding industries and thus contribute and support the private sector in an orderly and controlled manner both in scientific and organizational transformation.

Number of international bodies and institutions, including the Economic and Social Commission for Western Asia (ESCWA), as well as UNDP, other international institution, regional, will also participate in this effort.

The mechanism of this incubator, include the followings:

• Development of training programs and consultations followed by the selection of leading scientific wish to begin work in establishing a yield of profits.

• Coordination of incubators and then choosing them from among enterprises.

• The incubator during the incubation provides financial services, legal advice and support and develops plans around the dilemma of funding and the necessary investments.

Objectives

The most import objectives of the incubator according to the proposed technologies (medicines, food industry, IT … etc.)

• Helping graduates of universities and higher institutes to establish their institutions and their own business.

• Helping researchers to use the results of research carried out in technologies mentioned from the stage of laboratory work to the stage of practical application view production.

• Contributing to the resettlement of imported technologies and to assist in the transfer of technologies from developed countries.

• The incubator in the later stages to provide advisory services to the beneficiary institutions at work sites.

• The incubator provides advice in areas such as financial budgets discretion, and funding requirements needed to start production and organization of loans and payment methods.

• The incubator in the event of the availability of funds, provide soft loans for small enterprises.

• Incubators work mainly on developing a special relationship with local institutions, global development-related administrative and transfer technologies to local universities and research development.

• The incubator is usually implemented on intensive training courses for institutions incubated on some issues related to the success of the project.

• The incubator provides guidance on the new procedures and applicable laws entrepreneurs.

Management

The incubator is linked administratively by coordinating formulas with the National Commission for transfer of technologies and by the Iraqi universities and units that are consistent with the proposed technologies, including:

• Research Unit of drug/ college of Pharmacy / Baghdad University.

• Unit of common diseases/ college of Veterinary Medicine/ Baghdad University.

• Unit of medicinal plants/ college of Pharmacy/ Mosul University

• Unit of hemoglobin morbidity/ college of Medicine / Mustansiriya University.

• National Center for diabetes treatment and Research/ Medicine / Mustansiriya University.

• Center of blood diseases/ college of Medicine/ Mustansiriya University.

• Euphrates Unit for Research on Cancer/ college of Medicine/ Kufa University.

Those emanating from the other Ministries, including:

- Centre for the pharmaceutical industry.
- Center for Research and production of the diagnostic kits.
- Research Center for the veterinary medicines.
- Research Center pharmaceutical industry.
- National Center for Mobilization and packaging.

Therefore it requires the use of materials and instructions of existing laws to put the foundation or rules and procedure of the incubator from the laws we have mentioned above.

Moreover, passing laws may require the recall in the following basic features:

- Financial requirement of legal status and rights of individual property.
- Administrative requirements.
- Right of workers in the public sector when the loan was nurtured and how to leave his work in the sector.
- Issues of intellectual property rights for products.
- Legal features of the development of fund for incubator companies as they enter and when graduated and expanding production lines   .
Planning methods of benefit from the potential laboratory in the public sector and private sector.

The steps to implement the project
- Creation of a functioning business for the pioneers, examine the studying the legal aspects.
- Developing a plan of financing.
- Developing rule of procedure of the incubator.
- Agreement with the concerned parties.
- Organization of national symposium.
- Selection and training of nursing staff.
- Preparation of construction.
- Media and marketing
- Networking

• Follow-up performance

There is a number of proposed parties to finance this incubator project, including:

• Fund Development Planning Commission.
• United Nations Development program.
• Proceeds obtained from the 5% of the profits of companies that are allocated for research and scientific development.
• Cooperation mechanism.
• Incentives for creators.
• Consulting offices.
• Personal contracts for university professors.

Rules for admission to the incubator

The economic environment in Iraq determines some important rules to accept the products that will be adopted in this incubator:

• Product that has a relationship with proposed technologies that is currently marketing in the country (pharmaceutical and food industries ... etc.).
• Product that has the raw materials within the country.
• Product or service with high added value.
• Product that was developed inside the country (diagnostics kits, drug ... etc.).
• Product leading to the transfer of new technology (biotechnology, genetically modified organisms, genetic fingerprint)

New trends and phenomena
Of and scientific Incubators

Knowledge economy represents a new type of economy, different from the old economy, which was based on land, labour and capital as

101

factors of production while the new economy adopts the so-called knowledge economy based on factors, including technical knowledge, creativity, intelligence and information.

United Nations estimates accounts 7% of world GDP. Thus, the knowledge economy must be the main engine of knowledge for economic growth. The knowledge economy is characterized by innovation, education, and infrastructure of information technology.

The main forces that oppose to the knowledge economy are working to change the rules of trade and national capacity in the knowledge economy, including:

- Globalization.
- The information revolution.
- Proliferation of communications network.

Knowledge economy plays an important role in the knowledge society, globalization that is dependent on the economy; it is also contributed to the result of knowledge in technology developments, according to the following requirements:

- Establishments of organizations and new economic rules.
- Opening up world markets.
- Redrawing the map of the world economics.
- The emergence of new centers that depend on world trade.

The emergence of the knowledge economy has led to emphasis on the importance of education as a key to economic success and knowledge society which is closely linked to the knowledge economy. All these are dependent on creative mind generated from higher education, which contributes a significant role in the production of knowledge. Therefore, there is a relation between universities and knowledge economy and knowledge economy relies on knowledge production and the production of knowledge is one of the most important functions of modern universities.

According to the logical perception of the importance of the knowledge economy and adoption of standards, the UNESCO institute for statistics adopts the following indicators:

- Total expenditure.
- Expenditure intensity.

Comparison between countries of the world in research and their potential revolution, each rising in industrialized nations, falls in consumer countries for industry, which confirms the link between arbitrator and higher education.

Within the prospects of the knowledge economy, the government may support "multiple channels of higher education, including research and development" and in the area of health and medicine, in particular the increase in life expectancy during the last century 1900-2000 about 30 years, consequently resulted in an increase in the imports of society about 2 to 4 trillion dollars.

In order to play the Iraqi university prominent role in the knowledge economy, learning process is necessary as economic activity contributes essential role in the production of knowledge which is necessary in a series of knowledge society, and that the Iraqi university should resolve many of the problems such as:

- The link between higher education and the labour market.
- Strengthening the IT infrastructure and knowledge.
- The integration of contemporary techniques in the processes of learning and teaching.
- Trying to remove the traditional features of these universities.

The world economy also reminds us, that it is moving towards a knowledge based economy and this trend is explained by economic theories, including new growth theory. This theory says that sustained growth (rather than growth for a short period), is directly dependent on three factors:

- Technological level.
- Technological growth rate.
- Saving ratio.

The traditional factors of growth, in which capital and labour are involved in directly in the growth equation. These changes - which are

very important in the world economy - are considered as added value that comes from the high technological level, the technological growth of the state and not only from capital investment and work forces.

Economic growth depends certainly on the researchers, discoveries and inventions and to those who invest these inventions and creations. This is in addition to the good implementation of these creations that depends on skilled workers, who can deal with modern means of production.

Many countries are no longer depending solely on industrial zones and free zones, because this mechanism does no longer believe in acceptance of added value. These countries began to adopt new patterns since eighties, such as, technological areas, science and technological cities and areas of knowledge. The objective basis for these patterns is the maximum utilization of new and innovative ideas which emanate from research centers and universities. The link between research and development on one hand and industrial and service activities on the other hand, is the nucleus of these areas or new cities.

The technological incubators are those of new patterns that were adopted for the purpose of achieving the objective mentioned above. Technological innovators are effectively helping to move the idea of a new form of laboratory or experimental or academic to the model proposed for breeding technique. The incubator creates the company and owns shares of the company's budget; the technological incubators are the best means of developing countries or developed countries to encourage the establishments of the initiators of their companies and are product of proven economic.

The technological incubators are of the entrances adopted at the global level, to encourage and support small and medium industries, where there are today more than 1500 incubators operating in the world focused in the USA, Europe, Japan, and there are 500 incubators in developing countries. There are about 200 incubators in France and more than 100 in Britain and 200 in Germany. Furthermore there is Japanese experiment in the field of incubators and science parks.

The communities in general must use the modern technological developments and the appropriate environment form. These communities, which would deepen the work of free thoughts, contributing to industry change. Among these methods are business incubators and small projects. The business incubators is the integrated system of small projects that are, at the starting stage, in need of special support and protection so as to enable them later to move to foreign labour markets.

The overall objectives of the incubators are the development and creation of innovative projects, assisting owners of innovations and inventions, providing support and funding and providing services to destination funding for research and knowledge. One of the international experiences of such incubators is to implement the ambitious strategy for the developments of small projects; it requires a central body to manage, implement and follow up these strategies. The American experience is tracking U.S presidential administration but in France and Malaysia through specified ministry. In Egypt the incubators is represented at the social fund for development of the presidency of the council ministers.

There are currently in USA over six hundred of technological incubators such as Austin technological incubators, were used to reduce the failure rate for new projects, 50 projects have been graduated from the incubators, and 10900 new jobs were developed.

There are many types of incubators according to the objective for which they were established, including:

- Regional incubator
- International incubator
- Industrial incubator
- Specific incubator
- Technical incubator
- Research incubator
- Virtual incubator
- Internet incubator

The requirements for admission to incubators are place for the project, financial support, and technical support and skills developments. The incubator is preferably be located adjacent and not inside the campus of a university or research center in order to benefit from the resources and applied researches, laboratories and workshops, services and professors, but its presence within the university hinders the entry of customers because of security concerns.

Scientific incubators in the Arabic world

The incubators are working to accelerate economic growth by supporting the establishment of the main engine of the economy and its dynamic and high annual growth rate. The establishment and technology that produce goods with high added value requires an incubator for the care of these companies. These incubators provide opportunities to

accelerate the development of vocational skills for young people and specialists in the field of ICT incubator that was founded in Damascus between 2004 and 2006.

Technological Incubators in Egypt

The Social Development Fund adopted business incubators and technical mechanism to support the establishment of small projects and to develop the skills of self-employment among the initiators of technicians. Accordingly, the Egyptian Society for Small Projects introduced incubators in 1995 which approved the establishment of 30 incubators in Egypt. Then, it established 9 incubators that rely on simple technology in providing services, and light manufacturing projects which are dependent on knowledge and information such as the incubator of Mansoura, Asyout. The technical incubators are located near or inside the universities and centers of scientific research. The technological incubator of Mansoura University resembles the specialized informatics and biotechnology incubator in the Mubarak City of Alexandria. It is worth noting that one incubator accommodates about 40 projects to continue within incubator for 3 years. Statistics indicate that 520 associates will enjoy the services of incubators in 2006.

Science policies in Iraq

Science and Technology play a crucial role in shaping the challenges faced by individuals, organizations and nations constantly, (discoveries of genetic engineering, industrial human parties, mobile phone, biotechnology). The challenge facing mankind at the beginning of the twentieth century is how all countries could benefit from the strength of science and technology.

However, Iraq was unable clearly to improve the use of available science and technology, like other Arab countries, despite the availability of consulting firms and construction companies, millions of university graduates and about one million Arab engineers and hundreds of industrial companies and thousands of universities teachers.

The challenges facing Iraq, lies in the two groups, first resulting from major developmental problems, (food security, health, housing human rights, education, transport) and difficulty caused by the absence of the required scientific culture. The second is cultural in nature and include a special site independently. According to this scenario it requires the creation of systems of national science and technology take upon themselves the development of science and technology policies.

Iraq made over the past decades considerable progress in several areas, has increased the resources allocated to education, social services and infrastructure which has had a positive impact on the average per capita income and quality of life, followed by problems of concern (during the nineties). The per capita of the total GNP was decreased, the blockade halt efforts to diversify the economy and the adoption of the main sources of GNP on non- renewable mineral wealth.

There are some hypothesis for scientific and technological policies in the country which are limited in scope, effectiveness and ineffective strategies in the best of circumstances. So it was proposed to create new structures after some test on developed countries and developing countries.

The availability of financial resources in Iraq, especially before the nineties of the twentieth century has made great efforts in manufacturing, especially in the field of Military Industrialization. Iraq succeeded in building an independent military industrial base by enabling technology in modern manufacturing processes, however, strategies and manufacturing policies was clean from effective action to develp local capacity and providing appropriate incentives for local people to be able in modern industrial technology.

Despite this, Iraq still needs to pursue innovative methods to meet the daunting challenges of a large number of other sectors of production and services, as well as to develop scientific and technological capabilities of local traditional industries to modernize and to address a variety of social economic problems.

The scientific efficiency in Iraq itself has a capacity of innovative crucial role in facing challenges, in spite of standard conditions faced by the departure of many of them outside Iraq.

The limited scientific successes that have occurred in Iraq are the result of the efforts of some institutions of science and technology (Scientific Academy, the House of Alhikma and the institutions of higher education). On the other hand, important achievements were made in building the institutions mentioned, as well as in human resources development, but the institutions mentioned and others are still far from an enabling a distinguished role in development. The linkages and synergies between the scientific and technological institutions of governmental organization and the business world remain weak, despite the existence of some versions of contracting.

The spending on research and development in Iraq, at best, less than its counterpart in the Arab countries and more discouraging regarding the outputs of science and technology, so that scientific and technological publications in specialized areas and the number of patents granted to institution and individuals are much less than the average of the corresponding figures in Other developing countries.

As a result, the status of science and technology in Iraq needs a lot of attention. The input and output of scientific and technological point indicate the deficiencies in information networks, computers, advanced equipment, scientific research.

Scientific institutions

These include, institutions (universities, research centers universities, atomic energy, etc.), their shortcomings in Iraq are one of the reasons that led to the absence of a scientific and technological policies and the recognition of the limitations. The ineffectiveness of administrative practices and the existence of structural deficiencies are symbolic recognition of the need to develop capabilities in the next decade to operate in an environment different from recent years.

These institutions are currently working on:

- Production and dissemination of scientific research.
- Rating knowledge, covering a range of disciplines and areas of application.
- Training of some ranchers.

And, therefore it requires a complete reform of these institutions revitalization to support them, and identification of high-level priorities by increasing the competitiveness and environmental compatibility, creating an effective system of funding policies and linking them to industry and social and economic activities.

Scientific and technological cooperation with Arab countries, foreign states and international organizations

The current levels of scientific and technological cooperation between Iraq and Arab countries are very low, as well as with foreign countries which are almost non-existent as illustrated by the lack of joint scientific research and the outcome of joint publications. This refers to the need for Iraq in its quest to strengthen their scientific and technological interdependence.

To enhance communication and cooperation between Iraq with other Arab countries is a prerequisite in better determining the scientific problem and to obtain acceptable return of the available knowledge. Lounge of the basics of scientific cooperation is to avoid free turn key contains from any type of Technology, which is almost a priority involving scientists from two or more research fields, and incur the available possibilities to researchers to attend scientific meetings and make more use of international organizations.

The activity of science transfer

The term technology transfer indicates that the technology is acquired through the transfer of goods or services technology and therefore is not equipped for transportation and technological deficits.

The experience of Iraq in the transfer of technology is varied and appropriate in a large proportion, completed with foreign companies which provided comprehensive and complex technological deals in the framework of international market strategy, and the country suffered from indiscrimination of transfer that took place in the absence of a sound domestic policy in various technological fields.

There are two problems facing Iraq, the first is concerning the search, transmission, absorption, development and improvement of modern technology, and second is related to technology development. According to that, Iraq needs in the area of technology transfer the following:

- The search for technological alternatives.
- The selection of appropriate technology.
- Adapting the selected technology.
- Identifying the problems of adapting modern technology.

Research and development "R & D" activity

The research and development are both vital and active in maintaining the quality of scientific personnel, in ensuring access to advanced science and promoting technology transfer. In addition it is provide early warning preparation of technological progress, industrial, agricultural and health, whereas its investment is guaranteed.

The efforts in research and development in Iraq may differ from what made similar efforts in other countries in terms of outcome, it is still inadequate to meet the challenges posed by scientific and technological developments and the process of globalization despite the allocation of funds required in this area, and the last twenty years is good evidence.

- Establishment of an information society.
- Innovation of small and medium-sized enterprises participation.
- Development of human potential through the training of researchers.

Science policies in Iraq (Higher Education and other sectors)

There are no clear scientific and technology policies in Iraq, but may be the presence of strategies development that include the lines of long-term development of science and technology indirectly that deals independently within the development process. In Iraq private enterprises will invest in science and technology (Higher Education .... and others) in establishing a scientific and technological infrastructure.

The scientific, international cooperation in Iraq is limited and weak at present, while the efficiencies gained by scientific institutions in Iraq in coordination with existing competencies in the areas of social economic activity exists in society.

Under scientific siege, budgets reduced drastically, and scientific institutions reduced also their expenses strongly which led to the non continuation of the previous level of innovative capacity, and the inability of the infrastructure and science and technology to do their core functions.

The formulation of science policies

Iraq continued to practice, so far away from any genuine interest, the development of science and technology policy, due to many reasons already dealt with. It is worth mentioning here that any scientific and technology policies, in particular, depend on the quality of Iraq's exports. Petroleum Exporting Countries and Iraq, supplier of natural non-renewable sources reflected the policies of science and accordingly, it requires the decision- making process and scientific identification of reliable channels between scientific community and the political leadership. Moreover, the wording of policy drafting requires determining the objective of science and technology that includes:

• Promotion the growth of local companies specializing in services and manufacturing activities.
• Advancement of specialized institution.
• Increasing the movement of personnel in science and technology.
• Overlapping science policy and technology with a range of social and other economic activities.
• Development of institutions that will depend on science and technology that operates in a different environment.
• Strengthening the management structure of science and technology.
• Raising the level of resources.
• The effectiveness of R & D institutes.
• Development of technology transfer.
• Development of international cooperation.
• Improvement of researchers' wages and working conditions.
• The development of science and technology in long- term visions.

- The establishment needed in long term visions of all relevant institutions.
- Definition of the roles of effective government, private sector institutions, non- governmental organizations and professional associations.
- Adoption of progressive methods to build scientific capacity.
- Removal of duplication, overlapping and conflict in science organizations.
- Monitoring and evaluation and effective drafting in the relevant agencies in science and technology policies

It is proposed that a variety of science organizations should be related to the formulation of science and technology policies, including scientific societies and other professional such as industrial and technological organizations.

These organizations have to operate in an environment different from the classical environments in recent years (currently confined to the production, dissemination and application of knowledge covering a range of disciplines and areas of application), but must evolve and interfere with a range of social and economic activities and cooperate with other private sector organization. Moreover, these organizations propose concepts and scientific policy inputs.

Moreover, these scientific organization should involve the largest possible number of workers participates in the preparation of science and technology policies, including representatives of government departments concerned economists, chambers of agriculture, industry, trade, non-governmental organizations and scientific societies.

Institutions of higher education

The performance of institutions of higher education in Iraq is weaker than the performance of the countries that have the same resources and level of development. The reasons are due to organizational structure, prospects and understanding science policy.

It is noteworthy that all efforts made in the past to link universities with proposed scientific strategies were not successful for the same reasons. Therefore, it requires the involvement of these institutions in the channels that suggest implicitly of the scientific policy and development new scientific boards to discuss issues of science policy.

The efforts in research and development in Iraq may differ from what efforts made in other countries in terms of outcome and the challenges posed by scientific and technological developments and globalization. The linkages between research and development do not meet the need, as they are usually not based on cooperation, and are sometimes contradictory because of the lack of flexibility and bureaucratic practices.

The problems on research and development requires from its institutions to evolve, according to the ideas that have been developed. These relate to the maintenance of the quality of special scientific cadre. Further more then to access to renewable science in the world, promoting industrial development, technology transfer, contributing to social, and economic planning and accordingly proposed that the research and development institutions have special functions as well as:

- Proposals should be submitted through the channels when developing the new science policy.
- The possibility of providing early warning systems in preparation for preparation for technological change.

It is proposed in this area, that the scientific academy have a complex role in the development of science policy and is considered to be one of the main tributary of the scientific policy and may be a substitute for the supreme for Science Technology. The participation of specialized committees for example, could provide complex scientific projects, relating to environmental pollution, energy and natural resources projects

115

and areas of agricultural development, public health and natural resources.

The specialized scientific societies could propose several projects and comprehensive survey of scientific resources, human and various national materials. Also enhance the working groups that can be developed and networks of cooperation between scientists from various disciplines concerned, with the establishment of networks of information for selected sectors based on the priorities identified by policy. It can evaluate research projects and public awareness of science and technology and increased attention to scientific research.

These institutions are required to have the presence of a specific set of targets linked with science policy and technology, which are consistent with a coherent vision for the future.
The responsibilities to the views of specialized advisory functions include characterization and strengthening the linkages and knowledge flows and providing technical services.

Proposal to develop a higher council for science

Iraq's various institutions face difficulties in promoting scientific and technological capabilities and future planning of the scientific, issues to acquire the capacity of innovation. This can not be achieved unless being done within the framework of science policy interrelated. Accordingly, it is required to use new methods of science and technology policies, and to develop integrated growth strategies that take into account of local and external scientific conditions. To implement these, it is proposed to develop an academy or a higher council for science and technology. This Council (or academy) which is an institution with personal, moral, financial and administrative requirements characterized by autonomy should be linked to the Office of the Presidency.

The council carries out the followings:

- Development of science and technology policies in accordance with the demands of current and future science.
- Contributing to the scientific development of internal and external sources.
- Promotion of scientific studies and research in the country to keep abreast of scientific advances in the world.
- Establishment of scientific ties and close cooperation with Arab and international destinations.

The academy or the Supreme Council consists of:

- Members of not less than 35 not more than 40 including the President of the Council or the Academy.
- Secretary-General.

The member should be a scientist and researcher in one of the branches of knowledge (agricultural, industrial, treatments, medical, engineering) and has a broad access to one or another branch of knowledge, and has genuine scientific product.

- The academy members should be appointed by the Prime Minister and enjoys the rank of Deputy Minister.
- The Academy full-time secretary-general is appointed from among its members.
- The Academy has a number multiple specialized committees working in coordination with other scientific institutions in the country (Commission on Technology, the Committee of Water, Energy Commission and Commission for information).
- The Academy has specialized offices within the framework of scientific knowledge (agricultural, medical, engineering, pure science).
- The Academy creates the suggestion of science and technology policies and then filed for the presidency for the Adoption (after being revised, by its committees and services).
- It also works with the recommendation to grant material assistance to the centers and individuals, adoption of the establishment of various scientific centers.

- Development of labor contexts between scientific institutions and the beneficiaries and the mechanism of cooperation between scientific institutions of Iraqi and international institutions involved.

The Supreme Council for Science and Technology proposes a policy for science and technology in the country in accordance with the following tasks:

- Coordination of the efforts to formulate science and technology policies in Iraq at the institutional level.
- Clarification of methodologies used in policy formulation of science and technology.
- Modernization and integration of science policy with development policy.
- Analysis of scientific and technological capabilities in Iraq with a

focus on research and development.
- The need to inform policy makers of the methods used in the planning and programming of research activities
- Building local capacity through education and experimentation.
- Following up the implementation of these policies through the secretariat and a mechanism to provide on issues.

Formation of a Higher Council for Science and Technology

Detailed proposal:

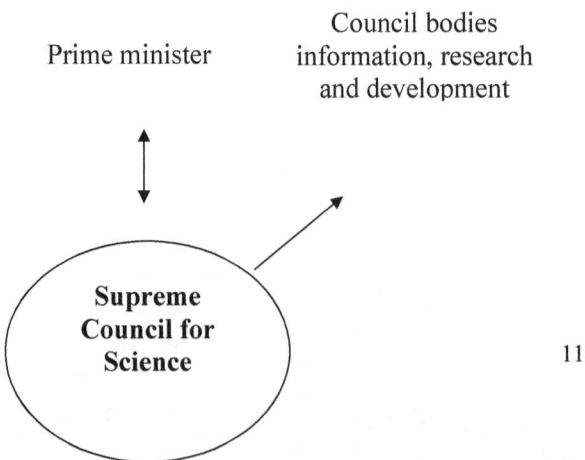

Prime minister

Council bodies information, research and development

Supreme Council for Science

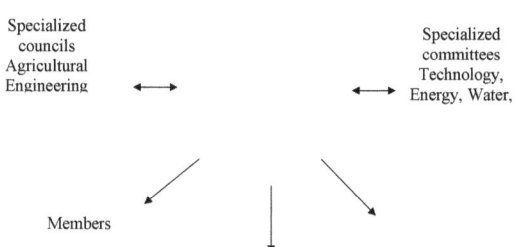

Specialized councils
Agricultural Engineering

Specialized committees
Technology, Energy, Water,

Members

-
- other countries, with balance between the two sides.

- Investment of scientific institutions of science and technology in creating the scientific and technological infrastructure.

- International scientific cooperation.

- Promotion of development of national technological capabilities in both the private and public alike. Coordination of competencies gained by scientific and technological system and their integration with national huge number of competencies in the areas of social and economic activity.

- The integration of science and technology policies with a set of national policies and programmers that meet this purpose.

- Continuation of production and dissemination of scientific and technological knowledge and maintain an effective level of innovative capacity.

- Continuous documentation of formulating policies and scientific technology.

-

General trends

119

Policies can be characterized by scientific and technological trends and are generally maintaining the balance between any movement toward the development of local scientific and technology and the establishment of links with external sources of technological knowledge that take place in several stages:

- Continuous assessment of the current status of science and technology.
- Development of the prospects of continuing to develop science and technology during any (year).
- Development of a strategy based on specialized studies related to the objectives of developmental policy.
- The preparation of a detailed five-year plan accompanying executive programs constitute the followings:

- Keeping pace with scientific and technological developments in the world (biotechnology, information technology, energy technology... etc).

- Keeping up with scientific and technological developments in the world through the follow-up scientific and technological capabilities such as (biotechnology, information and energy).

- Monitoring the change in scientific institutions and the Arab world and the extent of the involvement of scientists in Iraq with their peers in the Arab countries and the world.

- Following the changes in social and economic conditions throughout the world.

- Examination of human skills constantly has been much more important than raw materials and it leads to many possibilities, including:

- Achieving parity with other countries in science and technology.

- Identifying better scientific problems and understanding of the issues that are raised in a more comprehensive way.

Other organizational matters related

These include the input and output of science and technology policy with emphasis on the role of different institutions, including industrial, educational and private and scientific academy. It is also important to emphasize in this area on organizational matters that are between institution and how to submit proposals and receive guidance on science policy that includes:

- Providing specialists for ongoing assessment of the potential of science and technology.

- Involving the largest possible number of parties involved in the preparation of science policy as well as interaction with the production sectors and services through formal mechanisms.

- The participation of the private sector in financing scientific capacity building.

- Consideration of responsiveness to the requirements of development policies.

After gathering proposals for science and technology policy from various channels according to directions from the supreme authority, it is proposed, in this case, to adopt scientific policy objectives (competition, trade barriers, the environment, new technologies). Then the policy with the top destinations should be approved by political leadership.

Thus, according to this scenario it is needed to start work for the establishment and completion of institutional arrangements and accordingly the following are accompanied the proposal.

- Evaluation and forecast of scientific and technological advances.
- Assess the market demand for science and technology.
- Planning and management of science and technology.

The scientific policy decision should take into consideration the following:

- Be based on local capacity and scientific progress in other places and to balance them.
- Contribution to regional and international programmes for the development of science and technology.

The role of the Supreme authority:

- It is proposed to take measures immediately to develop a policy and scientific and technological integration in social and economic development plans in Iraq, and the establishment of linkages with the private sector through specific proposals.
- Creation of private channels and specialized committees to prepare the requirement of science and technology policy and guide these channels with the supreme Council or academic parameters of this policy.

Financing plans and activities of science and technology

It is required at this time highlighting the role of financial institutions and the mobilization of resources to allocate sufficient resources, to invest in technologies that have been obtained or that have been developed locally. By financial mechanisms it is necessary to implement policies, by increasing allocation of resources for scientific and technological activities, research and development budget in public and private sectors.

First: The state budget (current and investment).
Second: The socialist sector companies.
Third: The mixed sector companies and private sectors.
In order to establish a national fund for science and technology it is required to have feasibility study, allocated 0.25 per cent of Iraq's national budget, to finance projects of technological priority implemented through contracts awarded on the basis of competitive bidding.

The funding system in the private sector, which relies on the so-called policy of risk sharing by adopting the industrialized countries, ranging from tax incentives, grants and loans to encourage private investment in innovative activates

Chapter Three

Biochemical Markers in Diseases

The breast is constantly responding to changes in hormonal, nutritional, genetic, psychological, and environmental stimuli such as radiation that cause continual cellular changes. As a result of these changes, breast tumors (abnormal breast tissue) may develop either benign (noncancerous) or malignant (cancerous). The major significance of the benign processes less in the need to separate them from malignancies. The World Health Organization (WHO) classifies tumors of the breast (1981) according to histological aspects[) (Table 1).

Table (1): Histological classification of breast tumors

I. Epithelial Tumors
A. Benign
1. Intraductal papilloma
2. Adenoma of the nipple
3. Adenoma
a. *Tublar*
b. *Lactating*
B. Malignant
1. Non invasive
a. *Intraductal carcinoma*
b. *Lobular carcinoma*
2. Invasive
a. *Invasive ductal carcinoma*
b. *Invasive lobular carcinoma*
3. Paget's disease of the nipples

II. Mixed Connective Tissue and Epithelial Tumors	
a. **Fibroadenoma**	

Table (1.1): Continued.

b. **Phyllodes tumor (cystosarcoma phyllodes)**	
c. **Carcinosarcoma**	
III. Miscellaneous Tumors	
a. **Soft tissue tumors**	
b. **Skin tumors**	
c. **Tumors of haemopcietia and lymph tissues**	
IV. Unclassified Tumors	
V. Mammary Dysplasia / Fibrocystic Change	
VI. Tumor like Lesion	
a. **Duct ectasia**	
b. **Inflammatory pseudotumors**	

Benign Breast Tumors

. Fibroadenoma

This is the most common benign tumor of the female breast. It is a new growth composed of both fibrous and glandular tissue. These tumors are commonly found in younger women between the ages 20-35 years It increases in size, during pregnancy. It is less likely to develop after menopause. An epidemiological study suggests that fibroadenoma represents a long-term risk for breast carcinomas and that risk is increased in women with ductal hyperplasias, or a family history of breast carcinoma

Fibrocystic disease

This is an ill-defined condition of the breast where palpable lumps can be felt and is usually associated with pain and tenderness that fluctuates with the menstrual cycle. Fibrocystic changes are the most common, occurring in approximately 60% of premenopausal women. Women with this disease usually have a freely movable, palpable mass, at time it may cause pain, particularly when women are in the premenopausal phase of the menstrual cycle, however, breast pain can be caused by lesions other than fibrocystic changes. The palpable lesion may appear to increase and decrease is size cyclically; usually achieving its maximum size in the premenstrual phase of the menstrual cycle. Cystic disease is frequently accompanied by varying degrees of epithelial hyperplasia in adjacent ducts and lobules. In patients who have one particular form of fibrocystic disease (the proliferate form), the incidence of cancer increased very slightly.

. Malignant Breast Tumors

Incidence

Breast cancer is the most common malignant tumors in women, and it is the leading malignancy affecting women in North America and Europe. In 2000, approximately 184200 new cases of invasive breast cancer were diagnosed in the United States. The number of noninvasive breast cancer is hard to verify, but it probably account for and an additional 20000 to 30000 new cases; thus, the number of invasive and noninvasive breast cancer treated in 2000 approximately 200000

In Iraq, according to the results of Iraqi Cancer Registry (ICR), breast cancer accounting for (31.11%) and remained the commonest tumors in the year 2000[3], it was also shown that breast cancer was the first among the commonest ten cancers in Iraq. Figure (1) represents the population of breast cancer in Iraq for the last nine years. As shown in the same figure, the population of breast cancer increased more than double in the last

nine years.

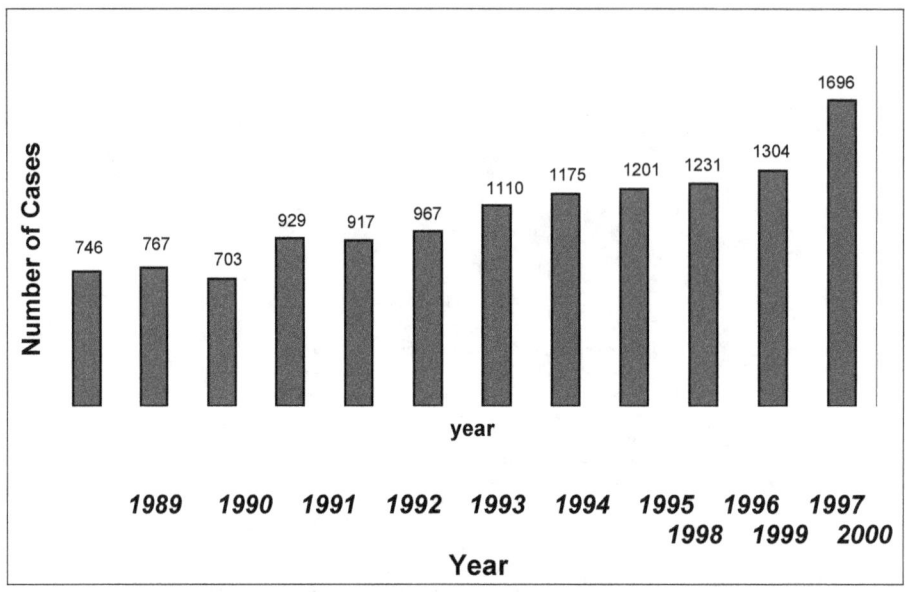

Figure (1.1): The population of breast cancer in Iraq through (1989-2000

. Etiology and Risk Factors in Breast Cancer

Numerous risk factors have been associated with the development of breast cancer, such as genetic, environmental, hormonal, and nutritional.

Despite all available data on breast cancer risk factors, 75% of women with this cancer have not exposed to any risk factors

Family History

Bence jones protein which is exhibits unusual solubility in water was the first tumor marker identified in 1848, it appears in large amounts in the urine of patients with multiple myeloma. More than 100 years after its discovery the Bence-Jones protein was identified as a monoclonal light chain of immunoglobulin.

Between 1928-1963, many substances including (hormones, enzymes, isoenzymes and proteins) were discovered and used as tumor markers useful in the diagnosis of individual tumors, but the general application of tumor marker for monitoring cancer in patients did not start until the discovery of α-fetoprotein (AFP in 1963 and carcinoembryonic antigen (CEA) in 1965. The production of such markers during fetal development as well as in tumors, led to the term oncodevelopmental markers. Monoclonal antibodies were developed in 1975. to detect oncofetal antigens and antigens derived from tumor cell lines such as CA125, CA 15-3, and CA 19-9.

More recent advances in molecular techniques with the use of molecular probes and monoclonal antibodies to detect chromosome or protein alteration, including the study of oncogenes, suppressor genes, and genes involved in DNA repair, have led to the rapid understanding and use of tumor markers at molecular level. Unlike earlier tumor markers, these new markers can be linked to specific biological processes related to the regulation of cell growth and tumor development including malignant transformation, proliferation, apoptotic cell death and metastasis.

Definition of tumor marker

A tumor marker is a substance that is present in or produced by tumor itself, or produced by the host in response to a tumor (6) that can be used to differentiate a tumor from normal tissue or to determine the presence of a tumor based on its measurement in the blood or secretions. Such a substance can be found in cells, tissue, or body fluids. It can be measured qualitatively or quantitatively by chemical, immunological, or molecular biological methods to identify the presence of a cancer.

Morphologically, cancer tissue has been recognized by pathologists as resembling fetal tissue more closely than normal adult differentiated tissue. Tumors are graded according to their degree of differentiation: as being well differentiated, poorly differentiated, or anaplastic (without form). Few markers are specific for single individual tumor (tumor-specific markers); most are found with different tumors of the same tissue type (tumor-associated markers). They are present in higher quantities in cancer tissue or in blood of cancer patients than in benign tumors or in the blood of normal subjects.

Tumor markers have been categorized as enzymes, isoenzymes, hormones, and oncofetal antigens, carbohydrate epitopes recognized by monoclonal antibodies, receptors, oncogene product and genetic changes. There are only a handful of well-established tumor markers that are being used by physicians. Many other potential markers are still being under research. Now there are many studies that are trying to find new genes involved in signaling molecules or proteins that "tell" cells to proliferate, invade or metastasize (9).

Classification of Tumor Markers

Tumor markers may be classified into chemical and genetic tumor Markers.

Chemical tumor markers

Table (1) Summarizes the classification of chemical tumor markers according to biochemical characteristics, and their associated malignancy.

Table (1) Chemical tumor markers

Marker type	Associated malignancy	Example
Enzymes	Liver	Alcohol dehydrogenase
	Bone, Liver, Leukemia, Sarcoma	Alkaline phosphatase
	Ovarian, lung, trophoplastic, gastrointestinal, seminoma, hodgkin's	Alkaline phosphatase placental
	Pancreas, Various	Amylase
	Colon, Breast	Aryl Sulfatase B
	Colon, Bladder, Gastrointestinal, Various	Galactosyl Transferase
	Lung, (small-cell) neuroblastoma,	Neuron-Specific

Hormone		
	Carcinoid, melanoma, pancreatic	enolase
	Prostate, Various (large bowel, lung, ovarian)	Prostate-specific antigen (PSA) Ribonuclease
	Colorectal, Breast, etc.	Telomerase
	Colon, Breast, Lung	Sialyl Transferenase
Hormone	Gushing,s syndrome, Lung (small cell)	ACTH
	Lung (small cell) adrenal Cortex, deudonal	Antidiuretic hormone
	Medullary thyroid	Calcitonin

Pituitary adenoma, Renal, Lung, Embryonal, choriocarinoma, Testicular (nonseminomatous)	hCG	
Torophoblastic, Gonads, Lungs, Breast	Human placental lactogen	
Liver, Renal, Breast, Lung, Various	Parathyroid hormone	
Pituitary adenoma, renal, lung, breast.	prolactin	
Oncofetal Antigen	Hepato cellular, germ line (non seminoma)	□-feto protein
	Colon	β- oncofetal antigen
	Liver	Carcino fetal ferritin
	Colorectal,	CEA

	Gastrointestinal, Pancreatic, Lung, Breast	
	pancreatic	Pancreatic oncofetal
	Cervical, Lung, Skin, Head& neck (Squamous)	Squamous cell antigen
	Colon,Gastrointestinal, Bladder	Tennesse antigen
Mucin	Ovarian, endometrial, Lung	CA125
	Breast, ovarian	CA15-3
	Breast	CA27-29
	Breast, ovarian	MCA
	Pancreatic, Ovarian, Gastrointestinal, Lung	Du-PAN-2
protein	Multiple Myeloma, β-Cell lymphpoma chronic	β- 2 microglobulin
	Insulinoma	C-peptide
	Liver, Lung, Leukemia	Ferritin
	multiple myeloma, Lymphomas	Immunoglobulin
	Pancreatic, Stomach	Pancreas associated antigen
	Trophoplastic, Germ cell	Pregnancy specific protein
	Hepatocellular	Prothrombin precursor
	Ovarian	Tumor associated trypsin inhibitor
Blood Group Related antigen	Pancreatic, Hepatic, Gastrointestinal,	CA19-9
	Pancreatic, Gastrointestinal, Ovarian	CA19-5

	Colon, Pancreatic Gastrointestinal,	CA50
	Ovarian, Breast, Colon ,Gastrointestinal,	CA72,4,CA242
Others	Breast	Estrogen&progester one receptors
	Brain, Various	polyamine
	Bone Metastasis (Breast), (multiple myeloma)	Hydroxy proline
	Neuroblastoma, pheochromocytoma	Catecholamine metabolites
	Gastroitestinal, Lung, Rhenmatoid	Lipid-associated sialic acid

Genetic tumor markers

A simple definition of cancer is "a relatively autonomous growth of tissue". Understanding the cause of autonomous growth would clearly facilitate the search for care. Advance in molecular genetics have provided a better understanding of the genesis of human cancer. The proliferation of normal cell is thought to be regulated by growth – promoting oncogenes and counterbalanced by growth – constraining tumor suppressor genes. The development of cancer appears to involve the activation or altered expression of oncogenes, and the loss or inactivation of tumor suppressor genes

Oncogenes (cell activation genes) are derived from proto- oncogenes (normal celluler genes) which may be activated by dominant mutations. The type of mutation might be point mutation, insertion, deletion, translocation, or inversion. Most oncogenes are associated with haematological malignancies such as leukemia and to lesser extent, solid tumors.

Suppressor genes (genes involved in the recognition and repair of damaged DNA) have mostly been isolated from solid tumors. p53 tumor suppressor gene is the most frequently mutated gene in human cancer, indicating its important role in the conservation of normal cell cycle progression. One of p53'S essential roles is to arrest the cells in G1 after genotoxic damage, to allow DNA repair prior to DNA replication and cell division. In response to massive DNA damage, p53 triggers the apoptotic cell death pathway. The loss of function of this gene may result in the inability of DNA repair process and may lead to the development of tumorgensis.

The exciting promise of using the detection of oncogenes and suppressor genes, for diagnosis, determining the prognosis, and predicting the response to the chemotherapy remains to be realized. Oncogens detection remains an experimental approach to human cancer.

Ideal Tumor Marker

An ideal tumor marker should be specific for a given type of cancer and sensitive enough to detect small tumors for early diagnosis or during screening, provide an estimation of tumor burden, and serve for monitoring effects of therapy and detecting recurrence of tumors. It can be measured qualitatively or quantatively by chemical, immunological, or molecular biological methods to identify the presence of a cancer.

Clinical Applications of Tumor Markers

Clinical applications of tumor markers depend on specificity and sensitivity. Specificity refers to the detection of specific tumors by specific markers. Sensitivity, in this instance, has to do with detecting all patients with the specific tumor.

The potential uses of tumor markers are:

- Screening in general population.
- Differential diagnosis of symptomatic patients.
- Clinical staging of cancer
- Estimating tumor volume.

- Prognostic indicator for disease progression
- Evaluating success of treatment.
- Detecting response to therapy
- Radioimmunolocalization of tumor marker.
- Determining direction for immunotherapy.

In general tumor markers may be used for diagnosis, prognosis, and monitoring effect of therapy, as well as a target for tumor localization and therapy. Monitoring treatment with tumor markers is an accepted application and generally indicates successful treatment; such monitoring iThe use of tumor markers for screening   the presence of cancer in asymptomatic individuals in a general population has been limited because most tumor markers are present in normal, benign and cancer tissues and are not specific enough to be used for screening cancer. However if the incidence of cancer is high among certain population, screening is feasible. Potential uses of some tumor markers are summarized in table (2).

Tumors of Ovary
Classification
The pathological conditions of the ovary may be classified as:
Non-neoplastic Functional Cysts
Follicular cyst
Corpus luteum cyst.
Theca lutein and granulose lutein cysts.
Polycystic ovarian disease.
Endometriomatous cysts.

Ovarian Neoplasm's.
The classification of ovarian neoplasm's given in table (3), is a simplified version of world health organization (WHO) histological classification, which separates ovarian neoplasm's according to the most probable tissue of origin

Table (3) Derivation of various ovarian neoplasms' and some data on their frequency and age distribution

Origin	Surface Epithelial cells (surface Epithelial – stromal cell tumor)	Germ cell	sex cord - stroma	Metastasis to ovaries
Overall frequency	65-70%	15-20%	5-10%	5%
Proportion of malignant ovarian tumors	90%	3-5%	2-3%	5%
Age group affected	20 + years	0-25 + years	All ages	Variable
Types	- Serous tumor - Mucinous tumor - Endometrioid Tumor - Clear cell Tumor - Transitional cell Tumor - Undifferentiated carcinoma	- Teratoma - Dysgerminoma - Endodermal sinus tumor - Chorio carcinoma	- Fibroma - Granulos-theca cell tumor - Sertoli – leydig cell tumor	

The most common group of ovarian neoplasm originates from the coelomic mesothelium that covers the ovary, which after neoplastic transformation seems to retain the capacity to recapitulate the epithelial components of the mullerian ducts. According to the (WHO) classification of ovarian tumors, surface epithelial-stromal tumors can be divided into serous tumors, mucinous tumors, endometrioid tumors, clear cell tumors, transitional tumors and undifferentiated carcinoma, table (3). Serous tumor is the most frequent of the ovarian tumors and the most common epithelial ovarian carcinoma, accounting for 40-50% of all such tumors. (26)

According to histopathological classification of ovarian tumors, serous tumors can be classified into.

Benign

- Cystadenoma and papillary cystadenoma.
- Surface papilloma
- Adenfibroma and cyst adenofibroma .

Borderline malignancy (of low malignant potential)

- Cystic tumors and papillary cystic tumor.

- Surface papillary tumor.
- Adenofibroma and cystadenofibroma.

Malignant.

- Adenocarcinoma, papillary adenocarcinoma.
- Cystadenocarcinoma.
- Surface papillary adenocarcinoma.
- Adenocarcinofibroma & cystadenocarcinofibroma.

Evidence is lacking about whether ovarian carcinoma may go through a borderline phase during its development and whether borderline tumors always shift into invasive ovarian carcinoma.

In the overall spectrum of serous tumors, about 60% are benign, 15% of low malignant potential, and 25% malignant. Benign serous cystadenomas occur slightly more often than benign mucinous tumors, but in their malignant form serous cyst adenocarcinomas are three to four times more common than mucinous cystadenocarcinomas. Serous and mucinous borderline tumors are seen but other types of epithelial tumors of borderline malignancy, such as the variant of Brenner and endometrioid tumors are rare.

Incidence

, the highest incidence of disease is found in America and northern Europe, the lowest incidence is found in Asia and Latin Amarica. In United States approximately 23000 cases occur annually leading to 13900 death each year, rate among blacks are lower than among whites, but rates for women of Chinese and Japanese are higher than rates in their countries of origin). In Iraq, ovarian cancer forms 38% of all gynecological malignancies, it was the seventh most common cancer among females with an incidence of 0.8 per 100,000 woman). It is the most common cancer to occur at an advanced stage.

Etiology and Risk Factors of ovarian cancer

Although the exact etiology of ovarian cancer is unknown, there are many risk factors which have been associated with the developing of ovarian cancer, such as Genetic, environmental, hormonal, and nutritional.

Genetic factors

The rare familial ovarian cancer syndromes are accounting for less than 1% of ovarian cancer cases. The most common hereditary syndrome is the breast-ovarian cancer syndrome. Most of these families have germ-line mutation in one of the breast cancer susceptibility genes, BRCA-1 or BRCA-2.

Increasing Ages

The incidence of ovarian cancer increases with age, the highest proportion of cases is diagnosed in women 50 to 59 of age. In women 50 to 75 years of age, the annual incidence is 50 per 100,000 (adjust for prior oophorectomy), approximately twice the rate in young women while benign tumors occur mostly in young women between the ages of 20-40 years old

Reproductive factors

Several   potentially   modifiable   reproductive   factors   appear   to   reduce the risk of ovarian cancer

- Pregnancy reduces the odds of ovarian cancer by 25 to 50 percent the decrease in risk is associated with an increasing number of pregnancies.

- Use of the oral contraceptive pill is associated with a 35 % reduction in the risk of ovarian cancer, increasing the duration of use is associated with decreasing risk, ten years of use by women with a positive fwomen with no family history who never used oral contraceptives

- Breast feeding is associated with a more modest effect on risk, reducing the odds of ovarian cancer by 20 % Certain gynecological surgical procedures are also associated with a lower likelihood of ovarian cancer. The risk of ovarian cancer is reduced by about 15% after tubal ligation or hysterectomy with ovarian preservation. The protective mechanism of these procedures may relate to impairment of ovarian function, causing an ovulation, or protection from exposure to exogenous carcinogens that enter the peritoneal cavity through the vagina. Talcum powder may be one of the carcinogen materials, studies have shown that woman who use talcum powder as part of their perineal hygiene are at increased risk. Talc is found in soap powders, and deodorants, and is used in packing of condoms and contraceptive diaphragms, talc might then migrate through vagina to reach the ovaries.

Infertility may increase the risk of ovarian cancer. An increased risk of ovarian cancer has also been reported with infertility treatment, particularly prolonged use of clomiphene citrate.

Staging

Staging of ovarian cancer is based on the finding at the time of surgery and pathological review. Because of the clinically occult spread, surgery is mandatory. The clinical staging ofamily history can reduce their risk to a level below that forcancer is intended to provide means by which information related to the progress of the disease, the methods and success of treatment modalities is obtained.

Ovarian malignancies are staged according to the international federation of gynecology and obstetrics (FIGO), basing on the finding of

surgical exploration

Treatment

There are treatments for all patients with ovarian epithelial cancer. Some treatment are standard, and some are being tested in clinical trials. A treatment clinical trial is a research study meant to help improve current treatments or obtain information on new treatments for patients
with cancer.

In addition, these tumors over express the HER2/neu (c-erbB2) thus certain targets for immunotherapy of cancer are already known and others
although remain undefined presumably exist.

Stage I: Treatment of stage I may include hysterectomy, unilateral or bilateral salping-oophoretomy and omentectomy. It also may include radiation therapy, chemotherapy and clinical trail conservative unilateral salpingo oophorectomy is adequate. It appears that ovarian preservation and women's fertility is safe and reasonable in women of reproductive
age

Stage II: treatment of stage II may include surgery to remove the tumor (hysterectomy, bilateral salpingo-oophorectomy, and omentectomy). Combination with chemotherapy or radiation therapy
gives approximately 85-90% five years survival.

Stage III: treatment of stage III may include surgery to remove the tumor (hysterectomy, bilateral salping - oophorectomy, and omentectomy) followed by chemotherapy or chemotherapy followed by
second look surgery.

Stage IV: Treatment of stage IV ovarian epithelial cancer is combination chemotherapy with or without surgery to reduce the size of the tumor. Extensive surgery is often insufficient to eliminate the intra-
abdominal tumor and
to chemotherapy is only partial in many of these patients

Ovarian Tumor Markers

Ninety percent of ovarian malignancies are epithelial. There are quantitative and qualitative changes in numerous circulating substances which have been associated with epithelial ovarian cancer. These may reflect an alteration in ovarian function, surface molecular structure or general responses to malignancy.

Expression of specific antigens associated with epithelial ovarian cancer is useful for establishing a diagnosis, classification and providing prognostic information. Monitoring the appropriate antigen titers is very useful in the identification of occult metastasis, monitoring of therapeutic response and detection of asymptomatic recurrence at an early stage. (The antigens defined on ovarian tumors are regarded as tumor-associated rather than tumor-specific. Several tumor markers have been investigated for one or more clinical use in ovarian cancer as shown in table (5).

Table (5): Tumor markers that have been investigated in ovarian cancer.
responsema-associated

Marker type		Example
Hormones		Progesterone), Estrogene , urinary gonodotrophin fragment.
Enzymes		Placental alkaline phosphatase creatine kinase, amylase glactosyl transferase, ribonuclease
Oncofetal antigens		Tissue polypeptide antigen alpha-fetoprotein ,carcinoembryonic antigen(CEA) .
Carbohydrate markers		A:Mucin tumor markers: CA125, CA15-3 B. blood group antigens related cancer marker. CA72-4 .
Genetic markers	Oncogene products	C- erb B-2 amplification HER-2/neu (
	Tumor suppressor	BRCA1(37) ,BRCA2

141

	genes	

There are several tumor markers that correlate with the incidence of ovarian cance important markers are:

CEA

Carcinoembryonic antigen (CEA), one of the onco-fetal proteins, is a cell surface glycoprotein, with a high molecular mass of 150-300 kDa. It is normally expressed in the early embryonic development and tends to disappear with the onset of differentiation of fetal tissue into adult ones. CEA has been studied extensively in ovarian cancer and has been reported to be elevated in 30-65% of epithelial tumors, mainly in patients with advanced stage disease. This antigen has been shown not to correlate well with status of disease.

CA19.9

CA19.9 is a carbohydrate antigen that is measured by a monoclonal antibody and can be found elevated in only 17-25% of patients with epithelial malignancies

CA 15-3

CA15-3 is a mucin-like membrane glycoprotein recognized by a pair of monoclonal antibodies: the murine antibody DF-3 and 115D8. Distinct epitopes of this high molecular weight antigen (300-400kDa) (84) is the carbohydrate side chain which accounts for about 50% of its structure.

CA15.3 is found in adenocarcinoma of breast, lungs, ovaries and pancreas(. Its level is elevated in 64% of ovarian cancer, it is most useful tumor marker for breast cancer.

r, but1.8.4 IL.6 and IL.10

The interleukins, IL-6 and IL-10, have been shown to be present in very high levels in the ascites and serum of women with advanced stage epithelial cancers. IL-6 correlates well with the stage and status of disease, but is elevated in only about 66% of patients, and its complementarily with CA125 is only modest.

M-CSF

Macrophage colony stimulating factor (M-CSF) has been found to be measurable in the serum of 68% of patients with clinically detectable disease.

Interestingly, some complementarities with CA125 has been documented. Patients with clinically evident tumor and a negative CA125 (< 35 u.ml-1), 56% had an elevated M-CSF serum level.

LSA

Lipid-associated sialic acid (LSA) can be measured in the sera of about 60% of patients with ovarian cancer, mostly those with advanced stage disease. A combination of LSA and CA125 improve sensitivity for detection of advanced disease but does not improve specificity.

OVXI

OVXI antigen is a high molecular weight mucin. The antigenic determinate of OVXI antigen was raised by immunization of mice with human ovarian elevated in 67%of patients with clinically evident ovarian cancer who are CA125 negative. The OVXI is elevated however, in only 45%of patients with ovarian cancer. In patients with residual disease at second-look surgery and a negative CA125, 27% had an elevated OVXI level in the serum

NB 70 K

NB70K antigen appears to be present in most major types of epithelial ovarian cancer, with an apparent molecular weight of 70 kDa (94). Among sera samples from ovarian cancer patients ,elevated NB70K levels were found in 87% of samples that contained elevated CA125

143

levels. No quantitative correlation was found, however, between levels of NB70K and CA125

TAG 72

Tumors associated glycoprotein (TAG-72) level is elevated in 50% of ovarian carcinoma cases and only in 4% of benign disease cases with the highest level of expression in mucinous cystadenocarcinoma and its measurement may be useful as a confirmatory tumor marker for the presence of ovarian cancer in those patients with elevated CA125 serum levels. Combined TAG-72 and CA-125 test increase the sensitivity for the detection of primary ovarian cancer to 73% with no significant change in specificity

Cancer Antigen 125(CA125)

Biochemistry

Cancer antigen 125(CA125) was first defined by monoclonal antibody (OC125) more than 20 years ago. It was associated with a family ofcancer cell line. OVXI antigen is the mosthigh molecular weight glycoproteins, that differed from classical mucins by means of carbohydrate conversion(less than 50%) and presence of both N and O linked carbohydrate residues. Size exclusion chromatography of native CA125 antigen material from body fluids results in at least two broad peaks of antigen reactivity with approximate relative molecular mass of 200 and >1000 kDa,(99) but lower molecular weight species have also been reported .

Chemical study has revealed sensitivity of CA125 to proteases; low pH, high temperature, and high ionic strength, properties consisted of conformational peptide determinant. However, CA125 activity can also be destroyed with relatively high concentration of periodate and blocked with different lectins, suggesting a close association with carbohydrate.

Structure

Although CA125 biochemical nature has long been elusive, its primary structure was established four years ago, indicating that it is trans-membrane protein with a short intracellular and a giant extracellular domain, the latter is with 22,097 amino acid residues. The extracellular part is composed of an amino-terminal part spanning 12,070 residues), followed by more than 60 tandem repeats of 156 amino acid motif and 229-residues linker to trans-membrane domain. Both the amino terminal part and the repeat domains are rich in serine and thereonine residues and arecontent was estimated to be 24-28%, with O-linked and N-linked glycans (102). Because highly O-glycosylated repeats are the landmark of the mucin family of glycoproteins, CA125 was also named MUC 16 to reflect the nature of CA125 as a new member of protein family of mucins. The mucin-like repeats contain a domain that was reported to be susceptible to proteolytic cleavage (104). An additional potential proteolytic cleavage site in CA125 was reported to be located immediately membrane-proximal. Figure (1) represents a proposed structure of CA125 antigen.

FUNCTION OF CA125

CA125 that may be of relevance for its biological function. First, because of its expression in embryonic membranes and adult derivatives of the fetal periderm, CA125 has been suggested to play a role as a lubricant, preventing adhesion of membranes. Anti adhesive properties have also been assigned to other mucins (106). Second, close analysis of glycans present on CA125 protein revealed the presence of several glycan structures that have been implicated in immune suppression raising the possibility that CA125 might help protect the embryo from maternal immune rejection and play an immunovasiverole in ovarian cancer. Furthermore mucin can bind to various sugar-binding molecules, such as galectins. CA125 was found to be a novel counter receptor for galectin-1. The known cellular responses to the cell-surface recruitment of galectin-1 include a change in proliferation activity, regulation of cell survival and regulation of cell adhesion. Depending both on the cellular context and its local concentration, galectin-1 exerts both inhibitory and stimulatory effects on these processes.

Third Gaetje et al. found that CA125 from human peritoneal fluid was shown to enhance the invasiveness of a benign endometriolic cell line EEC145, but it did not affect the invasiveness of a varietyof non-endometrioid cell lines, raising the possibility that CA125 plays a role in endometriosis .

Recently, Rump et al. in 2004 have demonstrated that mesothelin (a glycoprotein which is present in peritoneal fluid of ovarian cancer patients) is a novel CA125-binding protein and they (CA125 and mesothelin) are co-expressed in advanced grade ovarian adenocarcinoma, which indicates that CA125 might contribute to the metastasis of ovarian cancer to the peritoneum by initiating cell attachment to the mesothelial epithelium via binding to mesothelin

Expression

CA12pericardium), amnion and Mullerian duct during embryonic development. Trace amounts of CA125 are found in adult tissues derived from the epithelial lining of the pleura, peritoneum, pericardium, fallopian tube, endometrium and endocervix.

Relative to the expression levels of CA125 found in normal tissues, CA125 is often overexpressed from epithelial ovarian cancer tissue and other tumors of non-gynecological malignances.

Although CA125 is expressed both by normal and tumor cells, cell surface expression and release of soluble proteolytic fragments of CA125 into the extracellular space (115) appear to be associated with the conversion from benign to cancer cells.

5 is derived from celomic epithelium (pleura, peritoneum and1.9.5

Developing The CA 125 Assay

The development of an assay for the CA125 tumor marker grows out of attempts of Bast et al   which aimed to obtain monoclonal antibodies for serotherapy of patients in ovarian cancer. In this attempt, mice were repeatedly injected with a human ovarian cancer cell line and hybridomas were prepared from immune spleen cells and the P3NS-1 plasmacytoma. From these hybridomas, clones were isolated based on the production of antibodies that bound to the ovarian cancer cell line used for immunization, but not to a B lymphocyte cell line developed for the tumor cell donor. The one hundred twenty-fifth promising clone produced an IgG1 antibody of the desired specificity and was designated as OC (ovarian cancer).

Using immunohistochemical analysis, the OC 125 antibody was found to bind to antigen expressed by approximately 80% of epithelial ovarian cancer as well as by other gynecologic, breast, lung, and colon carcinomas: this antigen was designated as CA (cancer antigen) 125 The first monoclonal antibody radioimmunoassay for monitoring epithelial ovarian cancer, using OC125 antibody, was reported in 1983 by Bast et al.. After that several different formats for the assay have been developed using radiolabeled or enzyme-labeled OC 125 as a probe. Over the last decade, a number ofmonoclonal antibodies have been developed that react with one or two distinct epitopes on molecules expressing CA125. One of these antibodies, M11, has permitted the development of a second generation assay, CA125II, in which M11 is used to trap antigen, followed by OC125 to detect antigen that has been captured on a solid phase.

Clinical Applications of CA125

The best available marker for epithelial ovarian cancer is CA125. The normal range most frequently quoted for CA125 is 0-35 u.ml-1, although 99% of apparently healthy post-menopausal women have levels below 20 u.ml-1. In apparently healthy pre-menopausal women, levels of 100u/ml or higher canoccur during menses Elevation was also observed with the first trimester of normal pregnancy) Although elevated CA125 levels are found in approximately 80% of all patients with epithelial ovarian cancer, high levels are found in only about 50% of stage I disease.

This lack of sensitivity for early disease, and the fact that CA125 can be elevated in multiple benign disease such as endometriosis , limits the use of CA125 for the diagnosis of early epithelial ovarian cancer. Further

147

limitation is that CA125 can be elevated in adenocarcinomas other than ovarian cancer. Although CA125 can also be elevated in germ cell tumors of ovary, the markers of choice for this type ofovarian cancer are αβ-fetoprotein (AFP) and human chorionic gonadotrophin (hCG) and its β-subunite (β-hCG).

Screening

The lack of early symptoms means that approximately 70% of the patients with ovarian cancer present with advanced disease. While the overall five- year relative survival rate is of the order of 30%, the survival rate for stage III and IV disease combined is only 10% (122). In contrast, a five year survival of 90% may be achieved for patients with early stage disease confined to the ovary.

As a screening test, the main problems with CA125 are lack of sensitivity for early stage disease (only about 50% of patients with stage I have elevated levels) and lakeof specificity. Thus, a single measurement of CA125 is not an adequate screening tool for ovarian cancer. The rate of change in CA125 levels over time appears to be more specific screening method. In one study, the specificity reached 99.9% after redefining a positive test as CA125 concentration greater than 35 u.ml-1 was doubles within six months

CA125, however, in combination with transvaginal ultrasound may have the role in the early detection of ovarian cancer. This screening strategy achieved a specificity of 100%, and an apparent sensitivity of 81.7%. Other reports have found that the use of tumor markers complemspecificity of 99.9% and an apparent sensitivity of 80%. Measurement of complementary serum markers can be used as primary screening technique followed by transvaginal ultrasongraphy. This could provide cost-effective means of early detection and could significantly decrease the probability of surgical intervention for false-positive test results

Diagnosis

The diagnosis of ovarian cancer is usually carried out by surgery followed by histopathology. However, pre-operative serum levels of CA125 especially in post-menopausal women, may be useful in the differential diagnosis of benign and malignant pelvic masses. Among entary to CApost menopausal patients with a pelvic mass, a CA125 level greater than 65 u.ml-1 has distinguished malignant disease with greater than 90% accuracy. The accuracy of CA125 (cut-off concentration 35 u.ml-1) in differentiating between benign and malignant masses was 77%, which was almost identical to accuracy achieved with pelvic examination and Ultrasound (76% and 74% respectively). The combination of Ultrasound, CA125 and pelvic examination, however, improved the accuracy. Significantly, no cancer was found in any subject in which all three tests were negative.

Prognosis (chance of recovery)

The traditional prognostic factors for ovarian cancer   include125 (eg.

OVX1) is useful to achieve a

tumor stage, grade, histological type and size of residual tumor after primary debulking (cytoreductive surgery). However multiple studies have   shown that   CA125   levels after either 1,2 or 3 courses of chemotherapy is one of the   strongest available indicators of disease

outcome

A prolonged half life for CA125, or decrease in CA125 concentration of less than 7 folds of pretreatment concentration, during the early month of treatment, has been suggested to be an indicator for a poor outcome. CA125 concentration >70 u.ml-1 before the third course of chemotherapy was the single most important factor for predicting disease progression at

twelve months.

Monitoring

The most important application of CA125 is in the monitoring of patients with epithelial ovarian cancer. Serial CA125 levels can pre-clinically detect recurrent disease with lead times of 1-17 months (median 3-4 months, Doubling of initially elevated CA125 levels has been associated with   disease progression in more than 90% of cases. Furthermore, longitudinal monitoring with this marker has the potential to detect recurrent disease earlier and more cost-effectively than radiological procedures. While early detection of recurrent disease may lead to altered patient management, no study has yet shown that this lsurvival. The use of CA125 and other markers for monitoring, will attain greater importance, as more effective treatment becomes available for previously - treated ovarian cancer.

Treatment

Induction of specific immune responses by vaccination with murine monoclonal anti-idiotypic antibody (Anti-CA125), which imitates the tumor-associated antigen CA125, has a positive influence on the survival of patients with recurrent ovarian carcinoma. Patients subjected to this immunotherapy technique showed increased concentration of human anti mouse antibodies. Specific anti-anti-idiotypic antibodies, as a marker for induced immunity, were detected in 66% of eads to enhancedtreated patients. Survival of patients with a positive immune response was 19.9 ± 13.1 months in contrast with 5.3 ± 4.3 months in those patients without detectable Anti CA125-immunity

The explanation of this specific immuno response caused by vaccination with anti-ioditypic antibody is that the variable antigen binding regions of antibodies (Ab1) contain idiotypic determinants that are immunogenic and induce the formation of so-called anti-idiotypic antibodies (Ab2), some of these antibodies are able to functionally mimic the three dimensional structure of original antigen, thus selective immunization with Ab2 could induce specific immune reaction directed against the original antigen.

Antitumor vaccines were also developed by fusions of tumor associated antigens with dendritic cells. Human ovarian carcinomas express the CA125, HER2/neu, and MUC1 Tumor associated antigens which are potential targets for the induction of active specific immunotherapy. Fusions of ovarian cancer cells to dentritic cells resulted in the formation of heterokaryons that express the CA125 antigen and dendritic cells-derived costimulatory and adhesion molecules. The fusion cells have been shown to stimulate proliferation of autologous T cell that induce cytolytic T-cell activity and lysis of autologous tumor cells.

monitoring therapy and disease progression in metastatic breast cancer patients. A significant change must be at least (25%) and correlates with disease progression in (90%) of patients, with its regression in (78%). No change correlates with disease stability in (60%). CA 15-3 could replace CEA in metastatic breast cancer owing to its sensitivity and specificity.

Carbohydrate Antigen 19-9 (CA 19-9)

CA 19-9 is a carbohydrate antigen identified as a glycolipid-that is, sialylated lacto-N-fucopentose II ganglioside, which is a sialylated derivative of the Lewis a blood group antigen and is denoted as Le a. CA19-9 is synthesized by normal human pancreatic and biliary ductular cells and by gastric, colonic, endometerial, kidny, salivary gland, sweat gland and present in ductal epithelium of breast. In serum it exists as a mucin, a high-molecular weight (200-1000 KD) glycoprotein complete. The monoclonal antibody against CA19-9 was developed from a human colon carcinoma cell line, SW-1116 by Koprowski and associates.

. Methodology

CA 19-9 is measured with a double monoclonal immunoradiometric assay, using monoclonal antibodies raised against the SW-1116 cell line. The antibody reacts with CA19-9 found at low concentrations in sera from healthy individuals, but frequently increased in sera from patients with adenocarcinomas. The upper limit of normal for healthy subjects has been defined by the cutoff value of 37.0 (U.mL-1). CA 19-9 has become an established marker for pancreaticcancer, but it must still be regarded as a research test for colorectal cancer.

Another methods to determinate CA 19-9 were enzyme-linked immunosorbent assay. Both the capture and the enzyme-conjugated antibody use the CA 19-9 monoclonal antibody. It should be noted that this antibody is useless for cancer diagnosis when a patient is lacking the enzyme for the synthesis of sialyl Le a. In Japanese, about 5-10% of the population lacks this enzyme. Determination carbohydrate antigen CA

19-9 levels in serum were also measured by radioimmunoassay (RIA). Immunohistochemical technique used for the distribution of CA19-9 in tissues using an immunoperoxidase assay.By this technique the CA 19-9can be detected not only in cancerous tissues but also in non cancerous normal tissues.

. Screening

Numerous studies have addressed the potential utility of CA 19-9 in adenocarcinoma of the colon and rectum. The reported incidence of elevated serum CA 19-9 in colorectal cancer ranges from 20% to 40%. The incidence of elevated CA 19-9 in stage-related, with the highest sensitivity occurring in patients with metastases However, the sensitivity of CA 19-9 was always less than that of the CEA test for all stages of disease. The false-positive rate (>37.0 U.mL-1) is 15% to 30% in patients with non-neoplastibiliary tract. Consequently, CA 19-9 cannot be used for screening asymptomatic populations.

. Monitoring Response to Treatment

Kouri et.al compared CEA and CA 19-9 for predicting response to chemotherapy in 85 patients. Decreases in CEA more accurately reflect the response to therapy than did the decreases of CA 19-9. The pretreatment CA 19-9 value was, however, an important prognostic factor. Median survival was 30 months for patients with normal CA 19-9 values and 10.3 months for patients with elevated CA 19-9 values. CA 19-9 used to examined the serum levels and immunohistochemistry during the clinical course of female patientc diseases of the pancreas, liver andtreatment with idiopathic interstitial pneumonia (IIp) that had elevated serum levels of CA 19-9

. Clinical Application

Elevated levels (>37 U.mL-1) were seen in patients with pancreatic (80%), hepatobiliary (67%), gastric (40-50%), hepatocellular (30-50%), colorectal (30%), and breast (15%) cancer. Pancreatits and other benign gastrointestinal diseases show a 10 to

20% elevation; however, the levels are usually lower than 120 (U.mL-1). CA 19-9 levels correlate with pancreatic cancer staging (54). CA19-9 is useful in monitoring pancreatic and colorectal cancer. Elevated levels can indicate the recurrence before clinical finding by 1 to 7 months. Unfortunately, early detection of relapse may not be useful because of the lack of effective therapy for pancreaticcancer.

. CEA

Carcinoembryonic antigen is a marker for breast carcinoma, lung, gastrointestinal and colorectal (60). CEA is one of the older oncofetal protenis in use. CEA is a large family of related cell-surface glycoproteins with a highmolecular mass of 150 to 300 KD, it contains 45 to 55% carbohydrate with increase expression found in a variety of malignancies, including breast cancer(61) .CEA is not recommended for screening, diagnosis, staging or routine surveillance of breast cancer patients following primary therapy.

. TPA

Tissue polypeptide antigen is not a specific tumor marker (63). Antibodies that react with cytokeratin 8,18 and 19 identify it. TPA is a heterogeneous group of molecules with molecular weight range 20-45 KD (64). Both normal and cancerous cells produce TPA; it is useful in the monitoring of metastic diseases(

. TPS

Tissue polypeptide-specific antigen (TPS) is a new tumor marker defined by monoclonal antibody against the soluble tissue polypeptide antigen (TPA). First described as specific tumor marker by Bjorklund in 1957. In breast cancer patients TPS was especially useful in monitoring response to treatment and effectiveness of therapy in metastatic disease.

CA 549

CA 549 is an acidic glycoprotein and it is a marker for breast carcinoma. CA 549 is not useful in detecting early breast carcinoma but it

153

is useful is detecting recurrence of breast cancer in patients after initial therapy followed by adjuvant therapy .

CA 27.29 is detected by a monoclonal antibody B 27.29, this is produced against antigen in ascites of patients with metastatic breast carcinoma. CA 27.29 test above 37.7 KU.L-1 were considered positive, its most useful in monitoring metastatic breast carcinoma.

. CA 125

CA 125 is a high-molecular mass (>200 KD) glycoprotein recognized by the monoclonal antibody OC 125. The level of CA 125 is measured quantitatively by using immune radiometric assay. In healthy population, the upper limit of CA 125 level is 35 KU.L-1. CA 125 is elevated in ovarian carcinoma, endometerial, pancreatic, Lung, breast, colorectal and other gastrointestinal tumors. CA 125 is useful to detecting residual disease in cancer patients following initial therapy.

Mammary Antigen

Several new antigens have been recognized by monoclonal antibodies. Which have been identified in patients with breast cancer. They have been proposed as "tumor markers":

- MCA

Mucin-like   carcinoma   associated   antigen   (MCA)   is   a   mucin glycoprotein with a molecular mass of 350 KD. MCA was identified on the surface of a breast carcinoma cell line by the monoclonal antibody b-12. MCA level is elevated in 60% of metastatic breast cancer patients .

- MAM-6

MAM-6 an epithelial membrane antigen present on ductal and alveoli epithelial cells that is detected by monoclonal antibody raised against human milk-fat globule membranes.   Partial characterization of the antigen by SDS-PAGE showed that the antigen is a polymorphic epithelial sialomucin with a molecular mass over 400 KD.

- MSA

Mammary serum antigen (MSA) was detected by an antibody raised against a whole cell suspension of intraductal breast cancer.

Galectin-4

A protein Galectin-4 is expressed in non-invasive and invasive breast cancer but not in normal cell. An anti-Galectin-4 antibody was able todetect the presence of Galectin-4 very specifically. Galectin-4 is specific diagnostic marker of breast cancer whose patterns of expression at early stages of disease could identify those patients with a high risk of progression to aggressive cancer.

. Cathepsin-D

Cathepsin-D is a glycoprotein with molecular weight M.wt: 52 KD. It was discovered in 1979 in the culture medium of hormone dependent human breast cancer. It is a precursor to lysosomal acidic protease. This proteolytic enzyme can react against basement membranes.

Cathapsin-D may facilitate cellular actions such as migration, metastasis, and an invasion of other tissues. Estrogen has been shown to stimulate secretion of this tumor marker in certain hormone-dependent breast cancer cell lines. This antigen has been found to have potential application in breast cancer prognosis as its concentration appears to be related to the patients overall change for survival

. Carbohydrate Antigen 15-3 (CA 15-3)

CA 15-3 is a breast-associated antigen identified on the apical side of alveoli and ducts of mammary glands and as a circulating antigen. Distinct epitopes of this high molecular-weight mucin-like glycoprotein of 300-400 KD(83-85), which carbohydrate side chain

155

account for about 50% .

Also known as polymorphic epithelial mucin (87) (PEM), epithelial membrane antigen (EMA) or episialin (89). CA 15-3 can be identified by two monoclonal antibodies DF3 and 115 D8, in a double-determinate or sandwich-type immunoassay. The 115 D8 antibody was prepared against human milk-fat globulin membrane while the DF3 antibody was raised against a membrane-enriched fraction of a human breast carcinoma

. Structure of CA 15-3

CA 15-3 (Episialin) is synthesized as transmembrane molecule with a relatively large extracellular domain and cytoplasmic domain of 69 amino acids. The extracellular domain mainly consists of region of nearly identical repeats population, leading to substantial differences inmolecular weights of the CA 15-3 molecules from different individuals. The repeats together with adjacent degenerated repeats contain many serins and threonines that are potential attachment sites for O-liked glycans and constitute the mucin-like domain, which comprises more than half of the polypeptide backbone. The mucin domain of CA15-3 contains many prolines and other helix-breaking amino acids, resulting in a molecule with an extended structure and many β-turns. The extended structure is very rigid as aresult of the numerous O-linked glycans attached to the molecule. The CA15-3 extends 200 to 500 nm above the cell membrane.

. CA 15-3 Expression

- CA 15-3 Expression in Normal Tissues

CA 15-3 is predominatly found at the apical side of epithelial cells lining the acini alveoli, or lumens in various organs, i.e. in the mammary glands, salivary glands, sebacious glands, sweat glands, esophagus, stomach, pancreas, bile ducts, lungs, kidney, bladder, prostate, uterus, and rete testis .

- CA 15-3 Expression In Malignant Tissues

Relative to the expression levels of CA 15-3 found in normal tissues, CA15-3 is often overexpressed several-fold in many types of carcinomas derived from these tissues (101).   In these tumors, polarization of the cells is often lost, resulting in the presence of CA 15-3 at the entire cell surface. High levels of CA 15-3 are also detected on carcinoma cells present in pleural effusions on ascites from patients with breast or ovary carcinoma and on many breast carcinoma cell lines.

. Biosynthesis of CA 15-3

CA15-3 is synthesized as a large single polypeptide, in most cell lines approximately 200 KD or more. This precursor is rapidly cleaved by proteolysis in a small moiety, which contains thtransmembrane and cytoplasmic domains, and a larger part, which comprises most of the extra cellular domain. Both moieties remain non-covalently associated. This proteolytic processing step occurs in the endoplasmic reticulum and may be essential for further maturation. CA 15-3 is mainly processed by adding numerous O-linked glycans, which increases the apparent molecular weight on SDS-polyacrylamide gels to more than 400 KD. The extensive glycosylation protects the molecule against proteolytic degradation, since the precursors without O-linked sugars are degarded rapidly, while the mature molecule is extremely resistant to the action of proteases. The glycosylation also determines the rigidity of the molecule. The last step in the processing of CA15-3 is the addition of sialic acid to the glycans, which increases the mobility of the molecule on SDS-gels . The early proteolytic cleavage step is not directly responsible for the release of CA15-3 for the membrane, which suggests that CA15-3 is most likely released from the membrane by a second proteolytic cleavage step after arrival at the cell surface. The second proteolytic cleavage seems to be a slow and probably a random process, allowing the mucin to remain associated with the cell surface with a half-life of 16-24 hrs.

. Methodology

The CA 15-3 test from all sources uses both DF3 and 115-D8 antibodies. Serum is initially incubated with a polystyrene bead to which 115-D8 antibody has been attached. This antibody binds to antigenic sites on the glycoprotein, pulling it out of solution. The beads are then washed to remove unbound meterial and incubated with the radioiodine (125I)-labeled DF3 antibody. The radiolabeled DF3 antibody binds its antigenic sites and then the amount of radioactivity is quantitated. This is called Immunoradiometric Assay (IRMA).

. Biology of CA15-3

- CA15-3 and Cell Adhesion

Similar to mucins in mucus, membran-associated mucins might act as barrier molecules to protect cells against toxic substances, as in pancreatic and bladder ducts. The high densities of CA15-3, due to its extended and relatively rigid structure, might also interfere with the function of the adhesion molecules. In this way, CA15-3 might prevent interactions between opposing apical membrane of polarized normal cells and facilitate the formation and maintenance of the ducts during development

In carcinomas, the combination of overproduction and loss of polarization of CA15-3 expression might reduce cell adhesion and facilitate the invasion of tumor cells because CA15-3 might now interfere with the function of molecules required from tissue integrity.

- CA15-3 and Immune System

The putative function of CA15-3 in tumor progression may not only be restricted to inhibition of adhesion which will probably result in an increased invasive potential of cells, but CA15-3 overexpression may well be critical to the survival of tumor cells during dissemination (108). A completely different aspect of CA15-3 is its ability to act as a tumor-specific antigen. The underglycosylation of CA15-3 in various tumor cells exposes the protein backbone, leading to the generation of novel epitopes. This could elicit an immune response .

Chapter Four

Sialic Acids in Tumors

BREAST CANCER:

The breast cancer is the commonest tumor in women, but it may also occur in the male, accounting for almost 20% of all malignancies [1]. Over half a million women develop breast cancer every year [2]. Breast cancer has an enormous impact on the individual patient, and it often strikes in the prime of life. There is no proved method of primary prevention. Treatment may be physically disfiguring and emotionally disruptive. Breast cancer has an unpredictable course and the risk of metastases continues for 20 years or more. When breast cancer; results in death this is often after a prolonged, painful, and disabling period of disease [2].

The incidence of and mortality from breast cancer vary greatly around the world. In the late 1980s mortality in Britain was not only higher than in most other countries in Western Europe, it was among the highest in the world [3].
Incidence in Britain, however, was similar to that on other western European countries. Incidence has been rising in many parts of the world, including the United States, Canada, Europe, the Nordic countries, Singapore, and Japan, where the rates are the lowest in the world. Much of this rise may have resulted from increased diagnostic activity, and will accelerate with the introduction of screening. The corollary of high mortality coupled with average incidence in Britain is that survival is

worse than elsewhere in Europe [3]. As well as the probability of developing the disease increases through out the life and the mean age of women suffering from breast cancer is 60-61. The disease is more common in whites than nonwhites. The incidence of the disease among nonwhites women is mostly blacks however, is increasing specially in a younger women [4].

1.1.1 Clinical Types of Carcinoma of the Breast:
It is difficult to give any one growth a distinct classification, and clinical significance may be minimal. However, because the tumor may present in such a wide variety of ways it is relevant to recognize certain clinical types [21].

1. Invasive duct carcinoma: It is the commonest form and is met with principally in middle-aged or elderly women.

2. Medullary carcinoma: accounts for about 5 per cent of all breast cancer and affects a somewhat earlier age group than the average.

3. Colloid (mucinous) carcinoma and tubular carcinoma: These two variants account for about 5 per cent of all invasive duct cancers. They appear as well defined masses more common in the elderly patient.

4. Inflammatory carcinoma: Is a fortunately rare, highly aggressive cancer seen usually during pregnancy and lactation but may occur at any age unassociated with these events.

5. Paget's carcinoma: It is not common (about 1% of all breast cancers), usually multicentric in the nipple and breast ducts, but it is important because it appears innocuous.

6. 'Pseudo' lipomatous carcinoma: True lipoma of the breast is extremely rare. However, a carcinoma may sometimes develop a covering of the soft breast and subcutaneous tissue around itself to mimic a lipoma.

1.1.3 Early Detection and Diagnosis of Breast Cancer:
It is necessary to early detection of breast cancer before it has spread to axillary lumph nodes. A solitary lump in the breast must be regarded with suspicion until proved benign. Hardness tethering to skin or deep tissues, skin ulceration, nipple retraction or the presence of enlarged axillary nodes are all features pointing towards malignancy.

Mammography using radiological methods, thermography and needle biopsy are used in establishing diagnosis. Various systems of staging have been devised. They all grade the extent on criteria such as localization within the breast, extension to adjacent groups of lymph nodes, involvement of skin and deep structures, and metastases to distant sites. The aim of each classification is to indicate prognosis principally to provide an objective way of comparing methods of treatment.

Histology of the tumor is of prognostic significance. Recently there has been considerable interest in tumor oestrogen receptors as a guide to the suitability of oestrogen of anti-oestrogen therapy. Tumors that lack these receptors are unlikely to respond to hormone treatment[12].

1.1.3.1. Staging of Breast Cancer (4,21):

TNM classification: The international Union against Cancer has recommended a staging system known as **TNM** (tumor, nodes, and metastases). The details of a method of clinical staging in relation to the TNM classification is given in (Table 1.1).

Table (1.1): Staging of breast cancer by clinical examination.

Stage	Clinical extent
I	Tumor < 2 cm in diameter Nodes, if present, not felt to contain metastases without distant metastases
II	Tumor < 5 cm in diameter Nodes, if palpable, not fixed without distant metastases
III	Tumor > 5 cm or Tumor any size with invasion of skin or attached to chest wall Nodes in supraclavicular area without distant metastases
IV	With distant metastases

1.1.4 Treatment and Surgery of Breast Cancer:

Treatment may be curative or palliative. Curative treatment is advised for stage I and stage II, while treatment can be palliative for patients in stage III and IV and for previously treated patients whom develop distant metastases [13].

The extent of disease and its invasiveness are the major factors influenced the primary therapy [14].

Several approaches have been suggested to the plan of treatment of breast cancer [15]. However, radical breast surgery is less widely used than formerly.

Now endocrine and chemotherapy are increasing in popularity as adjuvants to the basic treatment. Schedules are continually evolving and there are no strict guidelines a part from reserving oophorectomy for premenopausal patients.

The presence of oestrogen receptors in the tumor increases the likelihood of response to castration and indeed to adrenalectomy. This latter manoeuvre is of greatest benefit to the premenopausal group who have responded to oophorectomy and then relapsed. Hypophysectomy is also practiced but less so than the other endocrine a blations possibly owing to the more restricted availability of the necessary surgical expertise [16].

1.1.4.1. Hormonal Therapy:

Oestrogens are the most commonly used hormonal agents and are particularly effective in postmenopausal women with oestrogen receptors in the tumor cell. Androgens have been employed but are currently unpopular because of their virilizing effects. Progestogens and corticosteroids have also been used but are generally thought to be of only minor value. Anti-oestrogens, of which the most used in tamoxifen, induce remissions in the majority of oestrogen receptor-positive patients both pre-and postmenopausal [17,18].

1.1.4.2. Chemotherapy:

It is used in metastatic breast cancer [19]. Cytotoxic therapy is usually reserved for advanced cases. The view that micrometastases are already present in many patients who on clinical grounds had been thought to have early local disease has widened the indications for chemotherapy, so that some centers are giving drugs with the primary excision whether or not there is distant spread. The list of agents employed is ever increasing and includes alkylating agents, antitumor antibiotics, antimetabolites, and the vinca alkaloids. These drugs may be given in various combinations, and may be combined with hormones as well as with surgery and radiotherapy [20].

1.1.4.3. Radiotherapy:

It is usually used after surgery (Particularly for tumors in stage I and II), palliative radiotherapy may be advised for locally advanced cancers with distant metastasis in order to control ulceration, pain and other manifestations in the breast and regional nodes. Irradiation of the breast and chest wall and the axillary, internal mammary, and supraclavicular nodes should be undertaken in an attempt to cure locally advanced and

163

inoperable lesions when there is no evidence of distant metastases. Radiotherapy is especially useful in the treatment of the isolated bony metastasis and chest wall recurrences [21,22].

1.1.5 Benign Breast Disease:

It is present with one or more of four symptoms and signs. They may describe a discrete lump, an area of lumpiness, nipple discharge or a pain in the breast. This disease represent (Fibrocystic Disease or Mammary Dysplasia, Fibroadenoma and Duct papilloma) [23].

1.1.5.1. Mammary Dysplasia (Fibrocystic Disease):

The disorder, also known as fibrocystic disease or chronic cystic mastitis, is the most frequent lesion of the breast. It is common in women 30-50 years of age, but rare in postmenopausal women; this suggests that it is related to ovarian activity. Estrogen hormone is considered a causative factor. The microscopic findings of fibrocystic disease include cysts (gross and microscopic), papillomatosis, adenosis, fibrosis, and ductal epithelial hyperplasia. Mammary dysplasia may produce an a symptomatic lump in the breast that is discovered by accident, but pain or tenderness often calls attention to the mass. There may be discharge from the nipple. Fluctuation in size and rapid appearance or disappearance of a breast tumor are common in cystic disease [24,25].

1.1.5.2. Fibroadenoma:

This common benign neoplasm occurs most frequently in young women, usually within 20 years after puberty. It is somewhat more frequent and tends to occur at an earlier age in black than in white women. Multiple tumors in one or both breasts are found in 10-15% of patients. The typical fibroadenoma is around, firm, discrete, relatively movable, nontender mass 1-5 cm in diameter. The tumor is usually discovered accidentally [26,27].

1.1.5.3. Duct papilloma:

It is usually occurs in women between 35 and 50 years of age, but rare before the age of 25. In the majority of cases, bright red blood or a serosanguineous discharge or, less often, a dark blood-stained discharge from the nipple is the only symptoms. On examination, a cystic swelling can sometimes be felt beneath the areola; pressure upon it will cause a discharge from the orifice of the affected duct on the nipple. Available evidence suggests that these lesions rarely undergo malignant transformation [21,28].

1.1.6 Biochemical Aspects of Breast Cancers:

Through the literature survey, it has been found that there are a several types of biomolecules may be vary in concentration and nature between the normal cells and tumor cells.

These differences include: enzyme activity, hormone levels and their receptor between normal and cancerous tissues [29].

Several enzymes and their isoenzymes are studied in breast cancer patients, they include: ribonuclease, sialyltransferase and galactosialytransferase and lactate dehydrogenase. Most of these enzymes revealed variations of clinical significance [30,31].

Also hormones investigated in breast cancer patients, they include: FSH and LH, progesterone, oestradiol and HCG. These hormones showed marked

variations and may used in the clinical evaluation of the disease [32]. Many properties of mammalian cells are expressed at, or mediated through, the cell surface. Among these properties are those, which distinguish a malignant cell from a normal cell. As neoplastic changes are expressed at the cell surface, altered surface characteristics are essential for the abnormal growth and behavior of malignant cells [33]. Sialic acid is thought to be important in determining the surface properties of cells and has been implicated in cellular invasiveness, adhesion and immunogenicity [34].

1.2 Tumor markers:
Definition:
Several definitions of tumor markers exist in the literature [35]. A restricted and classical definition of tumor markers pertains to the measurement of certain analytes either using chemical, biochemical or immunochemical methods in conveniently obtainable body fluids such as urine and blood. However, this narrow definition excludes the important class of tissue and cellular markers. Not all tumor markers are secreted into body fluids such as (**CA170, CA174**) membrane bound antigens and several intracellular antigens including aberrant nucleic acid sequences. However, at the fifth international conference on tumor markers (Stockholm, 1988) a consensus definition of one category of tumor markers was adopted: "Biochemical tumor markers are substances developed in tumor cells and secreted into body fluids in which they can be quantitated by non-invasive analysis. Because of a correlation between marker concentration and active tumor mass, tumor markers are useful in the management of cancer patients. Markers, which are available for most cancer cases, are additional, valuable tools in patient prognosis, surveillance and therapy monitoring whereas they are presently not applicable for screening. Serodiagnostic measurements of markers should emphasize relative trends instead of absolute values and cut-off levels".

The general potential uses of tumor markers include: Screening, diagnosis, differential diagnosis and classification, staging and grading, prognosis and monitoring treatment [36].

1.2.1 Measurement of Tumor Markers:

Different assay techniques have been used for the measurement of tumor markers. The in vitro measurement of tumor markers is in two realms: histochemical and body fluid analysis. Current probes for such measurements are largely based on monoclonal antibodies and polyclonal antibodies although some assays based on the total absence of immune reactions still exists. While immunohistochemical analysis of tumor markers generally are qualitative, the availability of image analysis techniques, software and digital signal acquisition methods provide a degree of quantitation of the intensity of staining and the degree of heterogenicity of tumor marker expression in a tumor mass. Almost all in vitro immunoassays for body fluid analytes are quantitative [36].

Today, most immunoassays of tumor markers are based on monoclonal antibodies using the dual monoclonal sandwich assay technique.

Further refinements in assay technology include the development of homogeneous assays wherein there is no separation of the bound and free reactants: new non-isotopic signal generation such as time resolved, fluorescence, bioluminescence and chemiluminescence and dye based particles[37].

Recently a new technique called immuno-PCR (polymerase chain reaction) has been introduced that uses a short piece of DNA as the tag in an immunoassay[38].

The in vivo identification of tumor mass needs a special mention here. Anti-tumor polyclonal antibodies and now monoclonal antibodies have been radiolabeled with a variely of diagnostic isotopes such as ^{131}I, ^{111}In and ^{99m}Tc and infused into cancer patients for in situ detection by and external gamma camera of primary and recurrent metastasis exploiting tumor markers as targets. Although this technique of scintigraphy is largely a qualitative in vivo measurement of the tumor marker, some estimate of the quantitative uptake in tumor markers has been made for dosimetry and eventual radiotherapeutic applications [39].

1.2.2 Classification of Tumor Markers:

Tumor markers can be broadly classified into tumor specific antigens and tumor-associated markers. Most tumor markers were often heralded as highly tumor specific, but subsequent studies demonstrated their presence in normal tissues of the adult or in various stages of ontogeny.

As a result, very few tumor-specific antigens can be recognized. The idiotypes of immunoglobulins of B cell tumors and certain neo-antigens of virus induced tumors are two examples that are strictly tumor specific. The vast majority of tumor markers are in reality tumor-associated antigens and can be classified into two types based on their size. The low-molecular weight tumor markers (- < 1000 Daltons) include some nucleosides, lipid associated sialic acid, polyamines, pseudouridine, pigment derivatives, and other metabolites. The macromolecular tumor antigens are the most important sub-type useful in the clinical management of cancer patients.

The large cancer antigens are either enzymes, growth factors, hormones, receptors, biological response modifiers, oncogenes and their products, or glucoconjugates which include glycoproteins and glycolipids. The classification of tumor markers into its various categories are summarized in (Table 1.2) [40].

Table (1.2): Classification of tumor markers.

Category	Examples
I. Tumor –specific markers	B-cell tumor immunoglobuline idiotype: virus induced antigens e.g.: SV40T antigen, T-cell receptor of T-cell leukemia.
II. Tumor-associated markers Low molecular weight markers	Polyamines, nucleoside derivatives; sialic acid (lipid associated) Vanillylmandelic acid and catechoamine. Van metabolites.
Macromolecular markers Enzymes, Isoenzymes	Placental alkaline phosphatase: prostate specific antigen, prostatic acid phosphatase, Thymidine kinase: Neuorone specific enolase. HCG: 11.2: EGI: estrogen and progesterone receptors.
Hormones cyctokines, growth factors soluble and receptors.	C-myc: src: ras: crb: neu: sis. CEA, AFP, lewis X; lewis Y.
Oncogenes and oncoproteins	CA125; CA15-3; SIA; CA19-9; TAG72; Matrix protein; N-CAM.
Oncofetal proteins Complex glycoconjugates: i- Glycoproteins and glycosamino- glycans. ii- Glycolipids 6. Cellular markers	Lewis X; Lewis Y; GM2; GD2; CA19-9 glycolipid Philadelphia chromosome; pre-cancerous cells in PAP smear

Some of Tumor Markers Used in Breast Cancer:

Tumor markers may be used to indicate the risk presence status, or future behavior of cancer. However, it is more valuable to use tumor markers for discrimination between malignant and benign tumors. New markers are frequently introduced into clinical practice without rigorous analysis, with the assumption that any information available to the clinician will help the patient[41].

1.3.1 CA 15-3 As A Marker For Breast Cancer:
The CA15-3 test measures the serum level of a mucin-like membrane glycoprotein, which is shed from tumor cells into the bloodstream. The CA15-3 epitope is recognized by two monoclonal antibodies in a double-determinant or sandwich radioimmunoassay.

1.3.2 CEA As A Marker For Breast Cancer:
CEA belongs to family of cell-surface glycoproteins with increased expression found in a variety of malignancies, including breast cancer. CEA is not recommended for screening, diagnosis, staging, or routine surveillance of breast cancer patients following primary therapy. Routine use of CEA for monitoring response of metastatic disease to treatment is not recommended. But in the absence of readily measurable disease, an increasing CEA level may be used to suggest treatment failure.

1.3.3 Estrogen Receptors and Progesterone Receptors As Markers For Breast Cancer:
The estrogen and progesterone receptors are intracellular receptors that are measured directly in tumor tissue. These receptors are polypeptides that bind their respective hormones translocate to the nucleus [42,43], and induce specific gene expression. There are three domains on these polypeptides: a C-terminal hormone binding domain, a central DNA binding domain, and an N-terminal domain that is important for transcription [44].
When the hormone binds to its respective receptor, the DNA binding domain is modified so it binds to DNA quite avidly and initiates transcription. This process clearly affects the growth of the cell. However, the intricacies of how the hormone and receptor complex affect cell growth are only partially understood[45,46].

1.3.4 DNA Flow Cytometrically Derived Parameters As Markers For Breast Cancer:
DNA diploid tumors are those in which a single peak containing an amount of DNA similar to normal control cells is generated by flow cytometry. DNA aneuploid tumors have additional peaks on DNA histogram. Presumably representing cells containing more or less nucleic acid than is found in 46 normal chromosomes [47].

1.3.5 C-erbB-2 (HER-2/neu) As Marker For Breast Cancer:
The C-erbB-2 gene encodes a transmembrane tyrosine kinase that is the receptor for a family of peptide hormones.

1.3.6 P53 As A Marker For Breast Cancer:
P53 is a tumor suppressor gene on the short arm of chromosome 17 that encodes a protein that is important in the regulation of cell division. The

P53 gene product appears to regulate transcription of several other genes. The full role of P53 in the normal and neoplastic cell is unknown. There is evidence that the gene product is important in preventing the division of cells containing damaged DNA. P53 gene deletion or mutation is a frequent event along with other molecular abnormalities in colorectal carcinogenesis.

1.3.7 Cathepsin-D As A Marker For Breast Cancer:

In 1979, a glycoprotein was discovered in the culture medium of hormone-dependent human breast cancer. It had a dependence on estrogens in that it could be increased by estrogens and inhibited by antiestrogens. It was discovered to be a 52-Kd protein, which is a precursor to a lysosomal acidic protease. Cathepsin-D, this proteolytic enzyme can react against basement membranes. Cathepsin-D also has mitogenic activity on MCF-7 cells that are estrogen-depleted. Further studies showed that cathepsin-D was relatively low in resting mammary cells but was elevated in malignant and benign proliferative breast diseases. These findings raised the suspicion that the Cathepsin-D could both promote abnormal growth of cells as well as contribute to the metastatic potential of malignant cells through its disruption of the basement membrane and therefore might be a marker for a poor prognosis in breast cancer [48].

1.4 The Sialic Acids:

Definition:

The term sialic acids represent a group of nine-carbon sugar collectively called neuraminic acid. Sialic acids, are the N-acetyl or N-glycolyl derivatives of the parent D-neuraminic acid (Fig. 1.1). They contain carboxyl, acetamide, ketone, deoxy group, as well as hydroxyl group [49,50].

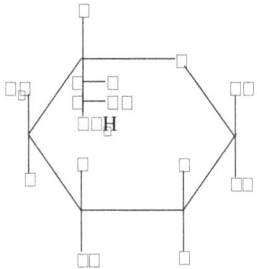

$(C_9H_{17}O_8N)$ D-Neuraminic acid

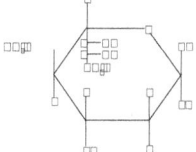

(C$_{11}$H$_{19}$O$_9$N) N-Acetyl Neuraminic acid

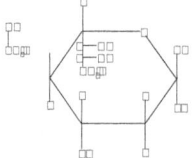

(C$_{11}$H$_{19}$O$_{10}$N) N-glycolyl Neuraminic acid

Fig. (1.1): Structure of the Sialic acids

Some of these sialic acids are known to carry o-acetyl substituents located at carbon No. 4 (C$_4$) and/or at the various position of the polyhydroxy side chain which are carbon No. 7, 8 and 9 (C$_7$, C$_8$, and C$_9$), (Fig. 1.2) [51].

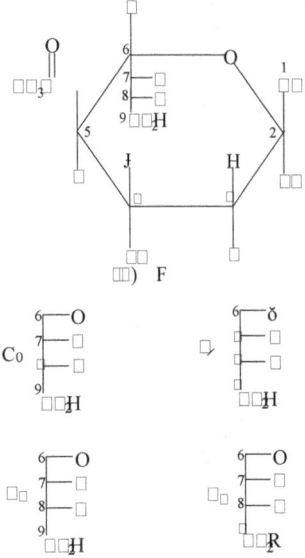

C_6 = unsubstituted sialic acids

Fig. (1.2): Structure of O-acetyl substitute sialic acids.

Sialic acids are usually located terminally and they are non-reducing residue of the carbohydrate prosthetic group of numerous glycoproteins and glycolipids [52].

1.4.1 Types of Sialic Acids:

Ten sialic acids were isolated, they differ in having various degrees of O-acetylation and N-glycolyation [53]. (Nana) which is N-acetyl neuraminic acid is the most common in mucous glycoproteins and in glycolipids [53]. The major derivatives of neuraminic acid as components of glycoproteins and glycolipids are N-acetylated or N-glycoloylated and frequently also O-acetylated [54]. O-acetyl groups were found at C-4, C-7, C-8 and most frequently at C-9 of Neu5Ac or Neu5Gc; in some cases O-lactoyl groups are also present at C-9 [55]. Mono-and oligo-O-acetylated sialic acids were isolated in pure form e.g. from glycoproteins of submandibular glands and horse erythrocyte membranes [56]. In rat, rabbit and mouse erythrocyte membranes 9-O-acetylated sialic acids, and in horse erythrocytes 4-O-acetylated neuraminic acid derivatives were identified [57]. It is difficult to identify the particular type of sialic acids present in certain tissue because, the two common analytical methods used, the Erlich and the Resorcinol method, are carried out in strong acids and under such condition the acyl groups are removed [53].

1.4.2 Physical and Chemical Properties of Sialic Acids:

Purified sialic acids are colourless; it is only after heating at 100°C for several hours that they turn yellowish. They do not melt, but decompose with discoloration over a range of several degrees, discoloration usually preceding decomposition. The sialic acids are rather strong acids (α-keto-acids) with a pK_a value of 2.6 [58].

The sialic acids and methoxyneuraminic acid are easily soluble in water. Bovine O,N-diacetylneuraminic acid dissolves readily in methanol, the other acids are only sparingly soluble in methanol. All sialic acids and methoxyneuraminic acid are insoluble in ether and light petroleum. The sialic acids are very unstable to both acid and alkali; aqueous solutions decompose already when kept for some time at room temperature due to their acidity. All sialic acids, but not methoxyneuraminic acid, reduce Fehling's solution on heating. The sialic acids consume in the oxidation by hypoiodite an amount of iodine varying with time between 33 and 90% of that calculated for the presence of one aldehyde group per molecule [53].

1.4.3 Methods for Determination of Sialic Acid:

A variety of procedures have been used for the measurement of total sialic acid. These can be broadly classified as colorimetric, fluorometric, enzymatic and highly sensitive high performance liquid chromatographic (HPLC) procedures[58].

1.4.3.1. Colorimetric procedures:

Two classical procedures have stood the test of time. One uses resorcinol and the other uses periodic and thiobarbituric acids. The resorcinol based assay uses heat and strong acid to hydrolyze glycosidic bonds. The released free sialic acids are reacted with resorcinol and copper ions to give a colored compound, which is extracted and measured at 580 nm. While the procedure described by Warren is typical of the periodic and thiobarbituric acid procedure, which measures only free sialic acid that is released after an initial hydrolysis step. In this procedure, formyl pyruvic acid formed as a result of periodic acid oxidation of free sialic acid is reacted with thiobarbituric acid to yield a red color, which is measured at 549 nm [59].

1.4.3.2. Fluorometric procedures:

In a typical and more specific assay formaldehyde that is formed upon oxidation of free sialic acid by periodic acid is reacted with acetyl acetone. The yellow product is excited at 410 nm and the resulting fluorescence is measured at 510 nm [60].

1.4.3.3. Enzymatic procedures:

Enzymatic assays are based on conversion of free sialic acids released by the enzyme neuraminidase to pyruvate and acetyl monnosamine with the aid of the enzyme acetyl neuraminic acid pyruvatelyase or neuraminic acid (NANA) aldolase. The resulting pyruvate can be coupled to the lactate dehydrogenase NADH system to measure the oxidation of NADH to NAD at 340 nm. Alternatively pyruvate can be coupled to pyruvate oxidase, flavine adenine dinucleotide (FAD), and thiamine pyrophosphate (TPP) to form hydrogen peroxide, which in turn is coupled to peroxidase in presence of 4-aminoantipyrine and a toluidine derivative to form a red chromogen, which is measured at 550 nm. The reactions associated with the NANA-aldolase-pyruvate oxidase-peroxidase system [61], as shown

1.4.3.4. High performance liquid chromatographic (HPLC) procedures:

The HPLC procedures provide the ultimate sensitivity. In one such procedure, sialic acid released from the sample by acid hydrolysis is converted to highly fluorescent derivatives by reacting with a fluorogenic agent for alpha-keto acids such as 1,2-diamino 4,5-methylene dioxybenzene in dilute sulfuric acid. The fluorescent derivatives are separated on an octadecyl (C18) bonded silica column using a reverse phase solvent system. The chromatographic step takes only 12 minutes allowing detection of levels as low as 25 femtomoles (F.mol) or 7.7 picograms (pg) of N-acetylmeuraminic acid and 23 F.mol or 7.5 (pg) of N-glycolylneuraminic acid, in an injection volume as small as 10 microliter. The procedure is capable of analyzing precisely sialic acids in a 5 μL of serum sample [62].

1.4.4 Functions of Sialic Acids:

Sialic acids are widely distributed in the human body and they perform important functions [63]. The plasma glycoproteins are soluble and they have a hydrophilic character, it is believed that these two characters are due to the presence of sialic acids as a terminal sugar residues in these plasma glycoproteins [64]. In addition to the role of sialic acids in protection of the plasma glycoproteins from splitting by proteolytic enzymes, they also play a role in the turn over of some plasma glyscoproteins; for example ceruloplasmin, which its removal from the circulation is believed to occur when sialic acids has been removed from its molecule; so it will be recognized by the liver cell plasma membrane [65].

The human red blood cell is studied with nearly 20 million molecules of sialic acid on the outer cell membrane which contributes to its electronegative charge, and by cell to cell repulsion prevents red blood cell from aggregating. Owing to its negative charge, sialic acid can bind positively charged molecules and thus play a role in the transport of such molecules [58]. RBC aging process is due to the removal of sialic acids from its plasma membrane, so RBC will be taken up by the endothelial system to be destroyed [66]. Similarly, the injection into rabbits of a desialylated preparation of ceruloplasmin resulted in the removal of the desialoglycoprotein from the circulation within a few minutes after injection, in contrast to the intact glycoprotein, which exhibited a normal survival time [66]. Sialic acids are believed to decrease the immunogenicity of the glycoproteins, for example, human orosomucoid (which contain 11.8% NANA) was found to be a poor immunogenic in the rabbit but the removal of NANA by neuraminidase enhance the immunogenic properties of this glycoprotein at least five folds [67]. In the same way the removal sialic acids from feutin enhances its combination with the antibodies. In RBC, the removal of sialic acids from its surface enhances the binding of influenza viruses to the RBC. Thus, sialic acid seems to protect self protein from self immune response and unfortunately it also seems to mask a foreign protein from rejection caused by host immunogenicity [67].

The presence of sialic acids in the sera of patients with various tumors inhibit the attack of immune lymphocytes to the tumor, so they cause masking to the tumor cells. However, the increased amount of sialic acid on the tumor cell surface can, by increasing adhesiveness, contribute to the formation of larger tumor emboli. Metastatic spread is also facilitated by sialic acid molecules increasing the adherence of tumor cells to vascular endothelium at secondary sites of implantation and by increasing the ability to aggregate platelets [68].

In glycohormones sialic acids perform important function, and their biological activity affected by the removal of sialic acids, example of these hormones are Human Chorionic Gonadotropin (HCG) and Follicular-Stimulating Hormone (FSH), this effect is presumably because sialic acids removal destroys the ability of these hormones to reach the target cells, so sialic acids seem to posses a hormone-receptor recognition function [69,70].

In mucin, sialic acids known to give the mucin it's viscosity and protect it from proteolytic splitting. Colonic mucin are predominantly neuraminidase resistant and contain O-acetyl substituent in the polyhydroxy side chain of the sialic acids, and it was found that the reduction in this substituent associated with diseases of the colon like ulcerative colitis and Crohn's disease [71,72].

1.4.5 Role of Sialic Acids in Disease Conditions:

McNeil et al [73], stated that the determination of sialic acids in serum is a sensitive, accurate method of estimating the glycoproteins content of the blood. Thus, sialic acids level increase in the same diseases that cause glycoproteins level to increase. Carter and Martin [74] demonstrated an increase in the level of sialic acids in serum of the patients with rheumatic arthritis, bacterial infection, cirrhosis, myeloma and macroglobulinanemia. They suggested that this increase is due to increased production of abnormal glycoproteins with normal sialic acids.

175

Elevated serum sialic acids has been shown to increase in patients with variety of malignant diseases including, melanoma, breast cancer and lung cancer [75-77]. Furthermore, patients with metastatic cancer had significantly higher sialic acids level than cancer patients without metastatic[78]. Increase in the level of serum sialic acids is usually due to bound sialic acids, which is bound to lipids or proteins, causing increase concentration of total serum sialic acids [79].

Brozmanova and Skrovina [80], studied serum sialic acids level in patients with bon tumors. They observed significant elevation among sarcoma patients as compared to those with benign tumors, therefore sialic acids level was suggested to be useful for comparison and diagnosis of bone tumors.

Serial determination of serum sialic acids has found to be useful monitor of tumor burden [76], and it had been shown to be proportional to the tumor stage [81-84].

Again the relation between sialic acids, tumor stage and clinical course indicates that serum sialic acids analysis could prove clinically important as a monitor of tumor burden in diseased patients, specially as sialic acids correlate both with disease progression and remission, and it may provide the earliest indication of tumor response to drugs [76]. One of the interesting facts about sialic acids is that it tend to increase in smokers and with age [85]. The study of side chain O-acetyl substitution of sialic acids is important, it has a value in identifying mucin producing metastasis arising from carcinoma of the colon [86], important in studies of perianal Paget's diseases, in distinguishing between carcinoma arising from the anal gland and those arising from the rectal epithelium [71].

In addition, reduction in the side chain O-acetyl substitution pattern of these sialic acids has been found to be associated with colonic malignancy, Crohn's disease and ulcerative colitis [87]. However, detailed studies about the biological significance of O-acetyl groups in sialic acids have shown that the degree of O-acetylation and the position of O-acetyl groups in sialic acids play a significant role in the action of sialidases. O-Acetyl groups at the sialic acid side chain reduce the rate of enzymatic hydrolysis, while a corresponding residue at C-4 prevents the action of all sialidases tested so far [88]. It was furthermore observed that the degree of 9-O-acetylation exerts an effect on immunological and complement reactions [89]. Therefore, the distribution of N-acetyl and/or N-glycolyl, with or without O-acetyl substituent on different tissue or secretion differ appreciably and may express the special function of these sialic acids in that tissue, for example the presence of O-acetylated sialic acids confers some protection to the epithelial surface of colon against the fecal stream (Bacteria and Enzymes) and it was suggested that the substitution with O-acetyl at C-4 position is responsible for sialic acids vibrio cholera neuraminidase resistance[90,91].

1.4.6 Sialic Acid and Cancer:

There has been much discussion of the relation between sialic acid and cancer. The elevation of serum sialic acid levels has been reported in cancer patients [92]. It has also been reported that, in melanoma patients serum sialic acid levels are greater than those in normal donors and the levels are in proportion to tumor burden [93]. The increase of sialyated carbohydrates, such as sialyl Lewis ^{a} (CA19-9) and sialyl Lewis^x (CSLEX-1), on the cell surface is generally observed with malignant or transformed cells [94]. Plasma from cancer patients shows an almost uniform elevation in sialyltransferase activity [95]. The elevated sialylated carbohydrate level in the plasma of cancer patients may contribute to the pathological immunodepression by blocking leukocyte interaction with endothelial cell leukocyte adhesion molecule-1 [96]. These sialylated carbohydrates that are increased in cancer patients have a basic oligosaccharide structure in common, with blood group antigens (ABH, Lewis, etc.); thus, it is considered that the former is induced by modification of the latter with cancerization. It is reported that oligosaccharides with the structure of ABH antigenic determinants are present in normal human urine [97]. However, there has been no investigation of the nature of oligosaccharides in the urine of cancer patients. LASA levels have been reported to be useful in monitoring patients with malignant melanoma. In one study when tumor recurrence was correlated with elevated LASA levels, the increased level was found as early as 9.3 months (median value) prior to recurrence [98]. Higher levels of TSA and LASA have been reported in leukemia patients compared to patients with anemia [99]. The TSA levels were significantly higher in acute myeloid leukemia compared to chronic myeloid leukemia and acute lymphatic leukemia patients. The LASA levels were significantly elevated in acute myeloid leukemia patients as compared to other leukemic patients. The sensitivity of sialic acid as a marker for leukemia is high with the sensitivity of LASA approaching 85 percent. The TSA levels in patients with oral and maxilla facial malignancy were reported to be significantly higher in patients with stage III and IV cancer, when compared to patients with stage I and II cancer. During follow-up of response to treatment while TSA levels declined during remission of disease, they became elevated with recurrence and metastasis [100].

1.4.7 Proteins Containing Sialic Acid:
Glycoproteins:

177

Definition:

Glycoproteins can be best defined as "conjugated proteins containing as prosthetic group one or more heterosaccharides, the latter is usually branched, lacking repeating units and bound covalently to the peptide chain" [101].

1.4.7.1. Chemical characteristics and structure:

There are great variations in chemical and physical properties of glycoproteins according to their location and function [102]. Molecular weight of glycoproteins may vary from 15,000 to over 2 million Dalton, usually contain 15 or fewer sugar units which are attached to the protein back-bone [102].

Glycoproteins are isolated from most organisms including: plants, bacteria, fungi, viruses and animals, and their chemical structure differ in the different organs, for example: the submandibular salivary mucin has a simple composition, it is almost exclusively N-acetylneuraminic acid and N-acetylgalactosamine [63]; while the intestinal glycoproteins are more complex, they have no unique amino acid composition but they do contain a characteristic group of sugars that include D-galactose, L-fucose, N-acetylglucosamine, N-acetylgalactosamine, and furthermore the chemical structure of glycoproteins may differ even in the different parts of the same organ in the same individual, for example, mucin in small intestine contain both neutral fucomucin and acid non-sulphated mucin however, in large intestine acid-sulphated and acid non-sulphated mucin are present [103]. In addition to the variation in glycoproteins structures in the same individual, variation among different strains of the same species has been reported [104]. In general, mucus glycoproteins from various sources share the following features: (i) very high molecular weight, usually in excess of 10^6 Dalton: (ii) approximately 75% carbohydrate and 20% protein core, with the remainder consisting of variable amounts of sulphate and water: and (iii) isoelectric point below 4, due to charged sialic acids and sulphated groups [105].

1.4.7.2. Structure of the Oligosaccharides attached to Glycoproteins:

Nine different sugar residues are generally found in the oligosaccharides chain attached to the protein core, these sugars differ according to their site and function, for example; glucose is found only in collagen, while galactose and mannose are more common and widely distributed. The two most frequently found hexoses are N-acetylgalactosamine and N-acetylglucosamine. Fucose, which is 6-deoxygalactose, is a common constituent, and frequently located at the terminal site in the neutral glycoproteins.

Two pentoses; arabinose and xylose were isolated from different tissues like dermatine. The ninth sugar is the sialic acids, of which N-acetylneuraminic acid (NANA) is an example, these acids are terminally located non-reducing residue of the carbohydrate prosthetic groups in the acidic glycoproteins [102].

On the other hand the N-acetylhexosamine are the most common sugars present at the proximal end of the oligosaccharide side chain, attaching to the protein back-bone, through the amino acids asparagine, serine, therionine, hydroxylysine or hydroxyproline (the first three usually present in mucus glycoproteins, while the last two present in connective tissue glycoproteins).

There are two types of linkage between carbohydrate of the polysaccharides side chain and the above amino acids, these are (i) the O-glycosidic linkage; and (ii) the N-glycosidic linkage (Fig. 1.3) [102,106].

Fig. (1.3): The O-glycosidic linkage (i) and the N-glycosidic linkage (ii).

Although it is possible to dissociate the polysaccharides chain complex by changes in pH or ionic strength, yet it is not possible to separate carbohydrate from peptide portion of the glycoproteins without directly

179

degrading the entire molecule, therefore carbohydrates are integral part of the glycoproteins [107

1.4.7.3. Functions of glycoproteins:

Glycoproteins are thought to participate in many important functions. Glycoproteins may serve as a structural molecules in the cell, the major portion of the glycoprotein in the animal cell is associated with the cell surface, and approximately 70% of the sialic acid-containing glycoproteins are found in the surface membrane [108].

Glycoproteins also serve as a structural molecules in collagen, elastine, fibrine, and bone matrix. Concerning collagen Herp and Pigmen in 1958 found that rat skin contained an insoluble component; after the collagen fraction had been removed by intensive treatment of the collagen with hot alkali; this component showed to contain the sugar characters of glycoproteins [67]. The other important function of glycoproteins is that they act as lubricants and protective agents, one of the well known examples is mucin; mucin is a glycoproteins containing viscous fluid being continuously secreted by the wet mucosa like respiratory, gastrointestinal and urinary systems. An example of the protective function of the glycoproteins is that of the human fetus, in which the surface epithelium of the stomach secretes neuraminidase resistant acid-mucin to protect the stomach wall from digestion by hydrochloric acid and the digestive enzymes [109].

Not only gastrointestinal mucin have this lubricant and protective function, but other mucin also performs similar function, for example respiratory mucin which protect the respiratory epithelium from the external environment by providing a barrier to the epithelium. Furthermore, the immunoglobulin content of the respiratory mucin; which is recognized as a first line of defense against infection; is a glycoprotein [110].

Other important function of glycoproteins is to serve as a transport molecules for vitamins, lipids, minerals, trace elements and hormones. Example of those glycoproteins are transcobalamin (bind vitamin B_{12}), prealbumin and transferrin. Prealbumin, which is of a special biological interest because it is responsible for the transport of a hormone and a vitamin together, it appears to contain one binding site for one molecule of thyroxine and it also transports retinol (vitamin A), which is bound indirectly by the retinol-binding protein that forms a protein-portion complex with prealbumin [111,64]. The other example of glycoprotein as a transport molecule is transferrin, which transport iron, it contains 8-9% carbohydrate in its molecule [64].

Glycoproteins could serve as a defense mechanism molecule in the body for example immunoglobulins, histocompatability antigen, complement and interferon. Immunoglobulines form a set of glycoproteins that have the ability to bind other molecules with a high degree of specificity. These molecules are foreign bodies or non-self and they are called antigens [112]. Furthermore, the carbohydrate moieties of glycoproteins which are displayed on the cell surface act as immunogenic determinants (antigenic behaviour of the molecule).

Example of this immunogenic determinant is the blood group antigen; i.e. the four different types of the blood group (A, B, AB and O); which are determined by the sequences and arrangements of the sugar residues and the glycosidic bond. So the type of terminal sugars and their arrangement in the oligosaccharides side chain of glycoproteins, which are present in the RBC membrane, will determine the blood group, and it is specificity of the individual[113,114,115,66].

The other and important function of glycoproteins, is that same hormones are glycoproteins (glycohormones) for example Human Chorionic Gonadotropin (HCG) and Thyroid-Stimulating Hormone (TSH). Human chorionic gonadotropin appears in the urine and serum of women in significant quantities during the first trimester of pregnancy. Thus, pregnancy test based on the estimation of the level of this glycoprotien in urine and serum of pregnant women.

Not only hormones, but glycoproteins may be a part of an enzyme (glycoenzymes); these are widely distributed among animals, plants and microorganisms; and they are biologically active molecules for example proteases, nucleases and clotting factors. The last are essential glycoenzymes present in the blood, they are important in haemostasis (stop bleeding). Some of these clotting factors may be deficit in certain diseases causing defect in haemostasis, an example of such a disease is haemophilia, which is a congenital disease [69]. Glycoproteins may also act as cell attachment and recognition sites, for example cell-cell, virus-cell, bacterial-cell and hormone-receptors. In 1953 Coman, D.R., suggested that malignant cells were less adhesive than their normal counterparts. Adhesion is defined as the attachment of the cell to each other, leading to the formation of tumor or, under normal conditions, to organs. Concerning recognition, the presence of galactose on the serum glycoprotein was necessary for the latter to be taken up by liver cell membrane, which in turn require sialic acids for this function. On the other hand, the circulating glycoproteins rapidly leave the portal system after desialization [108].

In hormone-receptor recognition as a functions of glycoproteins, insulin and glucagon are excellent examples. The receptors of these two hormones have been recognized as glycoprotein [116]. One of the interesting facts in glycoproteins function, is that they act as antifreeze in Antarctic fishes [102].

181

1.4.7.4. Role of Glycoproteins in Disease Conditions:

Considerable interest has been focused toward the plasma glycoproteins in the past few years, centered largely around demonstration of increased level of glycoproteins in the plasma of individuals suffering from various disease conditions.

Most pathological conditions involve glycoproteins are due to defective degradation of glycoproteins rather than synthesis [65].

In a previous study [117], it was demonstrated that patients suffering from various malignant conditions postulated that, the increase in glycoproteins arises as a result of depolymerization of the ground substance adjacent to the tumor; with subsequent release of the glycoproteins to the circulation, on the other hand, many other workers suggested that this increase is due to tumor destruction, proliferation and repair [118].

However, other workers suggested that the major possibilities of the increased level of glycoproteins in malignant diseases are due to; (i) increase in carbohydrate content of normal glycoproteins, (ii) increase glycoproteins production by the tumor itself, (iii) increase glycoproteins synthesized by the liver or by the lymphoreticular tissue [85].

Glycoproteins, which increase in malignant diseases [119,120], are also known to increase in the acute phase of diseases (acute phase protein or reactant)[85], infections and inflammatory diseases like rheumatic arthritis [117].

It was found that continuous estimation of glycoproteins level in plasma may give a clue about the progress of the disease. The other interesting fact about glycoproteins was that their level is more in smoker than in non-smoker persons[85].

It has been found that, glycoproteins level decreased in vitamin A deficiency, and drugs like Glutamine also cause reduction in glycoproteins level because both affect glycoproteins synthesis [121].

In several congenital diseases, including mucopolysaccharidoses and sphingolipidoses, glycoproteins have been blamed. These diseases are due to defect in glycoproteins catabolism, causing abnormal storage of glycoproteins and increase their accumulation. These diseases are called inbora error of metabolism and affect mostly serum and membrane glycoproteins [65].

It is well known that one of the glycoproteins functions is to determine the blood group of the individual. Furthermore, there are some relation between blood group and susceptibility to certain malignant diseases, for example blood group A individuals are more likely to have salivary gland tumors and carcinoma of the stomach than are individuals who are O, B or AB blood group. This susceptibility is of unknown etiology but it is believed to be due to the alteration in glycoproteins secreted by salivary gland or stomach of those people[63].

Deficiency in certain glycoproteins cause a disease condition, for example deficiency in the clotting factors (which are plasma glycoproteins) cause a defect in clotting mechanism of the affected patient with defect in haemostasis [64].

The tow leading diagnostic markers in human cancer, carcinoembryonic antigen (CEA) and α-fetoprotein are both glycoproteins, they increase in malignant diseases and their level may return to normal after treatment (with surgery or radiotherapy), but their level starts to increase again if the tumor starts regrowth. From this point, it seems that their level is beneficial to estimate the progress and follow up of the disease if estimated in many occasions [122,64].

1.4.8 The Lectins:

Lectins are divalent or multivalent carbohydrate-binding proteins with the ability to agglutinate erythrocyte (RBC of certain blood group), bacteria and other normal and malignant cells [123].

A great variety of carbohydrate-binding proteins (lectins) have been isolated from plants and have proved to be very useful in investigations of glycoproteins, glycolipids and polysaccharides and in studies of cells. Many of these plant lectins are able to agglutinate erythrocytes or other cells and they have therefore often been termed phytohaemagglutinins. Lentil lectin is the haemagglutinaing lectine isolated from common lentil lens culinaris and shows a specific binding affinity towards α-D-dlucose and α-D-mannose residues [124]. The ability of lectins to interact with soluble glycoproteins has been used to isolate and fractionate glycoproteins, this ability is due to binding of lectin to the oligosaccharides moieties of glycoproteins. So it is used in chromatographic techniques for glycoproteins fractionation [125]. Most of the soluble lectins isolated from vertebrate tissues bind β-galactoside. The best studied are group of dimeric protein found in many organism including the electric eel, chicken and man [126].

Another group of vertebrate β-galactoside-binding lectins can be isolated as monomers [127], other soluble lectins are multimeric. The serum of the eel contains lectin composed or have twelve subunit per molecule [128].

1.4.8.1. Biological functions of lectins:

It is reasonable to expect that the known biochemical properties of lectins dictate their endogenous biological function. Some of these properties and the functions that might be inferred from them are summarized in (Table 1.3) [129].

183

Table (1.3): Some common properties of lectins that suggest biological functions.

Property	Function suggested
Specific binding sites: All of one kind Of different kinds	Recognition of complementary oligosaccharide receptors (range of specificities)
2. More than one carbohydrate- binding site	Cross-linking glycoproteins or glycolipids in membranes and/or solution High affinity (multisite) binding to molecules or a cell surface with multiple receptors
3. Agglutinin	Binding cells together: Like cells (promoting adhesion, fusion, etc.) Unlike cells (promoting symbiosis, infection, phagocytosis, etc.)
4. Abundant	Structural rather than catalytic function
5. Generally not integrated in membranes	Relative freedom of movement in or between cellular compartments

One major property of lectins is their specific saccharide-binding sites. In the many lectins that are multimers of an identical subuint these binding sites are the same. In contrast, some lectins are composed of subunits with different binding sites. These include the lectin from the red kidney bean, phaseolus vulgaris. It is composed of two different subunits combined into five different forms of noncovalently bound tetramers [130]. Since the subunits have markedly different specificities for cell surface receptors, each combination could be envisioned to have a different function. For example the homotetramer of one subunit might agglutinate cells with an appropriate receptor, whereas a tetramer that contains only one of these subunits per molecule might inhibit such agglutination.
The common finding of more than one lectin in seeds, slime molds and even vertebrate tissues [131], raises the possibility of concerted specific reactions due to concurrent display of these proteins on a structure like a cell surface. A highly specific interaction directed by the binding properties of more than one type of lectin molecule could result.

The specificity of the binding sites of the lectins suggests that there are endogenous saccharide receptors in the tissues from which they are derived or on other cells or glycoconjugates with which the lectin is specialized to interact. Unfortunately no endogenous receptor for a lectin has yet been unambiguously identified, despite the fact that their carbohydrate-binding sites may be specialized for association with highly specific complex oligosaccharides [132]. The other properties and functions of lectins included that the fact of lectins have more than one carbohydrate-binding site suggests that they could act to cross-link glycoproteins and glycolipids in membranes of the same cell for various organizational purposes. Agglutination activity suggests functions in binding like or different cells for a variety of purposes ranging from morphogenesis in embryos to phagocytosis of one cell by another. The marked abundance of lectins suggests that they play a structural role rather than an enzymatic or catalytic function. The fact that many lectins are readily isolated as water-soluble materials suggests that if they play a role in membrane function it is by association with oligosaccharides on membranes without the constraints imposed by being integrated within the membrane bilayer. It of course remains possible that some functions of lectins may be mediated by properties that have not yet been discovered [133].

1.4.8.2. Applications:

Lectins play an important role in research into a variety of cellular properties and processes.

Their major biological effects, such as cell agglutination and mitogenic stimulation, appear to be mediated initially through interactions at the level of cell surfaces and mimic various physiologically important processes. Since lectins can be obtained in a purified form and show well-defined interaction specificities, they have frequently been used in model systems. Boldt and Coworkers [134], used lentil lectin, to study the mitogenic responses of various populations of human lymphocytes. Lectins also provide convenient "markers" in cell surface studies. Lentil lectin was used by Scott and Rosenthal [135], to characterize plasma membrane vesicles shed by guinea pig macrophages on exposure to sulphydryl-blocking reagents.

185

Many glycoproteins and glycolipids from malignant cells differ in carbohydrate composition from those found in normal cells [136]. Since many of these glycoconjugates contain sialic acid, which can be shed into the circulation, total sialic acid (TSA) is of great interest as a marker of malignancy [137], although it has not been demonstrated to be specific for any type of cancer. There are many controversies regarding the quantitative changes in TSA occurring in cancer patients [138]. It can only be said that increase in TSA is associated with certain diseases, including cancer, and is roughly related to tumor size.

Some authors [139] have based their work upon the fact that alterations in glycolipid metabolism are well documented in many tumors, including human cancers. These authors have reported raised levels of lipid sialic acid (LSA) in sera of patients with various neoplasms, but others [140] have found raised LSA values in sera of patients with acute inflammatory disease.

This has led to the conclusion that the high levels of the so-called LSA in the sera of patients with cancer probably emerge from associated inflammation [141] and, hence, the acute phase reactant glycoproteins mainly build up the LSA fraction. Moreover, Dnistrian et al [142] and Katopodis et al [143] reported that excessive sialic acid levels are found frequently in carcinomas of the breast, pancreas, colon, ovaries and other organs. In actuality, some investigators believe that high levels of sialic acid are markers for neoplasms of these organs, but they are not thought to be very reliable.

In a previous study [144], it was demonstrated that patients with breast cancer had lower neuraminidase levels compared with subjects without a personal or family history for breast cancer. Consequently, it was suggested that inadequate activity of neuraminidase enzyme may be a marker for breast cancer.

The objective of this part was to investigate the diagnostic utility of serum levels of total sialic acid (TSA) and lipid-associated sialic acid (LASA) in breast and other cancer patients.

The host information of all patients and normal healthy subjects is summarized in Table (2-3).

Table (2-3): The host information, which are used in this study

Groups	Number	Type of tumor	Metastases	Age (range)
Controls: **Normal healthy**	25	-	-	25-40
Non-tumoral disease: **Chronic Asthma disease**	20	-	-	20-60
Breast cancer: **Premenopausal**	40	38 Infiltrative ductal carcinoma 2 Infiltrative labular carcinoma	Liver and axillary lymphnode	30-42
Postmenopausal	35	34 Infiltrative ductal carcinoma 1 Infiltrative lobular carcinoma	Liver and axillary lymphnode and bone	48-68
Benign	25	24 Fibroadenomas 1 Fibrocystic disease		21-45
Other cancers	20			30-50

2.5.1. Estimation of Total Serum Proteins:

The method of Lowry et al [145] was used to estimate serum total proteins, using bovine serum albumin as standard. Protein, concentrations are expressed as g/dL of sera. Fig. (2.1) shows the standard curve of protein, which was constructed by plotting the absorbance at 600 nm against standard protein concentration.

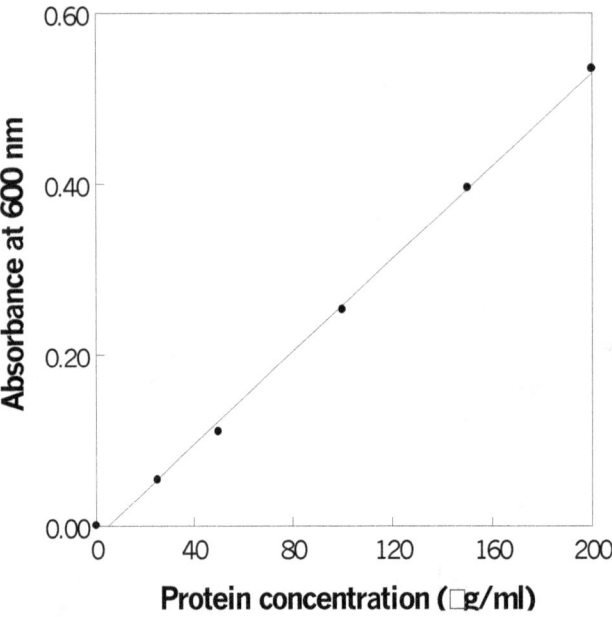

Fig. (2.1): Standard curve of protein determination in human sera by Lowry method.

2.5.2. Estimation of Total Serum Sialic Acid and Lipid-Associated Sialic Acid:

Serum LASA was estimated spectrophotometry by the method of Katopodis et al [143], with slight modification in the volume of sample used. Fifty microliters of serum was placed in test tube (triplicate) with 150 μL deionized water, then vortexed for five seconds and placed on ice. Three ml of cold (4°C) chloroform: methanol (2:1 v/v) was added, then again vortexed and 0.5 ml of cold deionized water was added, then also vortexed after that, centrifuged for 5 minutes at 3000 rpm, at room temperature. One ml of the resulting upper layer was transferred to another tube and 50 μL of phosphotungstic acid (1g/ml) was added, then vortexed and allowed to stand at room temperature for 5 minutes, then centrifuged for 5 minutes at 3000 rpm. The supernatant fluid was removed and the remaining precipitate was dissolved in one ml deionized water.

TSA levels were determined as follows:

Twenty microliters of sera and 980 μL of deionized water were placed in test tube, vortexed and placed on ice.

To each assay tube for LASA and TSA one ml of resorecinol reagent was added, and placed in a 100°C (boiling water bath) for exactly 15 minutes, followed by 10 minutes on a ice bath, two ml of butyl acetate: methanol (85:15 v/v) was added to each tube, then vortexed and centrifuged for 10 minutes at 3000 rpm. The extracted chromophore was read at 580 nm against distilled water.

Standard sialic acid: The standard sialic acid solutions with different concentrations (5, 10, 15, 20, 25, 30, 35, 40, 45) μg/ml were prepared by serial dilutions from a stock standard solution of sialic acid (1000 μg/ml). Fig. (2.2) shows the standard curve of sialic acid which was constructed by plotting the absorbance at 580 nm against the corresponding concentration of standard sialic acid solution, and was used to determine the TSA and LASA levels in the serum samples.

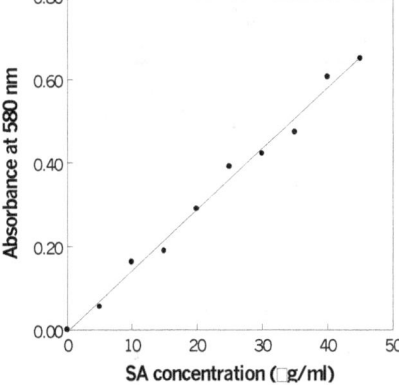

Fig. (2.2): Standard curve for determination of sialic acid concentration in human serum.

1. **2.6. STATISTICAL METHODS:**

The results for TSA, LASA, TP and TSA/TP ratio were analyzed statistically and values were expressed as mean ±SD. The level of significance was determined by student's t-test [146].

ResultS and Discussion

Determination of Total Sialic Acid (TSA) and Total Protein (TP) Concentrations in Sera of Patients With Breast Cancer, other Cancers and Non-C Individuals:

The individual and mean serum concentrations of TSA and TP for the normal healthy controls, pathological controls (chronic Asthma disease) and patients with breast cancer and other cancers are summarized in table (2-4). This table presents comparisons of the mean values of sera TSA an TP between different groups above, it shows that the TSA levels in breast and other cancer patients were significantly elevated (P < 0.001) as compared to the normal healthy and pathological controls (P < 0.001 and P < 0.01 respectively). However, comparison of serum TSA for different types of breast cancer was studied, the postmenopausal patients show a high level of TSA as compared to the premenopausal patients.

Table (2-4): Comparison of mean values for TSA, LASA and TP in sera of normal, pathological controls and in patients with breast cancer and other cancer.

Groups	No.	TSA (mg/dL) (mean ±SD)	LASA (mg/dL) (mean ±SD)	TP (g/dL) (mean ±SD)	TSA/TP (mg/g) (mean ±SD)
Controls: **Normal healthy** **Non-tumoral disease:** **Chronic Asthma disease**	25 20	56.7±8.2 80.8±1.25	17.86±1.59 21.57±4.02	7.03±0.83 7.06±0.91	8.27±0.73 11.54±0.7
Breast cancer: **Premenopausal** **Postmenopausal** **Benign**	40 35 25	100.29±17.38 128.25±21.43 85.6±0.16	32.13±10.01 30.93±10.16 19.29±1.84	7.1±1.02 7.16±1.13 7.08±0.93	14.23±1.45 18.01±1.71 12.28±0.8
Other cancer: **Endometerial carcinoma** **Sarcoma**	15 5	103.5±11.5 94.6±9.31	27.3±7.02 23.92±5.88	7.91±1.2 8.1±1.03	13.4±1.7 12.7±1.9

On the other hand, the mean values of total protein (TP) in sera of breast cancer patients did not find any significant differences when compared to the mean values with normal healthy and pathological controls, and on the contrary, the mean values of total protein in sera of other cancer patients were observed a significant differences (P < 0.01) than that in breast cancer patients, normal healthy and pathological controls (Asthma disease). It is clear from table (2-4) the mean values of total sialic acid to total protein ratio (TSA/TP) in sera of breast cancer patients (premenopausal and postmenopausal patients) were significantly elevated (P < 0.01) as compared to the normal healthy and patients with chronic Asthma disease, whereas, the serum levels of TSA/TP ratio in postmenopausal patients were significantly higher (P < 0.01) than those in premenopausal patients with regard to the mean values of TSA/TP ratio in sera of other cancer patients (endometerial carcinoma and sarcoma), show a significantly higher increase than those observed in normal healthy, patients with non-tumoral disease and benign patients (P < 0.01), but it is lower than in breast cancer.

Table (2-5) shows the specificity and sensitivity of TSA test in normal controls and in patients with breast cancer, other cancer and non-cancer (Asthma disease). The specificity was calculated as % of patients with cancer who had normal TSA values than normal while the sensitivity was calculated as % of patients with cancer who had higher TSA values than normal. Through table (2-5), the results show that 37 out of the 40 patients with breast cancer (premenopausal patients) 92.5% had elevated values of TSA. Of the groups of 35 patients with breast cancer (postmenopausal), 34 (97.1%) had elevated values for TSA. For benign patients, 22 out of the 25 patients included in group (88%) had elevated values of TSA. But in other cancer, test sensitivity of TSA was varied from 93.3 to 100%. However, in normal controls test specificity of TSA was 84% so that only 16% of those tested were falsely positive. Fig. (2.3) shows the distribution of the individual values of TSA in sera of cancer patients, non-cancer patients (Asthma disease) and normal healthy.

191

Table (2-5): Specificity and sensitivity of TSA in normal, controls and in patients with breast cancer, other cancer and non-cancer.

Groups	No.	TSA<65 mg/dL (normal)	Specificity % true negative	TSA>65 mg/dL (elevated)	Sensitivity % true positive
Normal	25	21	84	4	16
Breast cancer: Premenopausal Postmenopausal Benign	40 35 25	3 1 3	7.5 2.9 12	37 34 22	92.5 97.1 88
Other cancer: Endometerial carcinoma Sarcoma	15 5	1 0	6.7 0	14 5	93.3 100
Non-cancer: (Asthma disease)	20	4	20	16	80

Note: Sensitivity and specificity of TSA measuring as follows: Sensitivity was calculated as % of patients with cancer who had higher TSA values than controls (normal). Specificity was calculated as % of patients with cancer who had normal TSA values than controls (normal).

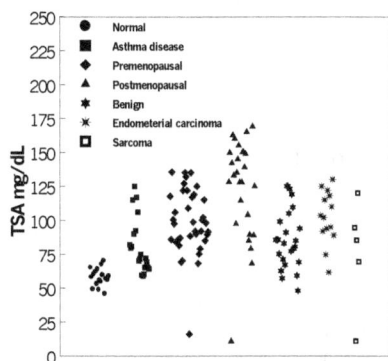

Figure (2.3): Distribution of the individual values of TSA in sera of breast cancer patients, other cancers, non-cancer (Asthma disease) and normal healthy.

Glycoproteins and glycolipids are present in membrane of malignant cells and differ in carbohydrate composition. This contribute to aberrant cell to cell recognition, cell adhesion, antigenicity and the invasiveness demonstrated by malignant cells [147]. Therefore, alterations in important glycoprotein constituents like sialic acid naturally assume importance in malignancy. Variations in serum TSA levels have been found to be useful for diagnosis, staging, prognosis and treatment monitoring of cancer patients [148]. TSA levels when normalized for TP variations and expressed as TSA/TP, become more tumor specific [149]. Increased glycolytic activity has been observed in malignant cells. During neoplastic transformation, the carbohydrate chains in glycolipids and glycoproteins are frequently altered. There is a close relationship between the expression of certain carbohydrate antigens and oncogenesis [150]. In an elegant study examining the significance of the linkage of sialic acid residues in cancer-associated carbohydrate antigens, by using specific monoclonal antibodies, it was demonstrated that not all sialic acids are specific to cancer. Indeed, this study demonstrated that there are significant variations in the cancer specificity depending on the difference in linkage in sialic acid residues [151]. However, the relevance of sialic acid to the tumor cell is apparent from the increased sialylation and

193

sialyltransferase activity observed in many cancer cells [70]. The aberrant glycosylation found in cancer cell membranes is presumably due to the activation of new glycosyl transferases that are characteristic of tumor cells and are absent or present only in small quantities in normal cells [152]. Thus, for instance, a relatively specific sialyltransferase is found to be present by as much as 2.5 to 11 times in greater amounts in transformed cells when compared to control cells [153].

Sialic acid bound to membrane glycoproteins and glycolipids apparently enters the circulation by either shedding or by cell lysis.

Approximately 98 to 99.5 percent of total sialic acid found in serum or plasma is bound to glycoproteins. Only a very small fraction of sialic acid is bound to lipids, which is mainly in the form of gangliosids. Normal levels of total sialic acid in serum are approximately in the range of 51 to 84 mg/dL. In contrast, the contribution of the pure lipid fraction to total sialic acid level is barely in the range of 0.4 to 0.9 mg/dL [154].

Since sialic acid is one of the component of glycoprotein and glycolipid, several investigators and our study concentrate on their levels in the sera or plasma or tissues of patients with cancer diseases. On the other hand, most of these studies have been concerned with TSA level.

Total sialic acid (TSA) level is increased in a variety of tumors, and this level is directly related to cancer burden and disease recurrence [154].

In a recent study on the usefulness of TSA in lung cancer, data obtained in this study show that the mean concentration of TSA was significantly higher in lung cancer patients when compared to benign and normal controls [155].

Erbil et al [75] reported on increased levels of TSA in genitourinary tumors, concluding that serum TSA levels were highly correlated with the stage and grade in patients with advanced urological cancer.

2. <u>Determination of Lipid-Associated Sialic Acid (LASA) Levels in Sera of Patients with Breast Cancer, Other Cancers and non-Cancer individuals:</u>

Serum lipid-associated sialic acid (LASA) levels were determined in normal healthy persons and in patients with non-cancer (Asthma disease) as a pathological controls and patients with breast cancer, other cancers, using the method of Katopodis et al [143].

Table (2-4) shows the individual and mean serum concentrations of LASA in different groups of cancer patients, non-tumoral disease (Astha disease) and in normal healthy, also this table presents comparisons of the mean values of sera LASA between these groups.

The results in this table reveal an overall elevation in LASA levels for each group of patients with cancer when compared to the normal healthy and pathological controls. This increased LASA values in sera of breast cancer patients except benign patients showed statistically significant differences than those values obtained from sera of normal control, patients with non-malignant diseases and other cancers ($P < 0.001$, $P < 0.01$ and $P < 0.01$) respectively.

It is clear from table (2-4) the level of LASA in both types of breast cancer patients (premenopausal and postmenopausal) show equivalent value.

Table (2-6) represents the percentages of LASA test specificity and sensitivity in normal individuals, patients with breast cancer, other cancers and non-cancer (Asthma disease), using the value of 19 mg/dL as the upper limit of normal.

The results presented in this table show that 35 out of the 40 patients with breast cancer (premenopausal) 87.5% had elevated levels of LASA. Of the groups of 35 patients with breast cancer (postmenopausal), 32 had elevated levels of LASA 91.4%.

Table (2-6): Specificity and sensitivity of LASA in normal controls and in patients with breast cancer, other cancer and non-cancer.

Groups	No.	LASA≤19 mg/dL (normal)	Specificity % true negative	LASA>19 mg/dL (elevated)	Sensitivity % true positive
Normal	25	22	88	3	12
Breast cancer:					
Premenopausal	40	5	12.5	35	87.5
Postmenopausal	35	3	8.57	32	91.4
Benign	25	5	20	20	80
Other cancer:					
Endometerial carcinoma	15	0	0	15	100
Sarcoma	5	0	0	5	100
Non-cancer: (Asthma disease)	20	2	10	18	90

Note: Sensitivity and specificity of LASA measuring as follow: Sensitivity was calculated as % of patients with cancer who had higher LASA values than controls (normal). Specificity was

calculated as % of patients with cancer who had normal LASA values than controls (normal).

For benign patients, 20 out of 25 patients included in group (80%) had elevated values of LASA. But in other cancer patients, test sensitivity of LASA had elevated values (100%).
On the other hand, in normal controls test specificity of LASA was 88% sothat only 12% of those tested were falsely positive. Figure (2.4) shows the distribution of the individuals values of LASA in sera of cancer patients, non-cancer patients (Asthma disease) and normal healthy.

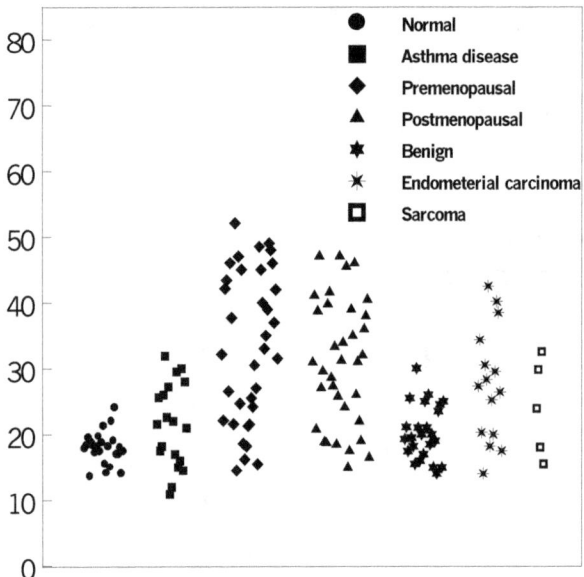

Figure (2.4): Distribution of the individual values of LASA in sera of breast cancer patients, other cancers, non-cancer (Asthma disease) and normal healthy.

Lipid-associated sialic acid (LASA) level is increased in a variety of tumors, and this level is directly related to cancer burden and disease recurrence[154].
In another studies LASA levels have been reported to be useful in monitoring patients with malignant melanoma [98]. However, LASA-P is a biomarker useful in a wide range of malignancies. It reflects alteration in the surface membrane of tumor cells. The LASA-P assay measures total gangliosides and glycoproteins[156]. Elevated LASA-P levels in breast cyst

fluid have been associated with increased risk of breast cancer [157]. Also, LASA-P levels are higher in women with benign or malignant breast tumors than in controls [158]. Some conditions other than cancer affect LASA-P. Among them, are myocardial infarction [159], infections, rheumatoid arthritis, and collagen degeneration. Polivkova et al [187], believe that the determination of LASA levels could be useful not only for cancer diagnosis but also prognosis.

In this investigation, it is established that the data for the TSA and LASA test confirms the previous observations, which have indicated that levels are significantly increased in the sera of breast cancer and other cancer patients, and both tests may prove to be of clinical value.

The increase of TSA are frequently modest in premenopausal patients and high in postmenopausal patients as compared to non-tumoral diseases and normal healthy controls and the demarcation between normal and abnormal levels is sufficiently sharp sothat with a 65 mg/dL cutoff (Table 2-5). The specificity and sensitivity data for the results was a favorable when compared to those of the most widely used immunodiagnostic test, CEA [160].

Sialic acid measurements appear to have a high sensitivity for a wide range of tumors.

However, the specificity of sialic acid measurements, especially the non-specific LASA measurements, is low since

The measurement of biochemical markers is being increasingly used for early diagnosis and monitoring the progress of cancer. Increased levels of protein-bound carbohydrates have been shown to occur frequently in patients with neoplasms [161]. Glycoproteins play an important role in the cellular phenomena that undergo alterations during cancerours transformation.

Barlow and Dillard [162] demonstrated that serum L-fucose could be helpful as a means of assessing disease status in patients with breast and cervical cancer.

Sugars in glycoproteins, glycolipids, glycosaminoglycans, oligo-and polysaccharides have been identified in a variety of animal tissues [163]. Moreover, various carbohydrate fractions bound to the plasma proteins

197

are elevated in patients suffering from cancer diseases and also certain non-cancer disease state [164].

Lawrence et al described a group of glycoproteins that are synthesized and released by human breast cancer maintained in organ culture and similar glycoproteins released by a human breast carcinoma cell line (BT-20). The electrophoretic mobility of these glycoproteins on cellulose acetate is consistent with increased glycoproteins staining material present in the α_2 to β-globulin region of serum glycoprotein electropherograms from patients with breast cancer[165].

However, the protein-bound carbohydrate and seromucoid of plasma have been demonstrated to be elevated in a wide variety of pathological conditions including spontaneous human carcinoma [166].

3.5 DETERMINATION OF BIOCHEMICAL CONSTITUENTS IN SERA OF PATIENTS WITH BREAST CANCER, OTHER CANCERS AND NON-CANCER (ASTHMA-DISEASE):
3.5.1 Determination of Seromucoid:

The method of Weimer and Mashin [167], was used to determine serum seromucoid. This method includes the following steps:

(1) Half milliliter of serum was added to 4.5 ml of 0.85% NaCl, then mixed and 2.5 ml of 1.8 M perchloric acid was added, after mixing by inversion, the assay tubes were allowed to stand at room temperature for 10 minutes, then centrifuged for 15 minutes at 3500 r.p.m. to obtain clear supernatant.

(2) To five milliliter of the supernatant, 1 ml of phosphotungstic acid reagent was added, after mixing the tubes were allowed to stand for 10 minutes.

(3) The tubes were centrifuged, after removing of the supernatant, five milliliter of 95% ethanol was added, then strie, centrifuged and the supernatant was removed.

(4) The resulting precipitate was dissolved in 0.5 ml of (0.1 N) NaOH, this was considered as the unknown.

(5) Set up blank with 0.5 ml of distilled water, and standard using 0.5 ml of working standard.

(6) To each unknown, blank and standard, added 1.25 ml of orcinol reagent and 7.5 ml of (60% v/v) H_2SO_4.

(7) All tubes were placed in a water bath at ($80\pm0.5°C$) for 20 minutes, cooled and read against distilled water at 520 nm.

Calculations:

$$\text{mg seromucoid/100 ml} = \frac{A_x - A_b}{A_s - A_b} \times 0.1 \times \frac{100}{0.333}$$

$$= \frac{A_x - A_b}{A_s - A_b} \times 30$$

Where:

A_x = The absorbance of unknown solution at 520 nm.

A_s = The absorbance of standard solution at 520 nm.

A_b = The absorbance of blank solution at 520 nm.

3.5.2 Estimation of Serum Protein-Bound Hexose:

The method includes the following steps:

(1) Hundred microliter of serum was added to 5 ml of 95% v/v ethanol and mixed carefully, then centrifuged for 15 minutes at 3500 r.p.m., after that the supernatant was decanted.

(2) The remaining precipitate was washed with 5 ml of 95% ethanol, then stired, after that centrifugation.

(3) The supernatant was decanted, the steps 4-7 was carried out as in section (3.5.1) [167].

Calculations:

$$\text{mg protein bound hexose/100 ml} = \frac{A_x - A_b}{A_s - A_b} \times 0.1 \times \frac{100}{0.1}$$

$$= \frac{A_x - A_b}{A_s - A_b} \times 100$$

Where:

A_x = The absorbance of unknown solution at 520 nm.

A_s = The absorbance of standard solution at 520 nm.

A_b = The absorbance of blank solution at 520 nm.

RESULTS AND DISCUSSION

The level of protein-bound hexose (galactose and mannose) was estimated in the sera of normal volunteers and in patients with breast cancer, other cancers and non-cancer (Asthma disease), using the method of Weimer and Mashin [167].

The mean concentrations of protein-bound hexoses in sera of all patients and normal healthy are summarized in table (3-1). Figure (3.1) shows the distribution of the individual values of protein-bound hexoses in sera of all cancer patients, non-cancer and normal controls.

Table (3-1): Serum protein-bound hexose (galactose and mannose) in normal controls and in patients with breast cancer, other cancers and non- cancer (Asthma disease) ± standard error.

Groups	Number.	Protein-bound hexose mg/dl ± S.E.
Normal	25	87.09 ± 1.82
Breast cancer:		
Premenopausal	40	111.9 ± 5.55
Postmenopausal	35	103.30 ± 4.48
Benign	25	90.7 ± 5.01
Other cancers:		
Endometerial carcinoma	15	127.75 ± 3.25
Sarcoma	5	131.5 ± 4.87
Non-cancer:		
(Asthma disease)	20	101.66 ± 4.1

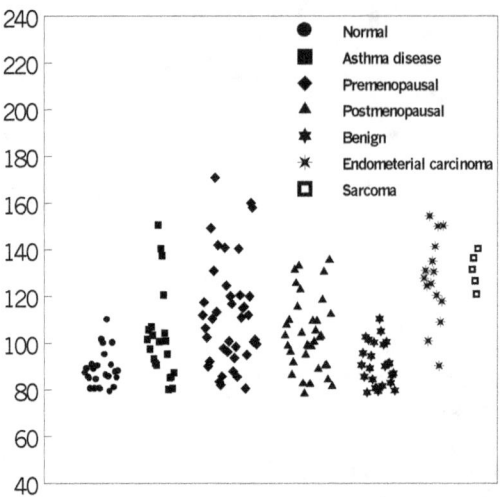

Figure (3.1): Distribution of the individual values of protein-bound hexoses in sera of patients with breast cancer, other cancers, non-cancer (Asthma disease) and normal healthy.

From the results presented in this table, reveal that the mean values of protein-bound hexose in sera of patients which suffer from breast and other cancers were elevated significantly in comparison to those of normal controls and patients with benign (P < 0.01).

The mean concentrations of protein-bound hexose reached to 111.9 ± 5.55 mg/dl in premenopausal patients, 103.3 ± 4.48 mg/dl in postmenopausal patients, whereas in other cancers it was 127.75 ± 3.25 mg/dl in endometerial carcinoma patients, 131.5 ± 4.87 mg/dl in sarcoma patients.

However, the mean level of protein-bound hexose in patients with non-cancer (Asthma disease) was significantly elevated when compared to those observed in normal healthy controls and with benign patients (P < 0.01), but the elevation was not significant when compared to the mean values of protein-bound hexose between patients with benign and normal healthy individuals (P > 0.05). The serum levels of protein-bound hexose in patients with other cancers were significantly higher (P < 0.01) than those in breast cancer patients and non-cancer, and also than those observed in normal healthy controls and benign patients (P < 0.001).

Table (3-2) shows the specificity and sensitivity of the protein-bound hexose in normal controls and in patients with breast cancer, non-cancer.

Table (3-2): Specificity and sensitivity of protein-bound hexose in normal controls and in patients with breast cancer and non-cancer (Asthma disease).

	No.	Protein-bound hexose ≤ 89 mg/dL (normal)	* Specificity % true negative	Protein-bound hexose > 89 mg/dL (elevated)	** Sensitivity % true positive
Normal	25	6	24	19	76
Breast cancer:					
Premenopausal	40	3	7.5	37	92.5
Postmenopausal	35	4	11.43	31	88.57
Benign	25	1	4	24	96
Non-cancer: (Asthma disease)	20	0	0.00	20	100

* Calculated as the number of cases having ≤ 89 mg/dl divided by the total number of cases by 100.

** Calculated as the number of cases having >89 mg/dl divided by the total number of cases by 100.

In this test using 89 mg/dl as the upper limit of normal, test sensitivity in those with breast cancer patients was varied from 88.57% to 92.5%, but this test had elevated in benign patients and non-cancer patients (Asthma disease) 96% and 100% respectively. The test was more sensitive for breast cancer patients and non-tumor disease (Asthma disease), as compared to the normal healthy controls.

Also, the results obtained revealed low specificity in different types of breast cancer.

On the other hand, the level of seromucoid was estimated in sera of normal healthy controls and in patients with breast cancer, other cancers and non-cancer (Asthma dusease).

The data obtained in this study are summarized in table (3-3). Figure (3.2) shows the distribution of the individual values of seromucoid in sera of all cancer patients, non-cancer and normal healthy controls.

Table (3-3): Serum seromucoid in normal controls and in patients with breast cancer, other cancers and non- cancer (Asthma disease) ± standard error.

Groups	Number.	Seromucoid mg/dl ± S.E.
Normal	25	10.29 ± 0.29
Breast cancer: Premenopausal Postmenopausal Benign	 40 35 25	 17.58 ± 2.08 15.92 ± 1.83 12.63 ± 0.33
Other cancer: Endometerial carcinoma Sarcoma	 15 5	 18.16 ± 1.3 19.78 ± 1.7
Non-cancer: (Asthma disease)	20	13.24 ± 0.73

However, the mean values of seromucoid level in other cancer patients show a significantly higher increase than in patients with breast cancer ($P < 0.01$) and also as compared with normal healthy controls, non-cancer and benign patients ($P < 0.001$).

The specificity and sensitivity of the seromucoid test are considered in table (3-4), using 11 mg/dl as the upper limit of normal, this test was sensitive for different types of breast cancer as compared to the normal healthy.

Table (3-4): Specificity and sensitivity of seromucoid test in normal controls and in patients with breast cancer and non-cancer (Asthma disease).

	No.	Seromucoid ≤11 mg/dl (normal)	*Specificity % true negative	Seromucoid >11mg/dl (elevated)	**Sensitivity % true positive
Normal	25	18	72	7	28
Breast cancer:					
Premenopausal	40	7	17.5	33	82.5
Postmenopausal	35	6	17.14	29	82.86
Benign	25	2	8	23	92
Non-cancer: (Asthma disease)	20	1	5	19	95

* Calculated as the number of cases having ≤11 mg/dl divided by the total number of cases by 100.

** Calculated as the number of cases having >11 mg/dl divided by the total number of cases by 100.

From these results, it possible to conclude that it was useful for differential diagnosis and disease monitoring, but not for the early diagnosis of these tumors.

Elevated levels of glycoproteins have been reported in the sera of patients with metastatic breast carcinoma [168]. Alterations in serum glycoproteins have been studied by determining the carbohydrate moieties, viz. fucose, hexose, hexosamine and sialic acid [169]. Variations in glycoproteins in human uterine cervical carcinoma has been reported [170]. These alterations are due to the exponential growth of malignant cells, which results in a rapid rate of membrane glycoprotein turnover and shedding of these excessive glycoproteins into the sera.

Patel, PS. et al [158] has observed significant increase in the levels of the protein-bound hexose and seromucoid in breast carcinoma patients compared with the normal controls, also the differences were significant when compared to the patients with benign breast diseases, it has also been suggested that the measurement of the two parameters be helpful in the diagnosis of breast carcinoma as well as in differentiating between lobular carcinoma and infilterating duct carcinoma patients.

Serum levels of tumor-associated glycoprotein-72 in patients with gynecological malignancies can be used as a clinical marker [171]. The potential role of sialic acid in the mechanism of tumor formation is indicated by the finding that sialic acid-rich glycoconjugates mask the surface of certain tumor cells by interfering with the immune response of the host [172], and that sialic acid content appears to be correlated with metastatic ability in a variety of tumor cells [173].

On the other hand, Yamamooto et al [174], reported that the increase in protein-bound hexose arises as a result of depolymerization of the ground substance connective tissue adjacent to cancer with release of these compound into circulation.

Bolmer et al [175] have suggested that the elevation of the plasma glycoprotein reflects merely the occurrence of tissue destruction, while Yaskhiko et al [176] have concluded that tissue proliferation or repair is a more probable etiological factor.

An enzyme which catalyzes the dismutation of superoxide free radicals $(O_2^{-\bullet})$ according to the reaction:

$$O_2^{-\bullet} + O_2^{-\bullet} + 2H^+ \rightarrow O_2 + H_2O_2$$

It has been purified by a simple procedure from bovine erythrocytes [177]. This enzyme, called superoxide dismutase, contains 2 equivalent of copper per mole of enzyme. The copper may be reversibly removed, and it is required for activity. Superoxide dimutase has been shown to be identical with the previously described copper-containing erythrocuprein (human) and hemocuprein (bovine)[177]. The enzyme has since been detected in a large number of tissues and organisms, and it is thought that it is present to protect the cell from damage by the highly reactive superoxide free radical [178].

Superoxide is formed by the one-electron reduction of oxygen, and has been identified as a product in a number of biological reactions [178]. It is particularly likely to be formed in the red cell and has been shown to be produced when oxyhemoglobine is outoxidized to methemoglobine [179].

$$Hb - Fe^{2+} + O_2 \rightarrow Hb - Fe^{3+} + O_2^{-\bullet}$$

Other likely sources include reactions initiated by ionizing radiation. Stable solutions of the superoxide radical were generated by the electrolytic reduction of O_2 in an aprotic solvent, dimethylformamide.

Slow infusion of such solutions into buffered aqueous media permitted the demonstration that $O_2^{-\bullet}$ can reduce ferricytochrome C and tetranitromethane, and that superoxide dismutase, by competing for the superoxide radicals, can markedly inhibit these reactions.

Superoxide dismutase was used to show that the oxidation of epinephrine to adrenochrome by milk xanthine oxidase is mediated by the superoxide radical[177].

The content and composition of glycoproteins and glycolipids are affected, with an increase in sialic acid on the cell surface membrane and in the serum [143,182]. Decreased activity of the enzyme superoxide dismutase (SOD) has also been found in all malignant tumors investigated so for [183]. Such changes in the content of glycolipids (LBSA) and the activity of SOD are not found in patients with benign tumors [143,184]. The present investigation was carried out to compare the content of LBSA and activity of SOD in sera of patients with breast cancer as compared to the normal healthy individuals.

4.5 ESTIMATION OF SERUM SUPEROXIDE DISMUTASE ACTIVITY:

Superoxide dismuatse (SOD) activity was estimated spectrophotometery by the method of Winterbourn et al [185], with our modification for serum. The method is based on the ability of the enzyme to inhibit the reduction of nitroblue tetra-zolium (NBT) by superoxide generated during the reaction of photoreduction riboflavin and oxygen.

Procedure:

1. Addition of 0.2 ml of EDTA/NaCN solution to 0.1 ml of serum sample was carried out, then 0.1 ml of NBT solution were added.

2. The assay tubes were brought to a standard temperature (20-22°C), after that 0.05 ml of riboflavin solution were added to each tube. The final assay volume of 3 ml was made up with phosphate buffer 0.067 M, pH = 7.8.

3. Subsequent exposure to bright lighting was controlled by placing the assay tubes in a white-light box where they received uniform illumination for 20 minutes with 18W fluorescent tube attached to the lid, then the absorbance was red at 560 nm against distilled water.

4. To determine the control value, the absorbance for another set of tubes containing the same mixture was read at 560 nm against distilled water immediately after the addition of riboflavin. (riboflavin was added after the addition of buffer).

5. To determine SOD unit, ten tubes containing (10, 20, 40, 60, 80, 100, 200, 300, 400 and 500 μL) of normal serum samples, and another tube containing no serum were treated as described in the steps 1, 2, and 3.

Calculations:

Percentage inhibition was calculated from each absorbance in the presence and absence of the enzyme:

Inhibition % = $\left(A_E - A_{NE}\right) \times 100$

Where;

A_E: The absorbance at 560 nm of the tubes containing different amounts of the enzyme.

A_{NE}: The absorbance at 560 nm in the absence of the enzyme.

The percentages of inhibition were plotted against the corresponding amounts of serum (Figure 4.1).

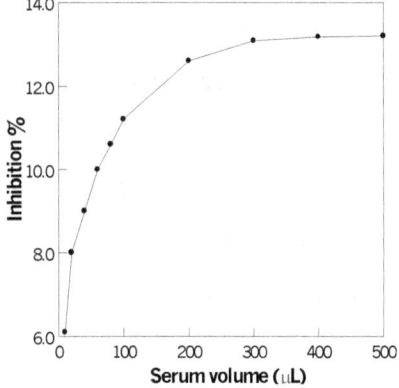

Figure (4.1): The Standard curve for the determination of SOD unit.

SOD unit was calculated from Figure (4.1) according to the following: the amount of serum (VµL) which gives half the maximum inhibition of NBT reduction (1 unit = 10.1 µL).

To calculate the SOD activity in sera of patients, the differences between absorbances before and after the light irradiation were, multiplied by the SOD unit.

4.6 DETERMINATION OF SERUM LIPID-BOUND SIALIC ACID:

Serum LBSA was determined by the method of Katopodis et al [143]. All details are

explained in section (2.5.2).

4.7 STATISTICAL METHODS:

Statistical analysis was performed by student's t-test [146].

Figure (4.2) shows the distribution of the individual values of SOD activity in different types of breast cancer patients.
SOD levels in sera of patients with breast cancer differ significantly ($P < 0.001$) from those of healthy and patients with benign tumor, but the SOD levels in sera of benign patients shows no significant differences from those of healthy individuals.

It is clear from table (4-1), patients with breast cancer had lower values of SOD activity compared with that of healthy individuals, (premenopausal, 1.29 ± 0.14, and postmenopausal, 1.05 ± 0.23). Very low SOD activity in comparison with healthy was observed in sera from patients with postmenopausal. However, a reliable decrease in the SOD activity was found in patients with breast cancer (premenopausal and postmenopausal) as compared to that of benign patients ($P < 0.001$), on the other hand, patients with breast cancer have a higher levels of LBSA (premenopausal, 29.32 ± 3.55 and postmenopausal, 27.35 ± 5.29), compared with healthy individuals and benign patients. No statistically significant difference was found between LBSA levels in patients with benign and healthy individuals, also there was no statistically significant difference among LBSA levels between the different subgroups of breast cancer (premenopausal and postmenopausal).

Furthermore, the ratio of LBSA/SOD was higher in patients with breast cancer compared with those with benign and normal healthy controls, the mean values of this index are shown in table (4-1)

211

Table (4-1): Comparison of mean values for the superoxide dismutase (SOD) activity and Lipid-Bound sialic acid (LBSA) levels in sera from healthy and patients with breast cancer. All details are explained in the text.

Groups	No.	SOD activity (mean±SD)	LBSA mg/dL (mean±SD)	LBSA/SOD (mean±SD)
Breast cancer:				
Premenopausal	20	1.29±0.14	29.32±3.55	22.74±2.25
Postmenopausal	20	1.05±0.23	27.35±5.29	30.05±5.87
Benign	20	1.53±0.17	18.73±2.29	12.34±3.64
Healthy (normal)	10	1.65±0.21	16.9±2.13	10.15±2.38

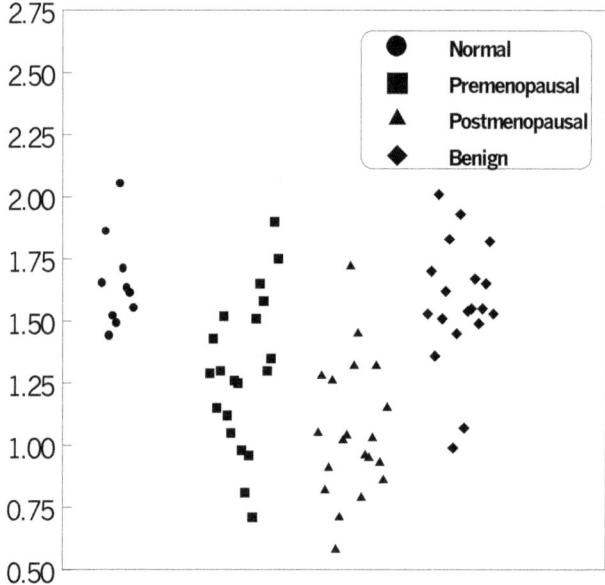

Figure (4.2): Distribution of the individual values of SOD activity in sera of patients with different types of breast cancer and normal healthy.

Knee et al [186] and Bolzan et al [187] reported that lower levels of SOD (especially the manganese dependent enzyme) are found in various malignant tumors compared with normal control cells.

High metastatic cell lines contain less SOD than low metastatic cell ones [186]. Prognosis for patients with low SOD levels in the leukaemic blasts is unfavourable [188], and a negative correlation has been established between SOD activity in the whole blood and the chromosomal sensitivity after x-ray irradiation of lymphocytes from patients with cancer of the mammary gland [187]. The results show that lower SOD activity in patients with tumors compared to the healthy controls (table 4-1), and the mean values for SOD activity in benign patients are near to those in healthy controls, these results are in agreement with the same results have been observed by Abella et al [189].

Table (4-2) shows the sensitivity and specificity of LBSA and SOD in normal controls and in patients with different types of breast cancer. Sensitivity and specificity of the determination of serum SOD activity in distinguishing patients with benign from premenopausal and postmenopausal patients are (85% and 95% respectively) for sensitivity, and it is possible that the lower specificity of this determination (15% and 5% respectively), while the sensitivity of LBSA for determination of benign from malignant is (95% for premenopausal and 100% for postmenopausal). Also, as with SOD activity measurement, the specificity of the determination (premenopausal 5%, and postmenopausal 0 %) is lower than its sensitivity.

Table (4-2): Specificity and sensitivity of LBSA and SOD activity in normal controls and in patients with breast cancer.

Groups	No.	Parameter	Negative results	Specificity % true negative	Positive results	Sensitivity % true positive

Healthy (normal)	10	LBSA	9	90	1	10
		SOD	8	80	2	20
Premenopausal	20	LBSA	1	5	19	95
		SOD	3	15	17	85
Postmenopausal	20	LBSA	0	0	20	100
		SOD	1	5	19	95
Benign	20	LBSA	12	60	8	40
		SOD	17	85	3	15

Note: Sensitivity and specificity of the SOD measuring as follows: sensitivity was calculated as % of patients with breast cancers who had positive results (lower SOD activity than healthy). Specificity was calculated as % of patients with breast cancers who had negative results (normal or higher SOD activity than healthy).

These results are due to the fact that patients with breast cancer have different diagnosis, also the differences in the serum activity of SOD in patients with malignant tumors and benign are probably due to the decreased enzyme level in the tumor cell [187]. Such deficiency appears, for example, when enhanced serum levels of gangliosides (e.g. LBSA) are released by the tumor cells. LBSA binds to the plasma membranes of the mononuclear cells and inhibits their functions, which may be an important mechanism for immunosuppression in malignant diseases [190].

However, from these results, it possible to conclude that the serum levels of SOD and LBSA reflect the changes in the content of membrane glycolipids and cellular activity of SOD.

Some authors admit that these changes in the tumor cell are in closed connection; the membrane of the malignant cell has an altered lipid content and structure organization, which leads to decreased antioxidant protection [191].

The loss of cell differentiation leads to an increase of the cell glycolipids, on the other hand, to decrease of the intracellular SOD [192]. Figure (4.3) shows a significant negative correlation between the two parameters in patients with breast cancer, and it is also indicates that patients with high levels of LBSA have low SOD content in the serum. Such negative correlation does not appear in benign. This is in accordance with the observations that changes in membrane glycolipids and cellular antioxidants occur in malignant, but not benign, tumors [193]. These findings suggest that SOD and LBSA are good tumor markers.

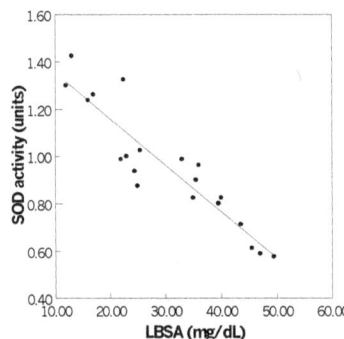

Figure (4.3): Correlation between superoxide dismutase (SOD) activity and the levels of lipid-bound sialic

Lectin, a general term applied to haemo-agglutinating substances presents in extracts of seeds of certain plants, which specifically agglutinate RBC of certain blood group, are also glycoproteins and glycolipids [125].

The ability of lectins to interact with soluble glycoproteins and glycolipids have been used to isolate and fractionate glycoproteins and glycolipids. This ability is due to binding of lectin to the oilgosaccharides moieties of glycoproteins and glycolipids [125]. Various lectins are known to be present in mammalian tissues and organs, the β-D-galactose and mannose-6-phosphate as a specific lectins from various tissues and organs have been studied extensively[194,195]. However, a few lectins with high specificity for sialic acid have been identified, such as limulin and carcinoscropine [196]. One major role of lectins, typified by the bacteria-legume symbiosis, appears to be to bind together cells of two different

215

species. There is evidence that lectins acting in this way participate in both the prevention of plant infection, by binding to saccharides on bacteria or fungi, and in the promotion of bacterial infection of vertebrate cells. Bacterial lectins apparently mediate the adhesion of these microorganisms to oligosaccharides on animal cells, which could be a prelude to infection.

Thus, Escherichia coli contains a lectin that binds D-mannose and its α-glycosides, and that presumably mediates bacterial attachment to cells. Another evidence for binding of Vibrio cholera to intestinal cell surfaces by a reaction inhibited by L-fucose has been presented [197]. Although a specific cellular function cannot yet be unequivocably assigned to any lectin, a large body of evidence indicates that lectins have been adapted for a variety of cell surface and intercellular functions in which the specific carbohydrate-binding site of the lectin binds a complementary saccharisde-containing substance as a prelude to one of a number of biological actions. Some lectins, such as those in root hairs, apparently bind complementary saccharides in a fairly discriminating way, which leads to highly specific symbiosis. In this case the lectin is apparently playing a highly refined recognition function, although its binding site is not so exclusive as to reject receptors on test erythrocytes. In contrast, evidence for different localizations and functions of the same lectin in different animal cells suggests that the specificity of lectin function is not dictated solely by the precise nature of its binding sites, but also by opportunistic factors that determine which of many receptors of adequate complementarity are available[129].

Furthermore, lectin which binds sialic acid residue of glycoproteins has also been isolated from wheat germ [198]. Sialic acid occupies an outstanding position both sterically and with respect to biological function in various glycoproteins and glycolipids.

Also, a lectin which specificity recognizes terminal sialic acids residue is likely to be a useful in studying the biological functions of sialoglycoproteins[199].

5.4.2 Preparation of Tissue Homogenate:

Three grams of frozen breast tissues were washed with 5 ml volume of 0.9% NaCl to remove surface mucus materials and contamination, then homogenized in 15 ml of 0.02 M phosphate buffered saline (0.075 M Na_2HPO_4/ 0.075 M KH_2PO_4 pH 7.2 containing 0.004 M of β-mercapto ethanol, 0.002 M EDTA and 0.075 M NaCl), using Tenbroeck ground-glass homogenizer to prepare the homogenate. The homogenate was centrifugated at 4000 r.p.m. for one hour. The supernatant was used as a source of lectin (crude or homogenate lectin) for binding (expressed as hemagglutination) studies. The supernatant was used through out study and stored at -20°C till using [200].

5.5 DETERMINATION OF BIOCHEMICAL CONSTITUENTS IN CANCEROUS BREAST HOMOGENATE:

5.5.1 Protein Determination:

Protein was determined by the method of Lowry et al [145], using bovine serum albumin as standard.

5.6 PRELIMINARY TEST FOR THE BINDING OF CANCEROUS BREAST LECTIN TO ERYTHROCYTE SUSPENSION:
5.6.1 Preparation of Standard erythrocytes Suspension for Hemagglutination:

Type A of human blood was obtained from physically normal volunteer. The erythrocytes were washed four times in 0.9% (w/v) NaCl and diluted with 0.9% NaCl to an absorbancy of about 2 at 620 nm [201].

5.6.2 The Hemagglutination Assay:

This assay is a modification of the procedure reported by Liener [202,203]. The binding of cancerous breast lectin to erythrocyte suspension was preliminary checked by hemagglutination according to the following modification.

1. Half ml of diluted cancerous breast lectin by ((Tris-Saline buffer, 0.02 M Tris-HCl buffer pH 8 containing 0.15 M NaCl and 0.02 M $CaCl_2$) was incubated with 0.5 ml of washed erythrocytes at room temperature for 30 min. Then the cells were pelleted by centrifugation for 3 min., the supernatant was decanted.

2. The cells were resuspended in the same buffer and aggregated cells allowed to settle for 5 min., then the absorbance at 620 nm of the upper layer (free lectin and cells) of the assay solution was measured.

Calculations:

Total binding (expressed as % hemagglutination) represents the amount of lectin, which binds the erythrocytes and causing hemagglutination.

$$\text{Hemagglutination activity \%} = \frac{A - A^*}{A} \times 100$$
(total binding %)

Where:

A = The absorbance of standard erythrocyte suspension at 620 nm.

A* = The absorbance of free (unbound) erythrocytes at 620 nm.

5.6.3 Determination of non-Specific Binding of Cancerous Breast Lectin Homogenate to Erythrocyte Surface Glycoconjugates:

The same steps mentioned in section (5.6.2) were followed to determine the percent of the non-specific binding, except, the whole blood were washed (3-4) times with normal saline (0.9% w/v NaCl), then two times with assay buffer (Tris-HCl buffer pH 8) and the suspension was prepared. Ten ml of this suspension placed in a test tube and 100 μL of neuraminidase was added (500 unit/ml) and the mixture was shaken for four hours at 25°C. Then centrifugation at 3000 r.p.m. for 3 minutes, was carried out. The supernatant was removed and the remaining blood cells were diluted with an appropriate amount of normal saline to an absorbancy of about 2 at 620 nm and then used for hemagglutination activity directly.

Calculations:

The percent of non-specific binding was calculated using the following equation:

$$NSB\% = \frac{A^\circ - A^*}{A^\circ} \times 100$$

Where:

NSB % = The percent of non-specific binding.

A° = The absorbance of neuraminidase-treated erythrocyte suspension at 620nm.

A^* = The absorbance of free (unbound) erythrocytes at 620 nm.

5.6.4 Determination of The Specific Binding of Lectin to Erythrocyte Surface Glycoconjugates:

The percent of specific binding of lectin to glycoconjugates was calculated by subtracting the percent of non-specific binding from the percent of the total binding.

SB% = TB% - NSB%

219

Where:

SB% = The percent of specific binding of lectin to erythrocyte surface glycoconjugates.

TB% = The percent of total binding of lectin to erythrocyte surface glycoconjugates.

5.6.5 Determination of Hemagglutination Activity Unit:

The hemagglutination activity unit is the level of test solution (hence breast tumor homogenate concentration) which cause 50% of the standard cell suspension to sediment in (0.5-2 hours) as determined by Lis and Sharon method [203], or by plotting the hemagglutination activity data against the concentration of lectin, (Fig. 5.1).

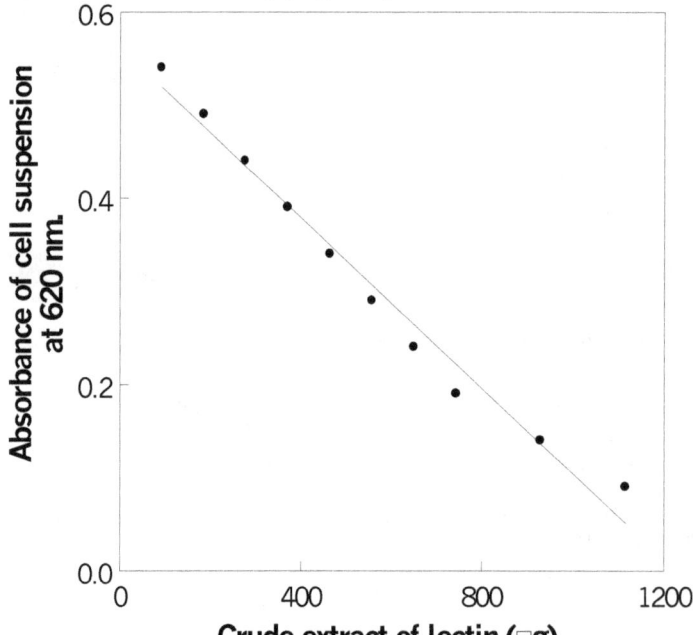

Figure (5.1): Hemagglutination assay of breast tumor homogenate lectin. All details are explained in text.

<u>**5.6.6 Factors Effecting on Lectin Binding to Erythrocyte Surface**</u>
<u>**Glycoconjugates in Cancerous Breast Homogenate:**</u>

5.6.6.1 The Effect of Different Lectin Amounts on Its Binding To Erythrocyte Surface Glycoconjugates:

Half milliliter of erythrocyte suspension was incubated with different amounts of crude lectin (93, 186, 279, 372, 465, 558, 651, 744, 930 and 1116 µg) dissolved in assay buffer for 30 minutes at 22°C. The final reaction volume was 1 ml, then the cells were pelleted by centrifugation for 3 minutes. After that the step 2, of the experiment (5.6.2) was repeated.

<u>Calculations:</u>

1. The same equation mentioned in experiment (5.6.2) was used to calculate the percent of total binding.

2. The percent of specific binding (SB%) was calculated by using the equation mentioned in section (5.6.4).

3. The percent of specific binding (SB%) was plotted against their corresponding lectin amount, as shown in Figure (5.2).

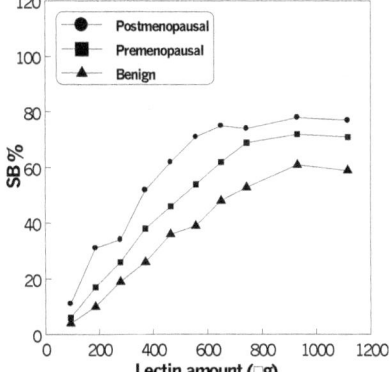

Figure (5.2): Effect of the amount of human breast tumor homogenate lectin on the hemagglutination activity. All details are explained in text.

5.6.6.2 Effect of pH on Hemagglutination Activity:

Fifty μL of human cancerous breast homogenate was incubated with 0.5 ml of erythrocyte suspension at 22°C for 30 minutes, using Tris-saline buffer of different pH from 7 to 9. The final reaction volume was 1 ml, then the cells were pelleted by centrifugation for 3 minutes. After that, the step 2 of the experiment (5.6.2) was repeated.

Calculations:

1. The same equation mentioned in experiment (5.6.2) was used to calculate the percent of total binding.

2. The percent of specific binding (SB%) was calculated by using the equation mentioned in section (5.6.4).

3. The percentages of specific binding (SB%) were plotted against their corresponding pH values, as shown in Figure (5.3).

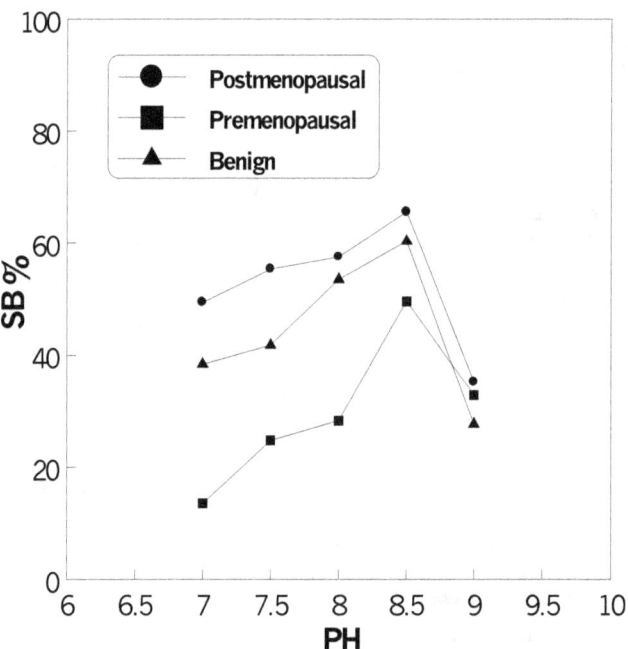

Figure (5.3): Effect of pH on the hemagglutination activity of human breast tumor homogenate lectin. All details are explained in text.

5.6.6.3 Effect of Temperature on Hemagglutination Activity:

Fifty μL of human cancerous breast homogenate was incubated with 0.5 ml of erythrocyte suspension for 30 minutes at different temperatures (5, 15, 20, 25, 30, and 35°C) using the assay buffer (pH 8.5). The final reaction volume was 1 ml, then the red cells were pelleted by centrifugation for 3 minutes. After that, the step 2 of the experiment (5.6.2) was repeated.

Calculations:

1. The same equation mentioned in experiment (5.6.2) was used to calculate the percent of total binding.

2. The percent of specific binding (SB%) was calculated by using the equation mentioned in section (5.6.4).

3. The percentages of specific binding (SB%) were plotted against their corresponding temperatures, as shown in Figure (5.4).

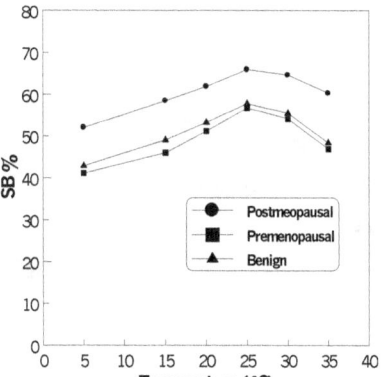

Figure (5.4): Effect of temperature on the hemagglutination activity of human breast tumor homogenate lectin. All details are explained in text.

5.6.6.4 Effect of Incubation Time on Hemagglutination Activity:

Fifty µL of human cancerous breast homogenate was incubated with 0.5 ml of erythrocyte suspension at 25°C for several time intervals (15, 30, 60, 90, 120, and 135 minutes) using the assay buffer (pH 8.5). The final reaction volume was 1 ml, then the red cells were pelleted by centrifugation for 3 minutes. After that, the step 2 of the experiment (5.6.2) was repeated.

Calculations:

1. The same equation mentioned in experiment (5.6.2) was used to calculate the percent of total binding.

2. The percent of specific binding (SB%) was calculated by using the equation mentioned in section (5.6.4).

3. The percentages of specific binding (SB%) were plotted against their corresponding times, as shown in Figure (5.5).

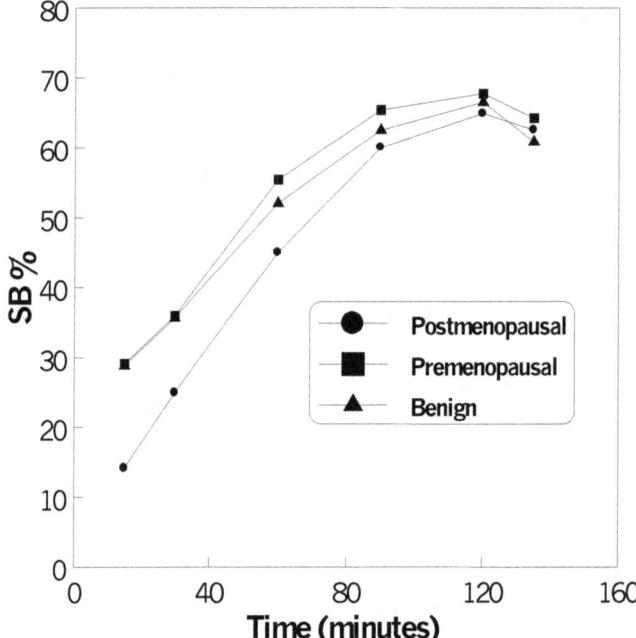

Figure (5.5): Dependence of hemagglutination activity of human breast tumor homogenate lectin on reaction time. All details are explained in text.

5.6.6.5 *Effect of Exogenous Ca++ ions on Hemagglutination Activity:*

Fifty μL of human cancerous breast homogenate was incubated with 0.5 ml of erythrocyte suspension at 25°C for 120 minutes using the assay buffer (pH 8.5), containing different Ca^{++} ions (2.5, 5, 10, 15, 20, 25, and 30 mM). The final reaction volume was 1 ml, then the red cells were pelleted by centrifugation for 3 minutes. After that, the step 2 of the experiment (5.6.2) was repeated.

Calculations:

1. The same equation mentioned in experiment (5.6.2) was used to calculate the percent of total binding.

2. The percent of specific binding (SB%) was calculated by using the equation mentioned in section (5.6.4).

3. The percentages of specific binding (SB%) were plotted against their corresponding Ca^{++} ions concentrations, as shown in Figure (5.6).

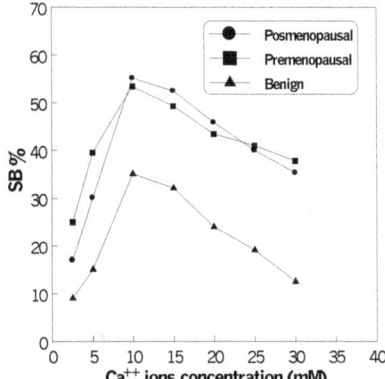

Figure (5.6): Effect of Ca^{++} ions concentration on the hemagglutination activity of human breast tumor homogenate lectin. All details are explained in text.

5.6.6.6 Effect of Denaturing Agents on Hemagglutination Activity:

Fifty μL of human cancerous breast homogenate was incubated at 25°C for 120 minutes with different concentration of denaturing agents (Urea, PEG, NaOH, and HCl), dissolved in the assay buffer (pH = 8.5), then 0.5 ml of erythrocyte suspension was added. The final reaction volume was 1 ml, then the red cells were pelleted by centrifugation for 3 minutes. After that, the step 2 of the experiment (5.6.2) was repeated.

Calculations:

1. The same equation mentioned in experiment (5.6.2) was used to calculate the percent of total binding.

2. The percent of specific binding (SB%) was calculated by using the equation mentioned in section (5.6.4).

225

3. The data of percent specific binding (SB%) were summarized in Table (5.1):

Table (5-1): Effect of denaturating agents on the hemagglutination activity of breast homogenate lectin. All details are explained in the text.

Groups	Type of test	Reagent added (M)	Specific binding %
	Control	-	100
Premenopausal	urea	3	74.59
		4	66.77
		5	57.13
		6	56.54
		3	75.46
Postmenopausal	=	4	71.65
		5	58.48
		6	47.58
	=	3	73.65
Benign		4	58.44
		5	29.17
		6	20.19
		0.5%	76.82
Premenopausal	Polyethlene glycol	1%	75.43
		2%	73.82
		4%	67.1
		0.5%	76.82
Postmenopausal	=	1%	75.65
		2%	74.27
		4%	71.59
		0.5%	75.35
Benign	=	1%	71.67
		2%	70.85
		4%	68.01
Premenopausal	NaOH	0.15	74.25
	HCl	0.15	71.38
Postmenopausal	NaOH	0.15	74.62
	HCl	0.15	71.59
Benign	NaOH	0.15	73.03
	HCl	0.15	70.98

5.6.6.7 Inhibition Studies of Hemagglutination Activity:

A number of carbohydrate were used as inhibitors (sialic acid, glucuronic acid, fructose, mannose and xylose) for the binding of lectin to glycoconjugates of erythrocyte surface.

The first step in this type of assay was carried out by addition of high concentration of lectin, which gives more of hemagglutination. Before addition the sugar, which used as inhibitor, 50 μL of human cancerous breast homogenate was incubated with 0.5 ml of erythrocyte suspension at 25°C for 120 minutes. The final reaction volume was completed to 1 ml by adding Tris-saline buffer (pH 8.5), then the cells were pelleted by centrifugation for 3 minutes. After that, the step 2 of the experiment (5.6.2) was repeated.

The second step in this type of assay was carried out according to the following:

Fifty μL of human cancerous breast homogenate was incubated with 0.5 ml of erythrocyte suspension at 25°C for 120 minutes The final reaction volume was completed to 1 ml by adding Tris-saline buffer (pH 8.5) which contain the desired concentration of sugar used (inhibitor). Then the cells were pelleted by centrifugation for 3 minutes. After that, the step 2 of the experiment (5.6.2) was repeated.

Calculations:

1. The same mathematical formula mentioned in experiment (5.6.2) was used to calculate the percent of total binding before and after addition of the inhibitor.

2. The percent of specific binding (SB%) was calculated before and after addition of inhibitor, by using the equation mentioned in section (5.6.4).

3. The percent of inhibition of hemagglutination represents the difference between the percent of specific binding (SB%) with lectin alone and that obtained with lectin plus the inhibitor. The data of % inhibition was summarized in table (5-2) and these data were plotted against their corresponding sugar concentration, as shown in Fig. (5.7).

Table (5-2): Inhibition of hemagglutination activity of human breast homogenate lectin.

All details are explained in the text.

Groups	Type of carbohy. test	Carbohy. conc. (mM)	Inhibition %
Premenopausal	Sialic acid	1	6.6
		1.5	10.4
		2	15.3
		2.5	19.7
		3	24.4
		3.5	29.1
Postmenopausal	"	1	15.45
		1.5	22.41
		2	30.6
		2.5	36.1
		3	44.85
		3.5	52.1
Benign	"	1	4.65
		1.5	6.61
		2	8.1
		2.5	10.55
		3	12.56
		3.5	14.65
Premenopausal	D-glucuronic acid	1	3.25
		10	6.1
		15	9.9

		20	12.2
Postmenopausal	=	1	4.1
		10	8.75
		15	11.1
		20	13.15
Benign	=	1	2.4
		10	5.9
		15	9.3
		20	11.9
Premenopausal	D-Fructose	30	59.15
	D-Mannose	30	55.8
	D-Xylose	30	51.05
Postmenopausal	D-Fructose	30	28.35
	D-Mannose	30	20.45
	D-Xylose	30	19.95
Benign	D-Fructose	30	.
	D-Mannose	30	.
	D-Xylose	30	11.6

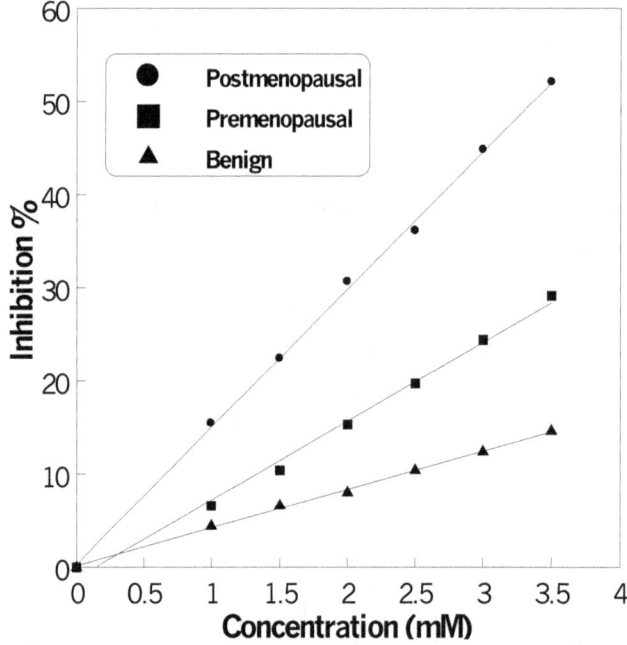

Figure (5.7): Effect of sialic acid on the hemagglutination activity of human breast tumor homogenate lectin. All details are explained in text.

5.6.6.8 Effect of Ionic Strength and Different Salts on Hemagglutination Activity:

5.6.6.8.1 Effect of monovalent salts on hemagglutination activity:

Fifty μL of human cancerous breast homogenate was incubated with 0.5 ml of erythrocyte suspension at 25°C for 120 minutes using the assay buffer (pH 8.5), which contains NaCl of various concentrations (0.05 M to 0.3 M). The total volume was 1 ml, then the cells were pelleted by centrifugation for 3 minutes. After that, the step 2 of the experiment (5.6.2) was repeated.

Calculations:

1. The same equation mentioned in experiment (5.6.2) was used to calculate the percent of total binding.

2. The percent of specific binding (SB%) was calculated by using the equation mentioned in section (5.6.4).

3. The percentages of specific binding (SB%) were plotted against their corresponding NaCl concentrations, as shown in (Figure 5.8 and table 5-3):

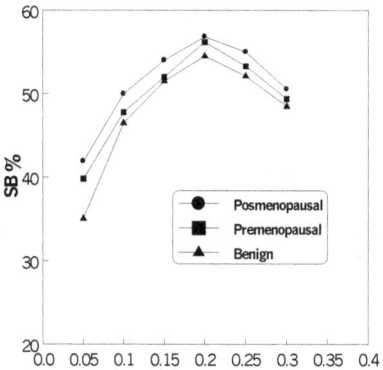

Figure (5.8): Effect of monovalent salt concentration on the hemagglutination activity of human breast tumor homogenate lectin. All details are explained in text.

5.6.6.8.2 Effect of divalent salts on hemagglutination activity:

Fifty µL of human cancerous breast homogenate was incubated with 0.5 ml of erythrocyte suspension at 25°C for 120 minutes in presence of 10 mM CaCl2 and different concentrations from (0.005 M to 0.02 M) of $MgCl_2$ (dissolved in the assay buffer pH 8.5). The final reaction volume

229

was 1 ml, then the cells were pelleted by centrifugation for 3 minutes. After that, the step 2 of the experiment (5.6.2) was repeated.

Calculations:

1. The same equation mentioned in experiment (5.6.2) was used to calculate the percent of total binding.

2. The percent of specific binding (SB%) was calculated by using the equation mentioned in section (5.6.4).

3. The percentages of specific binding (SB%) were plotted against their corresponding $MgCl_2$ concentrations, as shown in (Figure 5.9 and table 5-3):

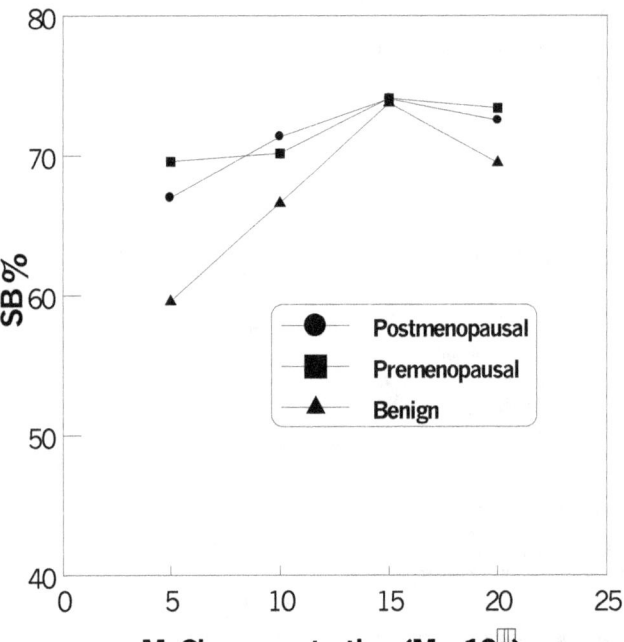

Figure (5.9): Effect of divalent salt concentration on the hemagglutination activity of human breast tumor homogenate lectin. All details are explained in text.

Table (5-3): Effect of mono and divalent salts on the hemagglutination activity of breast homogenate lectin. All details are explained in the text.

Groups	Type of salt test	Salt conc. (M)	Specific binding %
Premenopausal	NaCl	0.05	36.82
		0.1	47.78
		0.15	52.05
		0.2	56.17
		0.25	53.3
		0.3	49.39
Postmenopausal	-	0.05	41.93
		0.1	49.95
		0.15	54.01
		0.2	56.81
		0.25	55.03

		0.3	50.56
Benign	"	0.05	35.05
		0.1	46.5
		0.15	51.52
		0.2	54.96
		0.25	52.13
		0.3	46.19
Premenopausal	MgCl$_2$	5 x10^{-3}	69.58
		10 x10^{-3}	70.16
		15 x10^{-3}	74.09
		20 x10^{-3}	73.4
Postmenopausal	"	5 x10^{-3}	66.98
		10 x10^{-3}	71.35
		15 x10^{-3}	74.06
		20 x10^{-3}	72.52
Benign	"	5 x10^{-3}	59.8
		10 x10^{-3}	66.58
		15 x10^{-3}	73.76
		20 x10^{-3}	69.49

The homogenate of human tissue of breast cancer was characterized by significant hemagglutination activity toward human red blood cells (group A). Homogenization of breast tumor tissues was carried out in cold medium to protect of protein from denaturation due to proteolytic enzyme activity [200]. However, addition of β-mercaptoethanol and EDTA to the extracting solution were necessary to prevent the inactivation of lectin and to achieve the maximal extraction of the lectin [204].

The total binding of lectin to glycoconjugates was estimated according to the hemagglutination assay [202,203]. Hemagglutination assay is a semiquantitaive procedure and has been widely used as a laboratory test because of its ease and versatility. It depends on aggregating and sedimentation of the erythrocytes after reaction with the bivalent or multivalent lectin [205].

However, the non-specific binding was determined by using neuraminidase to be incubated with the erythrocyte suspension before the assay, this enzyme is responsible for the release of terminal sialic acid residue from the erythrocyte surface glycoconjugates, and hence, the penultimate N-acetylgalactosamine will be exposed for the lectin binding.

Until now relatively few sialic acid specific lectins [206] have been identified, among which, only one is commercially a available. Most of them show a broad specificity. Basu et al [207] have reported a novel sialic acid binding lectin Achatinin$_H$ from the hemolymph of Achatina Fulica snail. The types [208,209] of sialic acid found on the erythrocytes, a striking correlation has been found between the ability of the agglutinin to agglutinate cells and the presence of O-acetylneuraminic acid residue on the mammalian cell surface [210]. Indeed the lectin agglutinated only those erythrocytes which contain 9-O-acetylneuraminic acid residues. Furthermore, human erythrocytes which contain only nueraminic acid [211], but no 9-O-acetylneuraminic acid were not agglutinable even by enzyme treatment [209]. Similarly horse erythrocyte known to contain high amount of 4-O-acetylneuraminic acid [210] were not affected.

From these results it was believed that this active agglutination may be due to the O or N-acetyl group which is present on the structure of sialoglycoproteins present on outer surface of the red cells, figure (5.1) shows a rapid steep decline in absorbance with an inflection point appeared in the curve was due to the lectin concentration used [212], found in 93 μg, which has a good agglutination activity.

Optimum Conditions of Hemagglutination:

Through figures (5.3, 5.4 and 5.5), the results show that the maximum hemagglutination activity of lectin required pH 8.5, the temperature at 25°C and the time for 120 minutes and it is clear that the lectin binding is dependent on pH and temperature. It should also be noted that the percent of specific lectin binding decreases with the change of pH (below 7 and upper 9.5), this suggests that the abundance of H^+ ions in the acidic medium may inhibit the binding sites on both glycoconjugate and lectin molecules, OH^- ions in more basic medium may influence in the same manner, and that the sialic acid which involved in binding is unstable to both acid and alkaline pH [213].

In general the results has led to the conclusion that the high binding process of lectin with glycoprotein is pH dependent and any shift in the pH of environment my affect the stability of the macromolecules involved in the binding. This effect includes the induction of protonation-deprotonation process occurring within the ionizable groups of the amino acids present in the binding groups of these macromolecules [214].

Effect of Ca^{++} Ions Concentration on Hemagglutination Activity:

Figure (5.6) represents the effect of Ca^{++} ions concentration on the binding activity of human breast homogenate lectin. The results in this figure show that the highest binding of lectin was found in the presence of 10 mM Ca^{+2} ions. However, the Ca^{+2} ions plays an important role in stabilization the complex formed between the lectin and the glycoprotein present on the red cell surface, also the stabilization is due to the conformational changes in the protein due to the binding of Ca^{+2} ions [215]. Dolichos [216], observed that the Ca^{+2} ion will stabilize the native structure of the protein itself.

Furthermore, there are many isolated lectins requires Ca^{+2} ions in their binding or their physiological roles [217], also, different Ca^{+2} ions dependent lectins have been purified from various sources and most of these possess multimeric structures and are capable of forming cross-linked complexes [218].

Effect of Denaturating Agents on the Hemagglutination Activity:

The data presented in table (5-1) shows the effect of different denaturating agents on the binding activity of breast lectin (Urea, PEG,

NaOH and HCl). The results show that all of denaturating agents were effected on specific binding for lectin as compared to the control, but this effect was different between types of denaturating agents. An analysis of the data in table (5-1) shows that the percent of specific binding for lectin to glycoconjugates decreased with increasing urea concentrations, this effect can be attributed to the effect of urea on the hydrophobic forces between protein molecules.

Also, increasing concentrations of polyethylene glycol may results in precipitation of protein molecules which leads to decrease the interaction between lectin and glycoconjugates, and hence decrease the percent of specific binding.

Furthermore, the effect of 0.15 M of NaOH and HCl on the binding activity of breast lectin was investigated in this work, the results indicated that NaOH and HCl considerably reduce the percent of specific binding, their denaturating effect is due to great changes in pH of icubation medium.

Inhibition Studies of Hemagglutination Activity:

The inhibition percent of hemagglutination activity of human breast lectin by various carbohydrates (sialic acid, D-glucuronic acid, fructose, mannose and xylose) are summarized in table (5.2) and figure (5-7). The results in this table are classified according to their respective of group patients.

It is clear from this table, sialic acid and D-glucuronic acid were found to be the most potent inhibitors and gives high inhibition percent of hemagglutination at 3.5 mM and 20 mM respectively. However, the results obtained from this assay demonstrated that D-fructose, D-mannose and D-xylose tested at 30 mM in patients with breast cancer (premenopausal and postmenopausal) have the high activities to inhibit the binding of cancerous lectin, as compared to the benign patients. On the other hand, the inhibition of D-glucuronic acid suggests that it might be used as the eluting sugar in the purification of lectin.

Furthermore, 0.953 mM, 9.64 mM and 3.12 mM of sialic acid, sodium glucuronate and EDTA respectively were enough to produce 50% inhibition for lectin isolated from rat uterus [219,220].

Goebal et al [221], have suggested that the inhibition studies could be used as a technique for demonstrating and measuring the reactions occurred between lectin and its binding protein, for example, coupled disaccharides binds to protein via their p-aminophenyl glycosides and the terminal non-reducing hexose to play the predominate role in the specificity.

Effect of Mono and Divalent Salts on the Hemagglutination Activity:

The effect of NaCl and $MgCl_2$ as mono and divalent salts respectively on the binding of lectin to erythrocyte surface glycoconjugates were investigated. The results show that there is significant increases in specific binding percent in different types of breast cancer when using different $MgCl_2$ concentrations than those obtained in the presence of different NaCl concentrations, (table 5-3). However, an analysis of the Figures (5.8) and (5.9) shows that the highest binding of lectin was obtained in 0.2 M of NaCl and 0.015 M of $MgCl_2$. These data are in disagreement with the results reported by Nassir [222], who have found that there is no effect of such ions on the lectin binding in the presence of 15 mM Ca^{+2} ions in the range of concentrationd (LBSA) in sera

6.7 THE EFFECT OF C^{a++} IONS ON BINDING OF GLYCOPROTEIN TO PURIFIED HUMAN CANCEROUS BREAST LECTIN:

a. Fifty microliters of purified cancerous breast lectin was incubated with 0.5 ml of red cell suspension at 25°C for 120 minutes. Different concentration of Ca^{++} ions (5, 10, 15, 20 and 25) $x10^{-3}$ M were dissolved in the assay buffer (pH = 8.5) and were added to the sample. The final reaction volume was one ml. Then the cells were pelleted by centrifugation for 3 min. The step two of the experiment (5.6.2) was repeated.

b. Parallel incubations were performed to determine the non-specific binding of the lectin, as described in section (5.6.3).

Calculations:

The same mathematical formula mentioned in experiment (5.6.4) was used to calculate the % of specific binding of purified lectin. The % specific binding was plotted against their corresponding Ca^{++} ions concentration, as shown in Fig. (6.4).

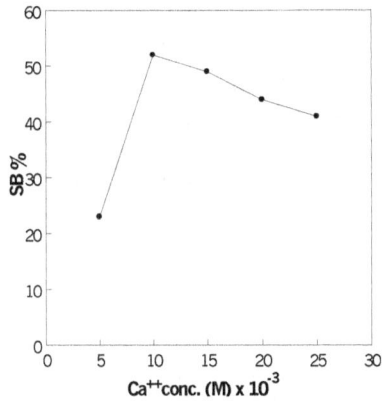

Figure (6.4): Effect of Ca^{++} ions concentration on the hemagglutination activity of human purified cancerous breast lectin. All details are explained in the text.

235

7.3 Kinetics of lectin binding to erythrocyte surface glycoconjugate:

7.3.1 The Time-Course of Cancerous Breast Lectin Binding to Erythrocyte Surface Glycoconjugates:

Figure (7.1) shows the time course of the formation of lectin binding to erythrocyte surface to glycoconjugate complex at four different temperatures (4, 11, 18 and 25°C), in breast homogenate sample.

The concentration of lectin-glycoconjugate complex that formed after time (t) was calculated from the following equation:

The concentration of lectin-glycoconjugate complex formed after time (t) in molar	=	The concentration of lectin involved in total binding (M)	−	The concentration of lectin involved in non-specific binding (M)

The results of time-course pattern at different temperatures indicated that the lectin binding to erythrocyte surface glycoconjugate is a temperature and time dependent process, since a maximum binding can be obtained at 25°C after incubation for 120 minutes, there is no analogous studies are available to compare our results.

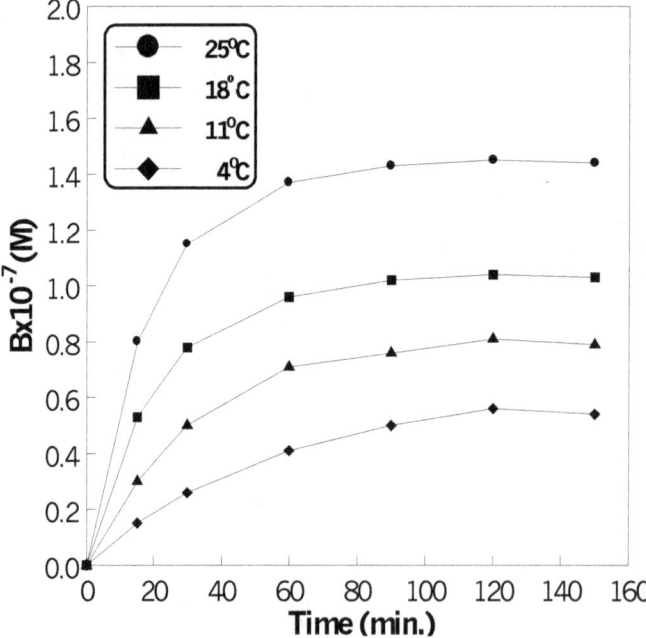

Figure (7.1): Time-course of lectin binding to erythrocyte surface to glycoconjugates at different four temperatures. All details are explained in the text.

Determination of Kinetic Parameters of Lectin-Glycoconjugate Complex Formation:

The time-course of lectin-glycoconjugate complex formation was carried out to describe the kinetic parameters of the binding (expressed as specific binding). The simplest proposed model representing this interaction was:

$$\text{Z 2 d 2 P (Z P Z P Z} \tag{1}$$

Where:

K_{+1}: is the association rate of lectin to glycoconjugate.
K_{-1}: is the dissociation rate of lectin-glycoconjugate complex.

At equilibrium:

K_a= [Lectin-glycoconjugate]/[Lectin][glycoconjugate]
(2)

K_d= [Lectin][glycoconjugate]/[Lectin-glycoconjugate]
(3)

Thus;

$$K_a = \frac{1}{K_d} = \frac{K_{+1}}{K_{-1}}$$

(4)

Where:

K_a: is the equilibrium constant (affinity constant).
K_d: is the equilibrium constant of dissociation of the complex.

The values of K_a and total concentration of lectin binding sites (B_{max}) were calculated from Scatchard and Eadie-Hofstee plots (Figures 7.2 and 7.3) respectively at four different temperatures (4, 11, 18 and 25°).

It is clear from table (7-1), the results show that the affinity constant (K_a) is depended on temperature (K_a increased from 0.847×10^7 M^{-1} at 4°C to 0.926×10^7 M^{-1} at 25°C). Whereas the value of dissociation constant (K_d) was calculated by using equation (4), and show that the lowest K_d value of lectin-glycoconjugate complex occurs at 25°C after incubation for 120 minutes.

237

Table (7-1): The kinetic parameters of lectin binding to erythrocyte surface glycoconjugates. All details are explained in the text.

	$K_d \times 10^{-7}$ (M)	$K_a \times 10^{7}$ (M^{-1})	$B_{max} \times 10^{-7}$ (M)
4	1.18	0.847	0.97
11	1.14	0.877	1.05
18	1.11	0.901	1.32
25	1.08	0.926	1.47

Figure (7.2): Scatchard plot of lectin binding to erythrocyte surface glycoconjugate at different four temperatures. All details are explained in the text.

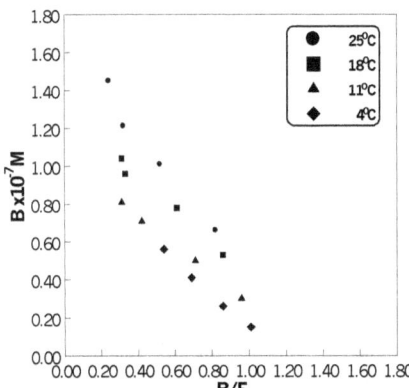

Figure (7.3): Eadie-Hofstee plot of data from Scatchard plot of lectin binding to erythrocyte surface glycoconjugate at different four temperatures. All details are explained in the text.

However, the time-course data shown in Figure (7.1) could be used to determine the reaction order of lectin binding to erythrocyte surface glycoconjugates using the following equation:

$$Ln[lectin\text{-}G]e \left[\frac{(lectin)_t - (lectin\text{-}G)_t (lectin\text{-}G)_e / (G)_t}{(lectin)_t [(lectin\text{-}G)_t - (lectin\text{-}G)_t]} \right] =$$

$$K_{+1t} \left[\frac{(lectin)_t (G)_t}{(lectin\text{-}G)_e} - (lectin\text{-}G)_e \right] \quad (5)$$

Where:

K_{+1}: is the kinetic association constant in M^{-1} $min.^{-1}$.

$(Lectin\text{-}G)_e$: is the concentration of the complex formed at equilibrium.

$(Lectin\text{-}G)_t$: is the concentration of the complex formed after time (t).

The equation (5) represents the second order kinetics, but in this work the percent of specific binding was in some cases, small and most of the lectin remains free and only small fraction binds even at equilibrium, i.e,

$(lectin)_t \gg (lectin-G)_e$ thus, $\dfrac{(lectin-G)_t (lectin-G)_e}{(lectin)_t} \gg \dfrac{(lectin-G)_t (lectin-G)_e}{(G)_t}$

and $\dfrac{(lectin)_t (G)_t}{(lectin-G)_e} \gg (lectin-G)_e$

So that the following equation could be used in order to fit the pseudo-first order kinetics:

$$Ln \frac{(lectin-G)_e}{(lectin-G)_e-(lectin-G)_t} = K_{+1}t \quad \frac{(lectin)_t (G)_t}{(lectin-G)_e}$$

(6)

On the other hand, Figure (7.4) shows the plot of

$$\ln \frac{(lectin - G)_e}{(lectin - G)_e - (lectin - G)_t}$$ against time (t) gives a straight line with a slope equal to the observed value of first rate constant (K_{obs}) in min^{-1}. The rate constant (K_{+1}) in M^{-1} min^{-1} was calculated at four different temperatures by using the following formula:

$$K_{obs} = K_{+1} \frac{[lectin][G]}{[lectin - G]_e}$$

$$\therefore K_{obs} = K_{+1}[lectin]$$

(7)

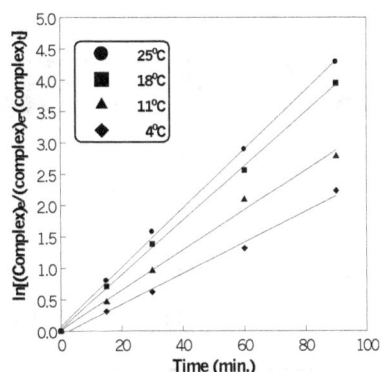

Figure (7.4): Kinetics of lectin binding to erythrocyte surface to glycoconjugate at different four temperatures. All details are explained in the text.

Also, the value of K_{-1} at four temperatures were calculated by using equation (4). Whereas, the half life time of association $(t^{1}\!/_{2})_{ass.}$, which represents the time needed for the formation of half amount of the complex at equilibrium, was determined from the concentration of the complex at equilibrium and the time-course curve. Also, the half life time of dissociation $(t^{1}\!/_{2})_{diss.}$, was calculated from the following relation:

$$(t^{1}\!/_{2})_{diss.} = \ln\frac{2}{k_{-1}} = \frac{0.693}{k_{-1}}$$

(8)

The values of $K_{obs.}$, K_{+1}, K_{-1}, $(t^{1}\!/_{2})_{ass.}$, and $(t^{1}\!/_{2})_{diss.}$ at four different temperatures are summarized in table (7-2). Data analysis of this table show that the highest rate for the association reaction occurs at 25°C, while the lowest rate occurs at 4°C, where the reaction temperature was

241

increased from 4°C to 25°C, the value of K_{+1} increased from $(0.676 \times 10^5$ $M^{-1}.min^{-1})$ to $(0.973 \times 10^5\ M^{-1}.min^{-1})$ which means the dependence of reaction rate on temperature. Also, the rate of dissociation of lectin-glycoconjugate complex (K_{-1}) is temperature dependent.

Table (7-2): The effect of temperature on the kinetic parameters of lectin binding to erythrocyte surface glycoconjugates. All details are explained in the text.

T°C	$K_{obs.}$ (min^{-1})	K_{-1} (M^{-1}. min^{-1})x10^5	K_1 (min^{-1})x10^{-3}	$(t\frac{1}{2})_{ass.}$ (min)	$(t\frac{1}{2})_{diss.}$ (min)
4	0.025	0.676	7.98	30	86.84
11	0.031	0.838	9.56	26	72.49
18	0.033	0.892	9.90	15	70
25	0.036	0.973	10.51	12	65.94

7.3.2 Scatchard Analysis:

Figure (7.2) shows Scatchard plot of lectin binding to erythrocyte surface to glycoconjugate in the presence of 10 mM Ca^{++} ions at different temperatures (4, 11, 18 and 25°C) after incubation for 120 minutes. This figure could be used to determine the kinetic parameters of lectin binding such as, the equilibrium constant of dissociation of the complex (K_d) and total concentration of lectin binding sites (B_{max}) of human cancerous breast lectin by using the following equation:

$$\frac{B}{F} = \frac{1}{K_d} \times (B_{max} - B)$$

The values of these parameters at different temperatures in presence of Ca^{++} ions are summarized in table (7-1). Through analysis the results in this table show that the total concentration of lectin binding sites (B_{max}) is temperature dependent, when the temperature was increased from 4°C to 25°C, B_{max} was increased from $(0.97 \times 10^{-7}$ M to 1.47×10^{-7} M), this fact could be explained according to the number of molecules possessing the activation-energy for interaction, increase with increase the temperature. On the other hand, the affinity constant (K_a) is also depended on temperature, this indicates that the reaction is slightly endothermic and explained by the fact that affinities of endothermic reactions enhanced by increasing temperatures. However, the values of B_{max} and K_d for human cancerous breast lectin at different temperatures obtained from Scatchard analysis were similar to those obtained from the Eadie-Hofstee plot (Fig. 7.3) [242].

7.3.3 Determination of Hill-Coefficient (n) of Lectin Binding to Glycoconjugates:

Figure (7-5) represents the Hill plot of lectin binding to erythrocyte surface glycoconjugate in the presence of 10 mM Ca^{++} ions at four different temperatures (4, 11, 18 and 25°C), The value of Hill-coefficient (n) equals the slope of the resulting straight line. The values were (1.54, 1.63, 1.71, 1.8) respectively. However, on application of the Hill equation [243,244] and using the results obtained from Scatchard analysis, it would be possible to evaluate the cooperativity of lectin binding sites through the determination of Hill coefficient (n). Furthermore, the results obtained in this work indicates that the cooperativity of lectin binding sites was low and affected by temperatures.

243

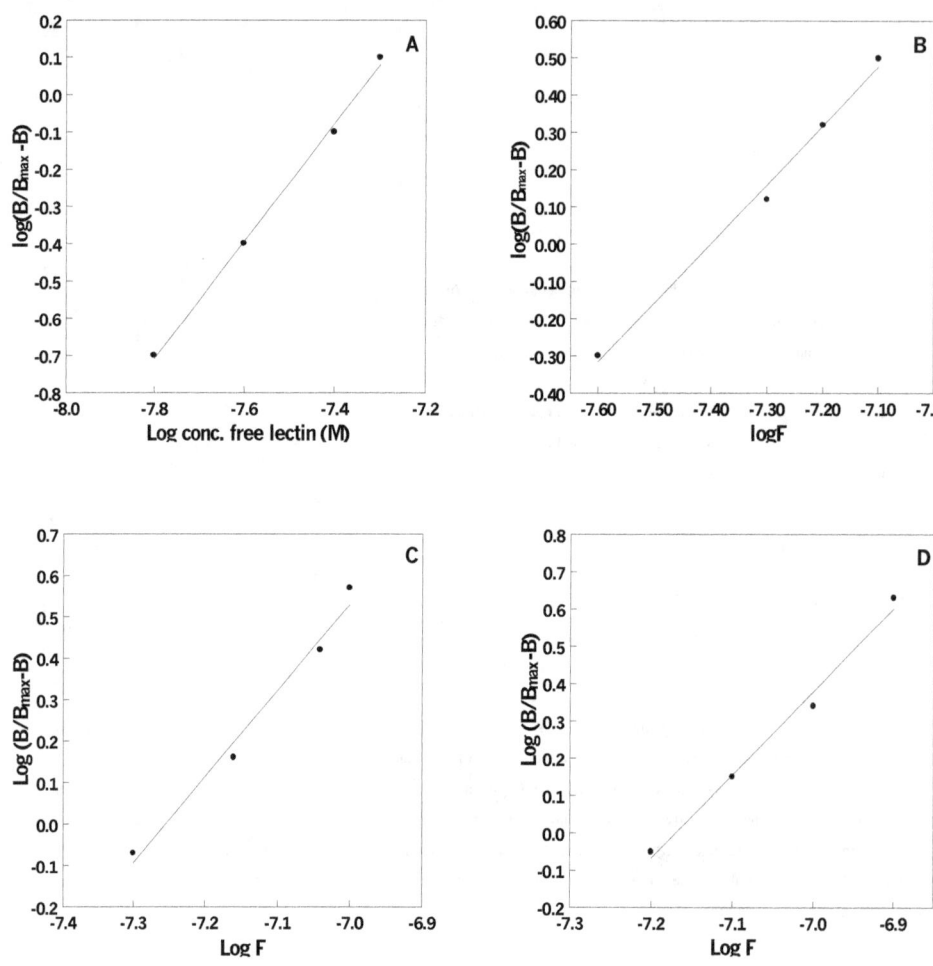

Figure (7-5): Hill plots of lectin binding to erythrocyte surface glycoconjugates at different temperatures, -A- 4°C, -B-11°C, -C-18°C, -D-25°C. All details are explained in the text.

7.4 THE THERMODYNAMICS OF THE LECTIN BINDING TO ERYTHROCYTE SURFACE GLYCOCONJUGATES:

A. Thermodynamic parameters of standard state:

Figure (7.6) shows Van't Hoff plot for the binding of lectin to erythrocyte surface glycoconjugates at different temperatures (4, 11, 18 and 25°). This figure revealed that the equilibrium binding constant (affinity constant) for lectin binding to glycoconjugates is temperature dependent. The results obtained from Van't Hoff plot indicated that $\Delta H°$ in general had a positive value of 9.15 KJ/mol, and that the reactions were nearly endothermic. However, the small positive value of $\Delta H°$ may indicate a favorable interaction between the lectin and glycoconjugate subgroups. These include the non-covalent interaction which are fundamentally electrostatic in nature such as charge-charge, charge-dipole, dipole-dipole, charge-induced dipole, dipole-induced dipole interactions and hydrogen bonds. The sum of these types of interactions can yield some stabilization to the folded structure of the complex.

The other values of thermodynamic parameters of standard state at four different temperatures (4, 11, 18 and 25°C), such as $\Delta G°$ values and $\Delta S°$ are summarized in table (7-3). From the analysis, the results in this table shows that the $\Delta G°$ values increases with decreasing temperatures, since the lectin binding to erythrocyte surface glycoconjugates needs higher energy at low temperatures. Whereas, the negative values of $\Delta G°$ indicates the stability of lectin glycoconjugate complex, subsequently the high affinity of the reactant.

Also, the high negative values of $\Delta G°$ indicates that the binding of lectin to glycoconjugates is a spontaneous reaction. Furthermore, these values are controlled by a high positive $\Delta S°$ values, table (7-3). The results show that the values of $\Delta S°$ decrease with increasing temperatures, this can be attributed to the more stable and more arranged status of lectin-glycoconjugate complex. On the other hand, the high positive value of $\Delta S°$ may be indicated that the binding spontaneity was enropically driven.

Entropy was the driven force for the occurrence of the binding, this shows that the hydrophobic interactions played an important role in the stability of complex formation [245].

Table (7-3): Thermodynamic parameters at standard state of lectin binding to erythrocyte surface glycoconjugates. All details are explained in the text.

T°C	$\Delta H°$ (kJ/mol)	$\Delta G°$ (kJ/mol.)	$\Delta S°$ (J/mol K)
4	9.15	-36.74	165.67
11	9.15	-37.75	165.14
18	9.15	-38.74	164.57
25	9.15	-39.74	164.06

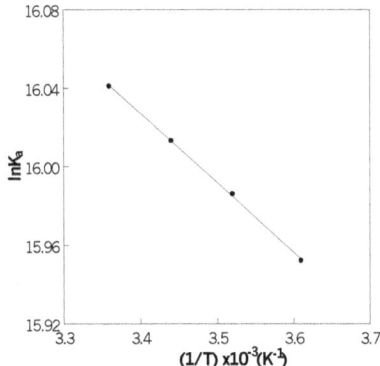

Figure (7-6): Van't Hoff plot for the binding of lectin to erythrocyte surface glycoconjugates. All details are explained in the text.

B. Thermodynamic parameters of transition state:

Through the transition state, the interaction of two substances leads to the formation of an activated complex (transition state), then the formation of the final product, i.e.: (the association of lectin with erythrocyte surface glycoconjugates) can be represented as follows:

Lectin + glycoconjugate ⟶ [Lectin-glycoconjugate]
an activated-complex

(transition state)

Lectin-glycoconjugate
(final product)

According to Arrhenius equation and kinetic constant, it could be calculated the thermodynamic parameters of the transition state (ΔH^*, ΔG^* and ΔS^*) at four different temperatures (4, 11, 18 and 25°C). Figure (7.7) shows Arrhenius plot for the binding of lectin to erythrocyte surface glycoconjugates, the slope of the straight line represents the activation energy (E_a) of the binding reaction.

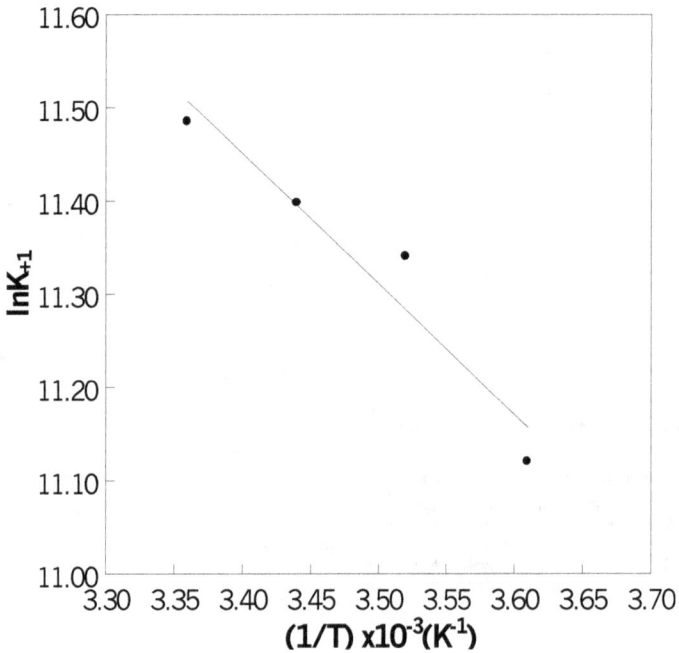

Figure (7.7): Arrhenius plot for the binding of lectin to erythrocyte syrface glycoconjugates. All details are explained in the text.

The values of thermodynamic parameters of the transition state (E_a, ΔH^*, ΔG^* and ΔS^*) are summarized in table (7-4). It is clear from this table, the high value of activation energy (13.05 KJ/mol) represents the required energy to overcome the transition state energy barrier and then giving the final product (lectin-glycoconjugate complex).

However, the value of activation energy is accordance with the high positive values of ΔG^* indicates that the formation of an activated complex is a non-spontaneous process.

Also, table (7-4) shows the values of ΔH^* at four different temperatures (4, 11, 18 and 25°C), the results revealed that the ΔH^* values decreased with increasing temperature. The slight changes in the values of ΔH^* at different temperatures could be attributed to the dependence on ΔH^* an activation energy (E_a) through the equation:

$\Delta H^* = E_a - RT$

Since the numerical value of RT is too small in comparison with the value of activation energy for the binding of lectin to glycoconjugates.

An analysis of the data in table (7-4), the results show that the ΔS^* values increases with decreasing temperature, was (-113.03 J/mol.K) at 4°C, -113.31 J/mol.K at 11°C, -113.44 J/mol.K at 18°C and –113.95 J/mol .K at 25°C). On the other hand, the high negative values of ΔS^* revealed that the activated complex had a more arranged structure than the reactants.

Finally, it could be concluded that the values of the thermodynamic parameters obtained from the study of lectin binding to erythrocyte surface glycoconjugates, give a distinct idea about the nature of forces that regulate the fromation of the complex.

Table (7-4): Thermodynamic parameters at transition state of lectin binding to erythrocyte surface glycoconjugates. All details are explained in the text.

T°C	E_a (KJ/mol.)	ΔH^* (KJ/mol.)	ΔG^* (KJ/mol.)	ΔS^* (KJ/mol.K)
4	13.05	10.75	42.06	-113.03

11	13.05	10.69	42.87	-113.31
18	13.05	10.63	43.64	-113.44
25	13.05	10.57	44.53	-113.95

In order to compare the values of transition state with those of standard state, it is suggested to have the thermodynamic model to describe the formation of the complex.

This model is illustrated in Figure (7.8). The thermodynamic model proposes that the formation of lectin-glycoconjugate complex undergoes three thermodynamic states.

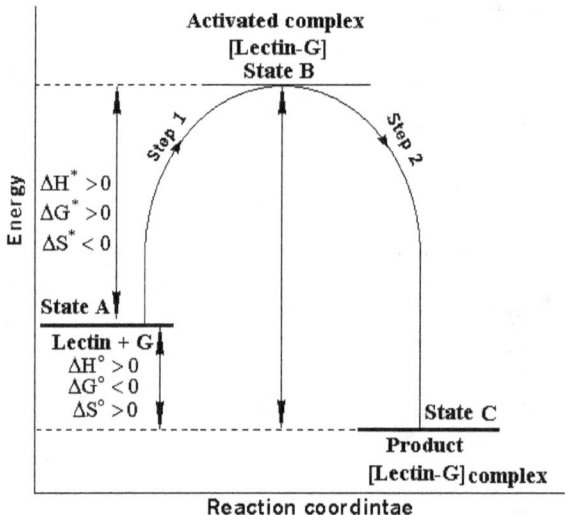

Figure (7.8): General energy diagram and thermodynamic model applied to the complex formation between lectin and erythrocyte surface glycoconjugates.

The thermodynamic state A, represents the initial energy level of lectin and glycoconjugate. The thermodynamic state B, represents the association of the two species to form the activated complex (lectin-glycoconjugate). The thermodynamic state C, represents the complete binding of lectin with glycoconjugate and formation of the complex. (lectin-glycoconjugate complex). However, this model involves two steps, in step 1 of the reaction, the binding of lectin to glycoconjugates is associated with positive ΔG^* value and thus requires external energy. Also, in step 1, the lectin binding, shows negative value for entropy change (ΔS^*), this negativity indicates the alteration in the structure of lectin-glycoconjugate transition complex to a more arranged structure. At step 2, the contribution of more interactions, gives a fully interacting complex (lectin-glycoconjugate). The formation of a protein-ligand complex is proposed to occur in two steps, the first is, the stabilization of the complex by hydrophobic interactions and the second is the stabilization by short range interactions, such as electrostatic interactions, protonation, hydrogen bonding and Van der Waals interactions [240].

Hydrophobic interactions contribute to the complex stability via high positive entropy ($\Delta S° > 0$), whereas, the electrostatic interactions, protonation, hydrogen bonding and Van der Waals interactions contribute to the complex stability via negative entropy change ($\Delta S° < 0$) [246,247].

It is clear from the thermodynamic data, the binding of lectin with glycoconjugate is entropy driven and it is in agreement with the concept that the hydrophobic interactions play an important role in such reactions.

Chapter Five

human chorionic gonadotropin (hCG) in gynecologic cancers

1.1 Gynecologic Cancers

The major malignancies of the female reproductive tract are endometrial, cervical, and ovarian cancer (Fig.1).Other gynecologic cancers, such as choriocarcinoma, fallopian tube cancer, vagina cancer, and vulva cancer are rare, but cancers metastasis to these female genitals are more common[1].

Ovarian cancer accounts for 4% of the total cancer in women worldwide. In Iraq, this cancer is the eighth most common malignant neoplasm in women (3.8-4.2% of the total cancer) behind cancer of the breast ,non-Hodgkin's lymphoma ,brain and other CNS, leukemia ,urinary bladder ,bronchus and lung ,and skin. The number of cases for the period (1992-1997) was 828[2].

The incidence rates of corpus uteri cancer (95% endometrial) were found to be higher in the richer countries and urban populations; it is the fifth leading cancer in women at these countries[3].However, there is evidence of some change in the socioeconomic determinants of the disease in developed countries. In Iraq, cancer of corpus uteri accounts for (0.9-2.2%) of the total cancer in women. The number of cases for the period (1992-1997) was 477[2]. The risk of uterine cancer is low before age 40 years and increases sharply thereafter [4].

253

Most cancers of the vulva, vagina and cervix are detected relatively early

because these organs are easily visualized and assessable for examination

by cytology and biopsy [1].Endometrial cancers are also detected early

because they normally heralded by vaginal bleeding. In contrast, cancers

of the ovary mostly present at a late stage with widespread intra-

abdominal metastases. Ovarian cancer remains the most lethal gynecologic

malignancy in women [5].

1.2 Endometrial Cancer

Endometrial cancer is the most common type of the corpus uteri

(Fig.1c), constituting about 95% of all malignant lesions of the uterine

cavity, while uterine

sarcomas accounts for fewer than 5 %[3].

The normal endometrium contains two major components: endometrial

stroma and glands. The glandular cell produces cytoplasmic receptors for

estradiol and, when stimulated, results in proliferation of glandular

epithelium, producing larger and more numerous glands.In the

premenopausal cycling endometrium, the maturational effects of

progesterone from the corpus leteum counter balance the proliferative

influence of estrogen. If conception does not occur, the lining is shed and

a new   cycle is initiated. When ovulation ceases at menopause, the

endometrial becomes quiescent and the glands atrophy. Tumors arising from the glandular epithelium, either de novo or as a result of abnormal estrogenic stimulation; are adenocarinomas[6]. The transition from benign proliferative endometrium to well differentiated adenocarcinoma probably proceeds through several intermediary steps, collectively termed hyperplasia. Hyperplasias are characterized by an overgrowth of the glandular component of the endometrial lining, whereas cancers are defined by the size of the cells, irregular nuclear membranes, coarse chromatin clumping, loss of glandular pattern, increasing nuclear atypia, and mitotic activity[6].

1.2.1 Histology

About 90% of endometrial cancers are endometriosis type (adenocarcinomas), which contain glands similar to those seen in the normal endometrium. These tumors are subclassified by their degree of differentiation into three grades:well (grade I, 50%), moderately (grade II, 35%), and poor differentiated (grade III, 15%). The International Federation of Gynecology and Oncology (FIGO) grading scheme is based on the growth pattern (relative proportion of glandular and solid areas):less

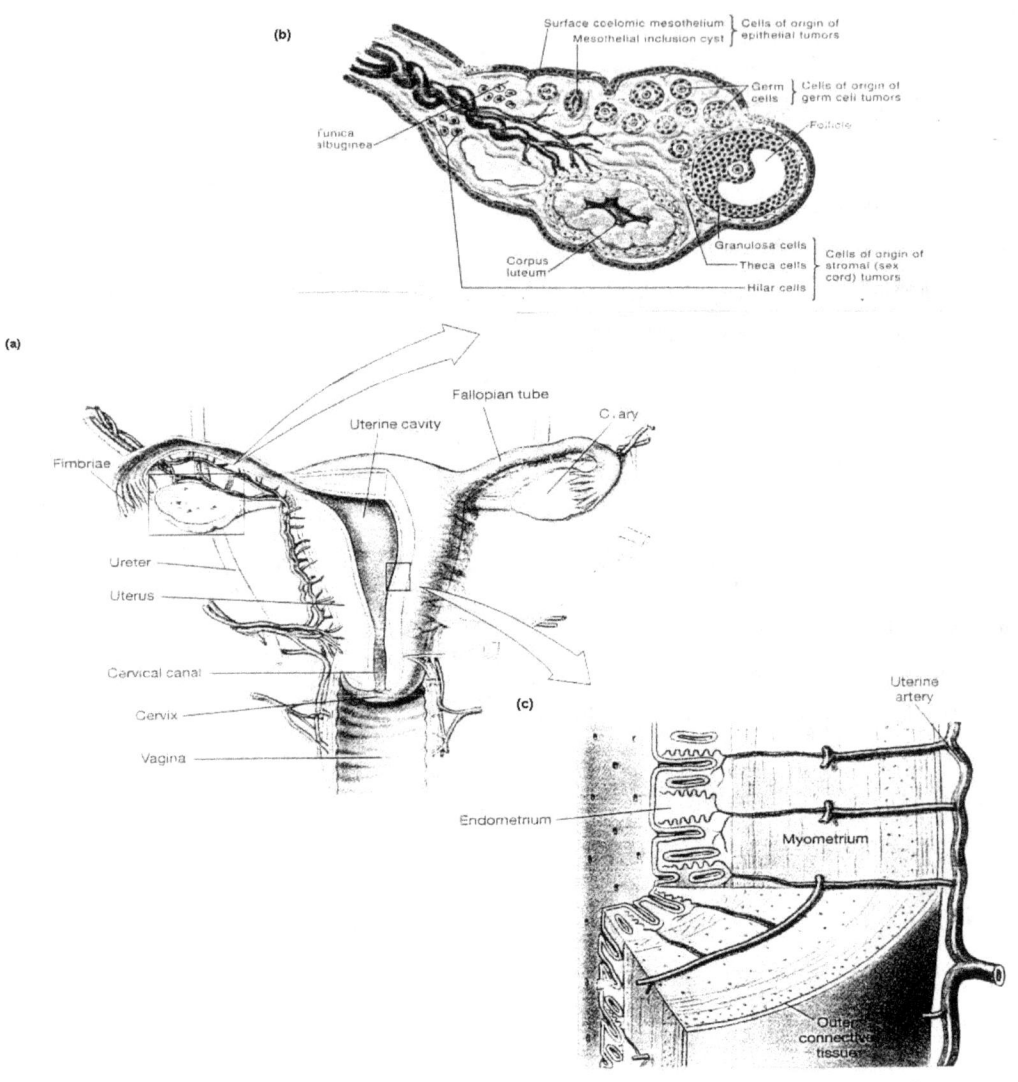

Fig.1 [(9)] **(a):Female reproduction tract**

(b): Embryologic origins of ovarian cancer.

(c):Tissue layers of uterus

than 5% solid growth is grade I, 6-50% is grade 2, and more than 50% is

grade 3[3].   Endometriosis adenocarcinoma accounts for 60-65% of the

adenocarcinomas, it is characterized by the disappearance of stroma

between abnormal glands, necrosis, and hemorrhage[1].Some typical

adenocarcinoma contains areas of squamous metaplasia, which can have

a benign or malignant appearance, such tumors are termed

adenocarcinoma with squamous differentiation[6].

A variant of endometriosis adenocarcinoma is the villoglandular type,

which appears to have more aggressive behavior [7].Uncommon cell types

(clear, papillary serous, mucinous, squamous and undifferentiated)

account for the remaining 10% of endometrial cancers [6].

1.2.2 Etiology

Endometrial cancer is one of the few malignancies for which the

etiology is well understood.Epidemiologic, endocrinologic, and clinical

studies have shown that the association between endometrial cancer and

most of the identified risk factors can be explained by increased exposure

to endogenous or exogenous estrogens.This hypothesis is supported by

the increased risk of endometrial cancer (related to obesity, early age at

menarche, late age at menopause, low parity or nullparity, certain types of

ovarian tumors, history of menstrual disorders, history of infertility, and

use of estrogen replacement therapy (ERT) or sequential oral contraceptives).It is also supported by the decreased risk of endometrial cancer (related to the use of combined oral contraceptives, early age at menopause, high parity, and smoking)[4].

Medical conditions such as diabetes, hypertension, and thyroid diseases have been suggested to increase the risk of endometrial cancer, but these finding are not consistent[8].It remains, unclear whether these finding are the result of the association of these medical conditions with obesity or with other biologic mechanisms.

1.2.3 Clinical Evaluation and Treatment

The initial growth phase of most endometrial cancers consists of polyploidy expansion within the endometrial lining .Small areas of necrosis or surface breakdown in the tumor produce abnormal vaginal bleeding. Consequently, the premenopausal women usually present with metrorrhagia, and the older woman has postmenopausal bleeding. Patient with advanced disease may have pelvic pain, bleeding, or bloating[3]. The diagnosis of endometrial can be reliably established by office endometrial biopsy. Dilatation and fractional curettage or hysteroscopy with biopsy may be helpful diagnostic procedures in cases in which out patient biopsy is non diagnostic[1].

The workup on the woman with endometrial cancer should include a physical examination, endometrial biopsy, laboratory studies, and a chest radiograph. Endometrial cancer is typically a disease of women in their sixties and seventies who frequently have coexisting medical problems, so the evaluation should focus on an assessment of operative risk. Additional more sophisticated studies such as proctoscopy, barium enema, ultrasound, computed tomography (CT), or magnetic resonance imaging should be reserved for clinical situations in which advanced disease is suspected[6].

Schematic approach to treatment endometrial cancer is illustrated in (Fig. 2)[6].

Surgical excision of the primary tumor via total abdominal hysterectomy with bilateral salpingo –oophorectomy (TAH-BSO); sometimes accompanied by removal of the pelvic and periaortic lymph nodes; is the mainstay of therapy for endometrial cancer. The selection of additional therapy is based on the result of the staging biopsies of uterine tumors, which was adopted in 1988 (Table 1) by FIGO surgical staging[3] .

1.3 Epithelial Ovarian Cancer

The ovary is composed of an outer cortex and an inner medulla. The cortex containing the coelomic surface mesothelium, germ cell (oocytes), specialized hormone producing stroma (granulose and thecal cell), and unspecialized supporting stromal cells. Primary ovarian cancers are classified; according to the structure of the ovary from which the tumor is derived (Fig.1b); into three major categories, epithelial, germ cell, and stromal[9]. The ovary may also be the site of metastasis spread from

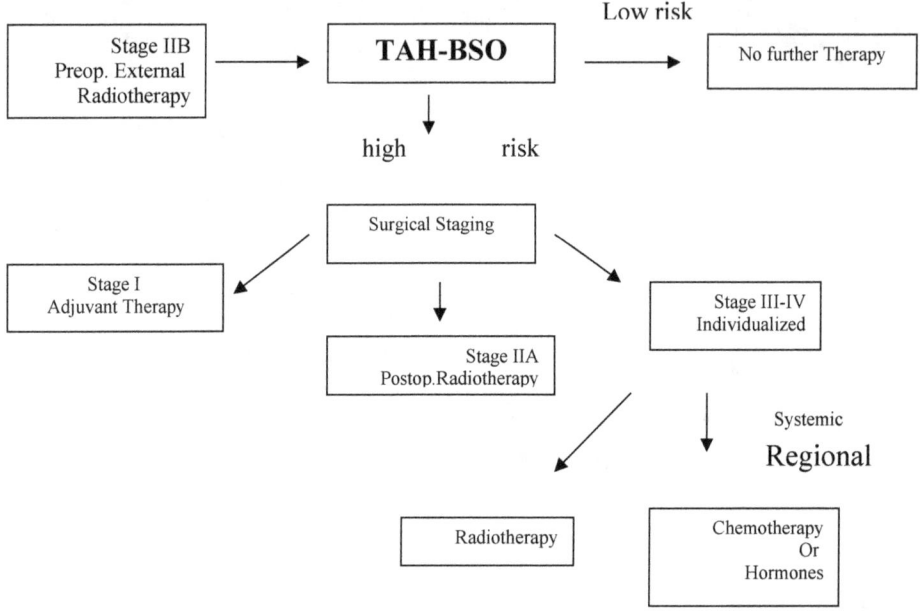

Fig.2 Basic treatment strategy for endometrial cancer[6].

Table (1) Surgical staging system for cancer of the uterine body[3].

Stage	Extent
I	**Cancer confined to the corpus**
Ia	Tumor limited to endometrial
Ib	Invasion to less than one half the myometrium
Ic	Invasion to more than one half the myometrium G_1:Well differentiated ($\leq$5% of a nonsquamous or nonmorular solid growth pattern) G_2:Moderately differentiated (6%-50%) G_3:Predominantly solid or undifferentiated
II	**Cancer involves corpus and cervix but does not extend outside the uterus**
IIa	Endocervical glandular involvement only
IIb	Cervical stromal invasion
III	**Cancer extends outside the uterus but not outside the true pelvis**
IIIa	Tumor invades serosa and/or adnexa or positive peritoneal

		cytology
IIIb		Vaginal metastases
IIIc		Positive pelvic and /or paraaortic nodes
IV		**Cancer extends outside true pelvis or invades bladder or rectal mucosa**
IVa		Tumor invasion of bladder and/or bowel mucosa
IVb		Distant metastases including intra-abdominal and/or inguinal lymph nodes

gynecologic and other tumors. Epithelial ovarian tumors are the most common, accounting for 80-90% of cases[5].

Epithelial ovarian cancers are derived from the coelomic surface mesothelium. During ovulation, the dominant ovarian follicle ruptures, releasing the ovum. To heal the ruptured follicle, surface mesothelial cells proliferate and fill the defect. Inclusion cysts may form and are lined with these mesothelial cells. Over years of repeated ovulation and repeated growth of mesothelia cells, the regulation of this proliferation may become disrupted, allowing the development of tumors (Fig.1b)[9].

Numerous factors can stimulate –or fail to control mesothelial proliferation including growth factors, oncogenes, and tumor suppressor genes[10].

1.3.1 Histology

Epithelial ovarian tumors classified according to cell type, pattern of growth (cystic, solid, and surface), atypia and invasiveness (benign,

261

borderlines, malignant). The ovarian surface epithelium, when involved in neoplastic conditions, often undergoes a mullerian differentiation as a result, it may produce any of the adult epithelia, including tube, endometrial and, endocervical mucosa, singly or in combination. So the histological types of the epithelial tumors are serous, mucinous, endometriosis, clear cell, Brenner, mixed epithelial, undifferentiated, and unclassified[3]. Serous tumors make up about 20% of all benign ovarian tumors and 75% of epithelial ovarian cancers. Malignant serous tumors are usually multicystic, bilateral and resembling fallopian tube epithelium. Serous carcinoma may have a complex mixture of cystic and solid areas with extensive papillations, or they may contain a predominantly solid mass with areas of necrosis and hemorrhage[11]. The second common type of epithelial ovarian cancer is endometriosis tumor (10%) which is histological indistinguishable from endometrial uterine cancer. About 6-10% of epithelial ovarian cancers are mucinous, which characterized by epithelial – mucin producing cell resembling those of the endocervix[9]. Clear cell tumors account for<5% of all primary ovarian cancers. The tumor cell is large and their cytoplasm is clear. These tumors have more aggressive behavior than other epithelial cancers. Brenner tumors, these unusual lesions are though to originate from the ovarian mesothelium despite their urothelial –like transitional cell structure. They are solid and almost benign.

1.3.2 Etiology

Several factors have been associated with an increased risk of epithelial ovarian cancer, while two factors appear to reduce the incidence of this malignancy – pregnancy and use of oral contraceptives – presumably because they suppress ovulation. The risk of epithelial ovarian cancer is high in ovulating nulliparous women, women using of fertility drug, women exposuring to hormones (particularly gonadotropins) and carcinogens, such as infectious agents and chemical carcinogens[12].

The large majority of ovarian cancer presumably related to environmental factors, but 5-10% of women with epithelial tumors have a predisposing familial syndrome. Three autosomal dominant syndromes have been identified: site –specific ovarian cancer, hereditary breast – ovarian cancer syndrome, and lynch syndrome II (adenocarcinomas of multiple sites, including breast, ovary, and endometrial, gastrointestinal tract). All three types of familial ovarian cancer develop at a younger age than sporadic ovarian cancer[9].

Other factors, such as obesity, high-fat diet, early menarche, late menopause, single women, may predispose women to develop this malignancy. The hypothesis is that the continual ovulation, uninterrupted by pregnancy may develop the disease[4].

1.3.3 Clinical Evaluation and Treatment

263

Epithelial ovarian cancer is seldom detected at an early stage; up to 80% of these tumors have metastasized by any of the four routes (peritoneal seeding, lymphatic embolization, direct extension and hematogenous dissemination). The first sign of early ovarian cancer is usually an asymptomatic mass found during a pelvic, rectal, or abdominal examination. A benign tumor or slow- growing cancer may grow quite large and cause abdominal distention and may compress the rectum or bladder, producing constipation, urinary frequency or nocturia. Ovarian tumor occasionally undergoes torsion, resulting in localized pain, nausea, and possibly low fever, and may also cause symptoms of inappropriate estrogen or androgen synthesis[9].

The diagnosis of epithelial ovarian cancer is surgical, usually by a laparotomy, but occasionally at laparoscopy. Ultrasound of adnexal pelvic mass is useful prior to the surgical diagnosis. Most patients with a pelvic mass require ultrasonography, chest radiography, CT, and aspiration of pleural effusion to check for metastases. Mammography should be performed to exclude primary breast cancer[3].

The management of primary epithelial ovarian cancer may be divided into three phases: primary definitive surgery, postoperative adjuvant therapy usually chemotherapy[13], and systematic follow up and reevaluation. The initial surgical procedure (usually TAH-BSO) is used to determine the extent of the disease (staging) and to remove as much gross disease as possible (cytoreduction). In ovarian cancer, metastases adhere superficially to peritoneal surfaces without deep invasion. Therefore, surgical resection of metastasis ovarian cancer is standard care[9]. The tumor must be staged to facilitate planning of adjuvant therapy, the FIGO staging system of 1987 (Table 2)[3] is based on the finding at surgical exploration. Following the cytoreductive surgery or debulking, patients should be treated, generally with chemotherapy and some time with radiation or endocrine therapy[14][15]. The majority of women with advanced epithelial ovarian cancer will ultimately relapse and develop drug-resistant disease. Thus, there is a common need for second-line treatment including cytotoxic drugs, or secondary cytoreductive surgery or palliative surgery[16].

Table (2) Surgical staging system for epithelial ovarian cancers[3].

Stage	Extent (proportion of cases)
I	**Cancer limited to ovaries (15%)**
Ia	Limited to one ovary, no ascites
Ib	Both ovaries involved, no ascites
Ic	Ia or Ib with ascites or positive peritoneal washings
II	**Cancer of one or both ovaries with extension limited to pelvic tissue(15%)**
IIa	Extension to uterus or tubes
IIb	Extension to other pelvic tissues
IIc	IIa or IIb with ascites pr positive peritoneal washings
III	**Cancer involving one or both ovaries with peritoneal implants outside the pelvis and/or positive retroperitoneal or inguinal nodes.Tumor is limited to the true pelvis but with histological proved extension to small bowel or omentum (65%)**
IIIa	Tumor grossly limited to the true pelvis with negative nodes but with histological confirmed microscope seeding of abdominal peritoneal surface
IIIb	Same as IIIa, but abdominal peritoneal implants do not exceed 2 cm in diameter
IIIc	Abdominal implants greater than 2cm in diameter and/or positive retroperitoneal or inguinal lymph nodes
IV	**Distant metastases present (including cytology-positive pleural effusion metastasis liver parenchyma or peripheral superficial lymph nodes(5%).**

1.4 Tumor Markers in Gynecologic Cancers

Tumor markers; which may be considered as any biological aberration that indicates the presence of a tumor; are required for primary diagnosis, histological   identification, assessment of the extent of the disease pre-

and post operatively, therapy guidance, and early detection of recurrence.

Ideally, the tumor marker assessed in serum, or in another body compartment, should accurately reflect the presence and the amount of residual tumor, and should also distinguish benign from malignant disease[17]. In gynecological practice, it is well documented that human chorionic gonadotropin(hCG), alpha-feto protein(AFP), estrogens, and androgens have been contributed greatly to the diagnosis and management of gestational trophoblastic disease, gram cell tumor,and granulose cell tumor, respectively[17][18].

By the introduction of polyclonal and monoclonal antibody technology, variety of tumor carbohydrate associated antigens have been identified as a result of glycosylation changes in the carbohydrate moieties of glycoproteins and glycolipids by tumor cells, some of tumor associated antigens also represent differentiation antigens and receptors that may reexpressed or over expressed[18][19].

1.4.1 Antigenic Markers

1- Squamous Cell Carcinoma (SCC) Antigen: The SCC antigen was described in 1977 as one of 14 subfractions of tumor associated antigen found in human cervical cancer tissue [20]. SCC antigen have been reported to be elevated (>2 ng/ml) in 35% of stage I patients, and increasing to 91% in stage IV for cervical cancer [21][22]. While serum SCC antigen level were increased in 8-29% of endometrial cancer. In vulvar

267

and vaginal squamous cell cancers, the reported frequencies of SCC antigen elevation are lower (42% and 17%, respectively) than in cervical cancer[17].

2- Lipid-Associated Sialic Acid (LSA): Elevated levels of LSA are found in a variety of malignancies, including cancers of the vulva, vaginga, uterus and ovary[18]. Due to its lack of specification, LSA used alone had not been useful in gynecologic cancers.

*3- **CA-125:*** Since its first report in 1983[23], CA-125 has been used widely for monitoring epithelial ovarian cancer. Among healthy individuals, 99% will have been serum level <35U/ml[24]. Approximately 85% of ovarian cancer patients have elevated CA-125 level (> 35 U/ml) for all histological types of epithelial ovarian cancers but more frequently for nonmucinous tumors than for mucinous types[25][26].It is also expressed in cancer of epithelium female reproductive tract[27] and can be detected in 22% of patients with nongynecological cancers (Breast, lung, Colon, Pancreas), also

detected in benign gynecological tumors (endometriosis, adenomyosis, ovarian cystadenomas)[28][29].

The low specificity hampers the use of CA-125 as a screening test for ovarian cancer. Combined with pelvic examination and/or ultra sound, the specificity can be increased[30]. The sensitivity of the marker might be also increased by examining peritoneal fluid, where the CA-125 levels are higher than in serum (Cutoff at 200u/ml)[31].CA-125 is very rarely elevated in endometrial cancer confined to the uterus, whereas elevation is found in 78-100% of cases with extra uterine spread[27].

4- Other Antigens Defined by Monoclonal Antibodies: Following the report of CA-125, a number of monoclonal antibodies such as CA 19-9 and CA 15-3 were developed in colorectal cancer[32], breast cancer[33], ovarian cancer and endometrial cancer[34] as immunnogens, and this explain their lack of specificity.

Various monoclonal antibodies have been raised against epithelial mucin like caner antigen MCA , CA M26 , and CA M29. These cancer antigens have been reported in cancers of breast, colon, ovary, endometrial and cervix [35][36],but non of them, either alone or in combination , has been shown to be as useful as CA-125 .

Another marker for ovarian cancer is NB/70K which seen to be a marker for all histological types of epithelial ovarian cancer[17].Serum NB/70K is elevated in all stages of ovarian malignancies, including more than 50% of early stage cases[37][38]. **5- Carcinoembryonic Antigen (CEA):** This oncofetal protein can be demonstrated in most gynecological cancers immunohistologically, while plasma levels are often too modestly elevated to be useful for diagnosis or for disease monitoring[17] . Slightly elevated plasma CEA levels are seen in

269

approximately 50% of ovarian cancer patients[39][26], and mucinous tumors tend to have highest levels. Measuring CEA with CA-125 and CA19-9 can be useful to differentiate between ovarian and colorectal cancer. In the uterus, adenocarcinomas that arise in the endocervix express greater amount of CEA than adenocarcinomas of the endometrial. This is reflected in the reported frequency of elevated plasma CEA levels : 68% in cervical cancer, and 34% in endometrial cancer[40]. Squamous cell cancer, which represent 85% of the cervical cancer, also express CEA, but at more modest level.In a study on 205 patients, only 28% had plasma level above 5ng/ml. High levels indicated advance disease or lymph node metastases[41].

1.4.2 Genomic Markers

By cytogenetic examination, using a chromosome spread technique or cell flow cytometry, general genetic alteration have been identifying. Aneuploidy is a common finding in endometrial cancer and ovarian cancer[42][43]. There is a correlation between DNA ploidy abnormalities and grade of differentiation (more common in moderately and poorly differentiated lesions). Trisomy of chromosomes 1,7 and 10 and allelic loss at loci on chromosomes 3p (71%), 9q(38%) 10q(35%) and 17p(35%) have also reported in endometrial cancer[44]. Most ovarian and endometrial cancers over express of macrophage colony stimulating factor (M-CSF) and c-fms which encode the M-CSF receptor[45][46]. The macrophages secrete cytokines (tumor necrosis factor α and interleukins 1 and 6) that stimulate the growth of tumors[47]. Epidermal growth factor (EGF) and polo-like kinase (PLK) protein (contribute to regulation of the cell cycle) have been found to be expressed in most ovarian tumor, while the suppressor gene p53 defective[9][48]. However, the clinical significance of these genomic markers has not yet been established.

1.4.3 Enzymatic Markers

Lactate dehydrogenase (LDH) and heat stable alkaline phosphatase (HSAP) have been also considered as potential tumor markers in gynecology cancers.

The glycolytic enzyme LDH aroused a considerable interest in oncology since Warburg[49] reported increased rate of glucose utilization producing more lactate by tumor cells. LDH is often elevated in epithelial ovarian cancer[50], as in many solid malignancies[51], making it a non-specific tumor markers. In germ cell tumor, the two isoenzymes (LDH-1 and LDH-2) are increased and their activity appear to parallel the response to therapy [52]. Serum LDH levels were documented to be elevated in cervical cancer even at the early stage of the disease and in combination with other biomarker was more beneficial for diagnosis and treatment monitoring of patients[53][54].

Alkaline phosphates (ALP) was one of the first examples of tumor associated enzymes[55]. The heat stable alkaline phosphatase (HSAP, Regan isoenzyme) has been found in a variety of solid tumors and in 6-64% of ovarian cancer patients[56][57]. The marker level did not correlated to tumor burden or prognosis and half of the patients lost the marker during progression.

1.4.4 Hormonal Markers

Gonadotropin hormones (LH, FSH) can function as tumor markers in gonadal stromal tumor in addition to estrogen and androgen[17]. Inhibins, which are produced in ovarian granulosa cells, cause a specific

suppression of pituitary FSH release. Radioimmunometric determination

of inhibin has proven to be reliable marker in the monitoring of granulosa

cell tumors[58].

1.4..4.1 Human Chorionic Gonadotropin (hCG)

Since the discovery of human chorionic gonadotropin

(choriogonadotropin) hormone by Hirose[59)] and Ascheim and Zondek[60],

its measurement has been the basis of pregnancy diagnosis and, a marker

for many trophoblastic and nontrophoblastic tumors.

This hormone is synthesized by the trophoblastic cells of the placenta

during the early weeks of pregnancy. Human chorionic gonadotropin

stimulates the ovarian corpus luteum to produce progesterone until the

placenta it self acquires the ability to produce this pregnancy sustaining

steroid[61]. An increasing evidence supports the synthesis of hCG in small

quantities by the pituitary[62].

Human chorionic gonadotropin belongs to the glycoprotein hormones

family (also includes hLH, hTSH, hFSH) whose members share a

common α-subunit (contains 92 amino acids) and vary in their β-subunit.

Each subunit is produced by a separate gene, the α subunit is encoded by

a single gene present on chromosome 6q21.1-q23 whereas cluster of seven nonallelic genes located on chromosome 19q13.3 encoded for β-subunit of hCG(hCGβ). (One or more of these genes may preferentially expressed during pregnancy and tumor genesis)[63][64]. The β-subunit confer biological specificity; in humans, hCGβ and hLHβ are closly related subunits with 82% identity, and this reflects a common biological function for these two hormones.The hCGβ (contains 145 amino acids) further differs from that of hLHβ (contains 114 amino acids) by the 24-amino acid carboxy terminal polypeptide extension (CTP). It has been suggested that this glycosylated extension may impart extra solubility and in vivo circulation life time to hCG[65)].

Human chorionic gonadotropin could be purified from pregnancy urine by a combination of organic precipitation, ion exchange chromotography, and gel filtration[66].

A- Chemical Structure of hCG

The primary structure of α and β subunits for hCG were determined in 1973[67][68]. There are five disulfide bridges in the α-subunit and six in the β-subunit (these are conserved across the family). Human chorionic gonadotropin (38,633 Dalton) is approximately 30% carbohydrate by weight and contains both complex biantennary N-asparagine linked and simple O-serine linked. Each carbohydrate moiety terminates in sialic acid, but considerable carbohydrate heterogeneity result in a wide isoelectric point (pI) distribution of the hormone (pI generally 3-6 and as high as 10 for asialo forms of the hormone). The hCG produced in trophoblaste disease exhibits greater carbohydrate heterogeneity (such as triantennary structures) and some cancers produce only asialo hCG[66]. Removal of the terminal sialic acid residues markedly reduce the half-life of hormone in the circulation by enhancing binding to hepatocyte lectin and thus clearance from the blood stream. The carbohydrate moieties of hCG also played a role in hormone secretion, stability, folding and subunit assembly[99]. In vitro, studies with deglycosylated hormone generally indicate a greater loss of biological response than receptor binding. It is believed that the carbohydrate chains bind to a lectin-like membrane component to give the biological response. It was further found that the carbohydrate in the α-subunit was more important in the hormone function than that present in the β-subunit, which seems to be important to maintain the proper conformation of the hormone[70][71]. Various attempts have been made to construct three dimensional (3D) model of hCG[72-78)]. Based on amino acid sequence and information; accumulated from chemical modifications (oxidization, deglycossylation, desialyation, reduction), enzymatic modifications (nicks, fragmentation and deletion of fragments), cross reactions, disulfide pairings, molecular biology studies (site directed mutagenesis, chimeric hormone constructs) with monoclonal antibodies(MAb) mapping of surface epitopes, spectral analyses (especially circular dichroism (CD)) and diffraction analyses (X-

275

ray diffraction of hydrogen floride-hCG crystals), multi wavelength anomalous diffraction (MAD)); the proposed structure of hCG is predominantly composed of β structure with three helical segments, two in the α and one in the β-subunit. The antiparallel β- strands in each subunits are joined by three hairpin loops. Both subunits structure like some protein growth factors (NGF, TGF-β and PDGF-ββ) contain the so-called cysteine knot motif by three disulphide bonds (cys I-IV, cys II-V, cys III-VI). The heterodimer is stabilized by a segment of the β-subunit which wraps around the α-subunit and is covalently linked like a seat belt by cys 26-cys110. This hetrodimer has a large area of interface with only a small hydrophobic core. The overall topology of hCG subunit is shown in (Fig. 3).

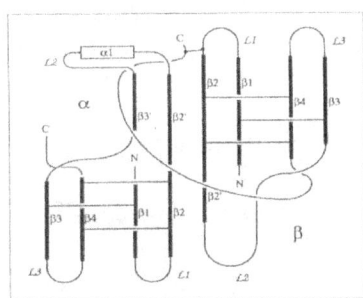

fig.3 A schematic drawing of the hCG dimer topology

B- Molecular Forms of hCG

Various molecular forms of hCG (intact or modified), free subunits (intact or modified), and degradation products are present in biologic fluid, tissues of normal and tumoral organs and reference preparations[79].

Intact hCG is defined as heterodimer comprising the two mature α and β subunits. Its levels in the sera of normal nonpregnant women increase with age, and higher than in men[80][81]. In women <50 year the upper reference limit is 8.6 pmol/l (2.9 Iu/L), and in those >50 years is 15-5 pmol/L (5.3 Iu/L), where the level of hCG in urine is < 2 pmol/mmol creatinine. In contrast, hCG levels are 2-6 pmol/L (0.7-2.1 Iu/L) in sera of healthy men. Plasma intact hCG rises exponentially during the first trimester of pregnancy, reaching a peak of 25-30 µg/ml at 8-10 weeks. Following a rapid decreases until 15 weeks, a slower but continuous fall is observed up to delivery. Interestingly, amniotic hCG levels are <20% of maternal serum level at all times of gestation[79].

Free hCGβ refers to the non-combined β-subunit consisting of a glycosylated 23KD single chain polypeptide. This form appears to be devoid of any biologic role during pregnancy (the peak level reaches 50-70 ng/ml between 8-10 week)[79]. In normal individuals, free hCGβ serum values are extremely low (never excceding 4.5 pmol/L) while this form is most often secreted in nontrophoblastic tumors[82].

Free hCGα refers to non combined α-subunit. Although it appears to have a structure identical to that of the combined α subunit of hCG, its carbohydrate composition is quite different which prevents combination[83]. This form may have a biologic role in pregnancy independent form that of hCG, where its level in serum slowly increase up to 18 weeks to reach a peak of 30-50ng/ml. In healthy individuals, levels up to 3000 pg/ml are present in sera originate in the pituitary gland[62]. Free hCGα may increase in pituitray tumors.

Beta -Core Fragment of hCGβ (hCGβcf), is small forms (10KD) immunoreactivity identify. Its two disulfide-bridged peptides lacking the amino acid sequences 1-5, 41-54 and 93-145 and corbohydrate structure changes of hCGβ[84]. It has been demonstrated that HCGβcf is primarily product of renal degradation of hCGβ, although some fragments may originate from either placenta or cleavage in the circulation. hCGβcf is the most abundant fragment of hCGβ in pregnancy urine and is also found in the urine of patients with a broad spectrum of malignancies and benign tumors. Circulating hCGβcf is almost undetectable, while levels of 0.51-1.25 pmol/mmol creatinine are found in urine of healthy women[69]

Nicked hCG (hCGn or hCGβn), are detectable in a significant proportion of both hCG and its free β subunit of normal and tumoral origins, as a result of intrachain proteolysis nicking within the β44-49 region [85][86]. The hCG appears to be uns Table and rapidly dissociates and weakly recognized by MAb. Furthermore, some results indicate that hCGβn is an intermediary form in the metabolism of hCG, and further cleavage to hCGβcf.

Several other molecules are detectable mostly in tumors, due to the modification of peptide structures both in hCGα and hCGβ such as N-terminal heterogeneity hCGα, mutant hCGα, large hCGα and CTP, hyperglycosylated hCG[87].

C- Production and Metabolism of hCG

Both normal placental cells as well as neoplastic trophoblastic cells,and sperm cells in the male synthesize and secrete hCG and its free subunits[88]. Human chorionic gonadotropin plays a critical role in the maintenance of the corpus luteum during the first 4 to 6 week of gestation to produce progesterone to keep the endometrial intact where the blastocyst is implanted, hCG also stimulates the testosterone production by the developing tests in males Fetuses[79]. The physiological processes regulating hCG production are not well understood. It is likely that its biosynthesis is dependent on the stage of differentiation of the trophoblastic cells and regulated by several autocrine and paracrine factors acting through cellular signals on the regulatory elements of the α- and β-subunit genes[89].

About 80% of hCG is metabolized in liver and renal tissue and excreted predominately as hCGβcf, whereas 20% of circulated hCG is excreted unmodified. In normal individuals, the plasma half-life of hCG is about 24-36 hours. Its clearance includes an initial, fast component ($t_{1/2}$ of 5-6h) and a second, slower component ($t_{1/2}$ of over 24 h)[69].

D- Clinical Use of hCG Determinations

Diagnosis of Pregnancy and Related Disorders: Immunochemical determination of hCG in serum or more commonly in urine, is the main method for diagnosis of pregnancy. In serum a discrimination limit of 10 Iu/L is often used [79].

Spontaneous abortion is the most common complication of pregnancy, and abnormally low serum hCG concentrations are often observed in these patients. Serial determinations of hCG in serum in combination with sonography are much used for diagnosis this condition [66]. Decreasing or slowly increasing hCG concentration during early pregnancy may also indicate ectopic pregnancy (implantation of the blastocyst outside the uterus)[66].

The potential usefulness of either hCG or its free subunits(in combination with AFP) in prenatal screening for chromosomal abnormalities (particularly Down's syndrome), was the subject of intense debate[90][91]. While the mean hCGβ value in cases of trisomy 21 is significantly higher than in unaffected cases, the median value in trisomy 18 was found to be significantly lower .

Placental and Testicular Trophoblastic Tumors: Infact hCG and free hCGβ are ideal tumor marker for gestational trophoblastic disease (GTD --choriocarcinoma,and hydatidiform mole[92]...)and testicular germ cell tumors[93].The ratio of hCGβ to intact hCG is higher in patients with malignant than with benign trophoblastic tumors, which used for diagnosis. Measurement of blood intact hCG can be utilized for the therapeutic monitoring of GTD . Molecular heterogeneity has been demonstrated in the carbohydrate structure of hCG in choriocarcinoma,

281

hCG is substantially diminished in sialic acid content and is composed of tri and tetra-antennary carbohydrate moieties[94].

Human chorionic gonadotropin or its free subunits presents in (80%) of sera patients with nonseminomatous testicular tumors, where hCG is elevated to more than 20,000 pg/ml[93]. Indeed, hCG, free hCG, AFP are the Most useful markers for the diagnosis, prognosis, and follow up of these malignancies[95]. Measurement of hCG in CSF is done when cerebral metastasis are suspected (ratios of hCG in CSF to hCG in serum exceed 1:60). In seminoma testicular cancer, hCG is elevated in 16% of patients[96].

Nontrophoblastic Tumors :The presence of hCG and its subunits in the tumor itself or in the serum and malignant effusions of patients with nontrophoblastic and nongonadal tumors were investigated. Numerous investigators, using immunochemical procedures, have demonstrated that cancers of the breast, uterus, lung, ovary, cervix, gastrointestinal tract, bladder, liver produce elevated concentrations of hCG or its subunits.

a-<u>Blood studies:</u> Early results employing radioimmuno assay(RIA) for hCG indicated that a great variety of malignant tumors expressed hCG[97-102]. The overall incidence was in the range of 19%-30% of all tumors studied. The levels of hCG were only moderately increased and shown variable correlation to tumor stage, histological grading or clinical course. Therefore, the clinical value of determine hCG in serum for diagnosing and monitoring patients with non-trophoblastic malignancies remains controversial. Studies with highly specific sandwich procedures and effective MAb showed that free hCGβ is mainly elevated while intact hCG and hCGα are slightly elevated or within the normal range in the sera of nontrophoblastic cancers.The malignancies that exhibited the greatest incidence are gynecologic cancers, tumor of the head,neck,lung,gastrointestinal tract tumors,and melanoma[102-111].

These studies suggested that free hCGβ is highly diagnostic of malignancy in general and defines a subgroup of aggressive nongonadal malignancies.

b-Urine studies: hCGβcf, free hCGβ, and asialo hCG have been reported in urine of different malignancies employing two soild phase capture antibodies[112][104][105]. Using a cutoff of 0.2ng/ml for hCGβcf,59% of the cervical and endometrial and 70% of the ovarian cancers patients exceeded this level[113]. It has been suggested that the hCGβcf in the urine of patients is due to the degradation of the free hCGβ produced by these cancers.

c-Effusion fluids studies:Free hCGβ immunoreactive material has been reported in ascetic and tumor cyst fluids of patients with non trophoblastic cancers (including gynecologic cancers) more than intact hormone[106][107].Free hCGβ levels have shown to be higher in malignant ascites as compared to the corresponding plasma values of the same

283

patients. Determining free hCGβ in malignant effusions enhanced the sensitivity of this marker as compared to serum.

d-Tissues studies: Human chorionic gonadotropin in the cell is present in two pools, a secretary pool and membrane pool. The latter becomes an intrinsic part on determination hCG on the cancer cell surface. Various investigations on cultured cancer cells (including cells form nasopharynx, lung, cervix, bladder, breast, endometrial, colon, prostate, oral cancers, leukemia's, lymphomas, and retinoblastomas), using flow cytomatry technique, demonstrated the expression of membrane associated hCG and its subunit[114-124]. These studies showed high expression of free hCGβ than intact hCG and there was no relationship between the hCGβ positivity and the histological type or morphological features of tumor, but a number of authors have suggested that tumor which expresses hCG will pursue amore aggressive course and has a worse prognosis[125].

Analyses also done on extracted of media of cultured caner cells, reflecting the secretary pool or total cell pools. Other techniques such as immunohistochemical techniques were used to identify hCG in tumor and normal tissues[126-137]. Positive staining for hCG were found in, ovarian, cervical , colorectal , gastric , hepatoblastoma , large bowel, urothelial and breast cancers tissue. Authors also reported the stimulation of the growth of several tumor cell lines by hCG[138-141]. These findings with other results which confirmed that hCG has also chemical and physiologic properties of growth factor[76][77], have provided a scientific

basis for studies of, prevention from, and control of the cancer by active

or passive immunization against hCG and its subunits[142]. Some studies

used anti hCG vaccines which originally was developed for fertility

control[143][144]. In addition to that, studies on cluster of genes encoding

the hCGβ demonstrated that five nonallelic genes are transcribed in vivo

with highly variable level of expression in first trimester placenta tissue,

whereas normal nontrophoblastic tissue express 2 allelic hCGβ genes. In

tumor tissue collected from patient with breast bladder, prostate, thyroid

cancer found that up to 61% of these tumors expressed four nonallelic

hCGβ genes different from that of normal tissue. These findings provide

the basis for a simple test that may be useful for the molecular diagnosis

of nontrophsblastic cancer[64][115].

E- Determination Methods of hCG

Immunological methods are nearly exclusively used for clinical

determination   of hCG[82], while assessment of the potency of

hCG preparations to be used for   pharmaceutical purposes should be

performed by bioassays.

Biological Methods

a-In vivo methods: These bioassays measure the response of gonadal

tissue to hCG in various animals (mice, rabbits,frogs). These methods are

no longer widely used because its susceptible to yielding spurious results

285

due to variation in the metabolic clearance rates of the forms of hCG being assessed and are based on animal –derived rather than Human chorionic gonadotropin receptor[69].

b-In vitro methods: Two methods have been widly used for assessing the hLH-like bioactivity of hCG, one is based on the rat interstitial cell testosterone response (RICT assay)[145] and the other on the mouse interstitial cell response (MICT assay)[146]. These methods have the advantage of the low detection limit but the limitation is their lack of specificity (hLH activity, factors modulate cellular responses) and heterologous nature of the systems.Homologous bioassays have been constructed with the modern techniques of molecular biology, where the human hCG receptor gene has been cloned and transfected into cells to produce human receptors[147].

Binding Methods

Binding assay can utilize antibodies or receptor as binding protein.

a. Competitive Immunoprocedures

Radioimmuno assay(RIA), and Receptor methods: Pregnancy test is the first specific immunoprocedueres (qualitative agglutination inhibition methods) in which, latex particles or sheep red blood cell coated with the hCG, mix with the urine sample and then with a solution containing antibodies to the hCG. Presence of hCG in urine inhibits agglutination. This method is still widely utilized, especially as in-house methods[69].

The quantitative specific immunoprocedures for hCG were typical competitive immunoprocedure in which the radio active iodine ^{125}I-hCG competes with sample analyze for binding to anti-hCG. Increased hCG in sample, decreased bound radio activity. These methods are still used widely for measurement of serum and urine hCG levels[148][69]. Another type of assays systems available for serum hCG determination is a radioreceptor assay (RRA). This method is based on the competition between the hCG in the serum and a ^{125}I-hCG for binding to hCG receptor present in tissue [69].

b. <u>Non – competitive immunoprocedures</u>:

Non competitive immunometric with labeled antibody (sandwich or two-site immunometric methods)are quantitative methods for hCG and its subunits with low detection limit, large measurement range. The labeled anti hCG reacts with sample hCG bound to solid phase anti hCG. Diffferent labels are used such as enzyme, fluorescent, and luminescent.

The specificity of sandwich methods is defined by the reactivity and recognition ability of the antibodies ($\beta \bullet \to \alpha, \beta \bullet \to \beta, \alpha\beta \bullet \to \beta, \beta cf \bullet \to \beta, \beta CTP \bullet \to \alpha, \alpha \bullet \to \alpha$) where $\bullet$-- capture antibody and $\to$ tracer antibody[79](Fig.4).

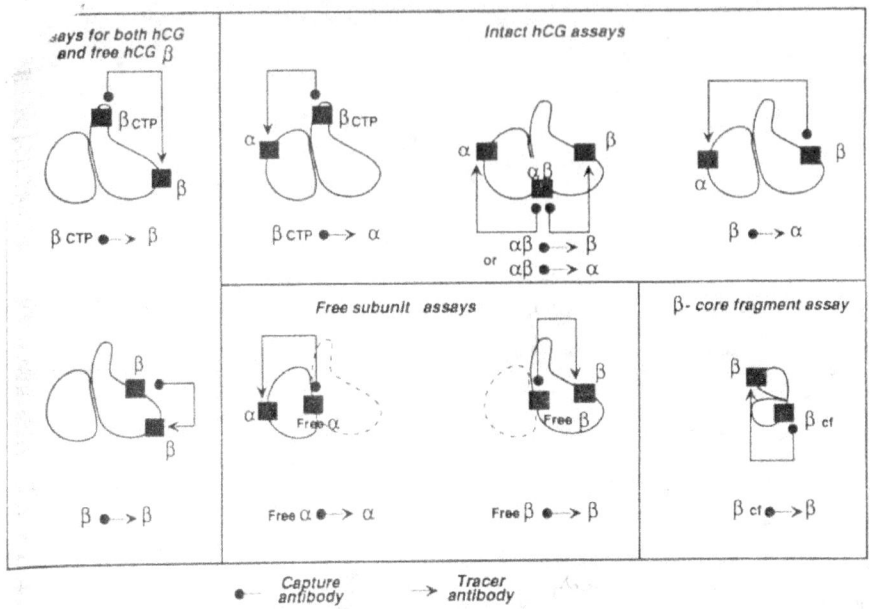

Fig.4 Schematic representation of the sandwich methods used for the

measurement of hCG, its free subunits, or hCGcf[79]

1.5 Human Chorionic Gonadotropin Receptor (hCG-R)

Human chorionic gonadotropin receptor is a cell surface protein ,

present on testicular leydig cells and on ovarian theca, interstitial,

luteal, and mature granulosa cells. In both males and females, the

hCG-R recognizes the pituitary hormone LH. In the pregnant female,

the same receptor also recognizes hCG[149].

The hCG-R belongs to a subfamily of glycoprotein hormone

receptor within the G protien-coupled receptor family (whose

members are characterized by the common structural feature of seven

transmembrance domains)[150].

Although there are differences in the response duration, affinity and dissociation rate of hCG for the hCG-R as compared to LH, it is generally believed that both hormones bind to and activate the receptor similarity. Studies to date indicate that the cAMP second messenger system is the predominant pathway stimulated by either LH or hCG. Yet, it has been reported that stimulation with LH or hCG leads to activation of phospholipase C ,resulting in formation of inositol phosphates and elevation in intracellular Ca^{2+} $[Ca^{2+}]$[151)(152).

The responsiveness of a given target cell to hCG or LH can be modulated by alteration in the number of cell surface receptor such as homologous and hetrologous down regulation, as a results of internalization and lysosomal degradation of hormone- receptor complex[149]. Desensitization (reduction in response intensity) has also been observed for hCG-R it has been hypothesized that the desentization occurs as a result of receptor phosphorylation[153].

1.5.1 Structure of the hCG-R and the Nature of Hormone – Receptor Interaction

Structural studies have been hampered by the low abundance of hCG receptor, nonetheless, researchers have made sufficient progress in this area. Data from chemical crosslinking of labed hCG to the receptor, immunoprcipitation of a biosynthetically labeled hCG-R,

289

purification of the receptor, have led to the estimation of the overall size and structure of this receptor[154-158]. Studies on the cDNA and genomic clones for hCG-R have yielded more detailed information on the structure and function[147][159-161]. The antibodies developed to the receptor have confirmed the topology of this receptor and are being used to address structure function relationship[149][154]. All these studies established that hCG-R is a single chain glucoprotien of 85-93 KDa. Its composed of two halves of equal size., the N-terminal extracellular hydrophilic, exodomain of ~ 350 amino acid residues and the membrane associated intracellular C-terminal endodomain of ~334 amino acids residues, which includes seven hydrophobic transmembrane helices and three cytoplasmic loops with three extracellular loops that link the seven transmembrane domains (Fig.5) The hCG-R is encoded by 11 exons located on chromosome 2 p21, the first 10 of which code for the exodomain and the 11th for the endodomain.

hCG Receptor

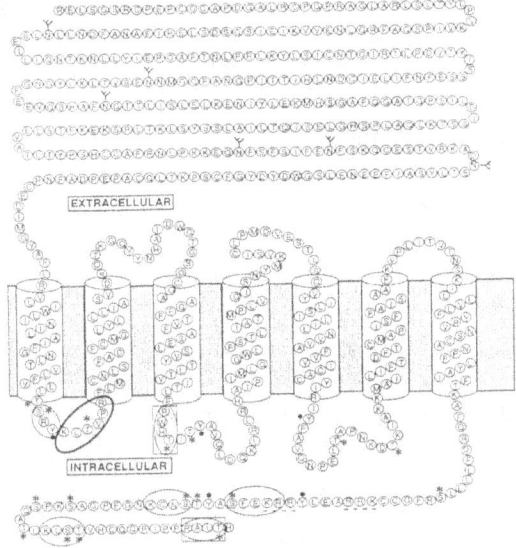

Fig.5 Amino acid sequence, orientation, and proposed topology of the hCG receptor in the plasma membrane.Potential sites for N-linked glycosylation are shown by the branch-like structures .The sequences underlined with dashes in the cytoplasmic tail mark two clusters of basic amino acids which might represent potential

tryptic cleavage sites.Potential intracellular sites for phosphorylation and denoted by asterisks (serine and threonine residues) or dark dots (tyrosine).The rectangles denote weak consensus sequences for cAMP-dependent protein kinase – catalyzed phosphorylation.The ovals and heavy ovals denotes weak and strong consensus sequences for c kinase-catalyzed phosphorylation[154].

Results from mutational analysis[162-164], chimeric construction[165], synthetic peptide studies[166] and chemical modification of the receptor[154] showed that the hormone binding and activation processes are separable.The large extacellular domain of hCG with six sites for N-linked glycosylation and (8-9) leucine –rich repeats (LRR) is responsible for high selectivity and affinity hormone binding without hormone action[167-170]. LRR are thought to form a crescent with concave inner surface consisting of β sheets which may bind hormone

(Fig.6)

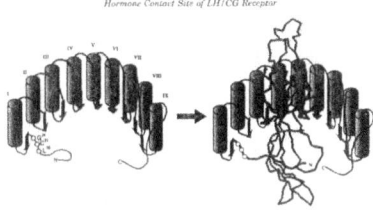

Fig.6 Schematic model for the interaction of the hCG receptor exodomain with hCG. Hormone interacts with the inner face of the crescent structure of the receptor[173].

Activation, in contrast, has been identified with transmembrance domain [171]. The molecular mechanism involves the initial high affinity contact of hCG with receptor exodomain, then the resulting complex (may not be thermodynamically stable) undergoes conformational changes and makes secondary low affinity interactions with exoloops of membrane associated domain(Fig.7), causing an allosteric structural change in the endodomain which leads to signal generation and hormone action[172X150].

Glycoprotein Hormone
(LH, FSH, hCG, TSH) Receptor

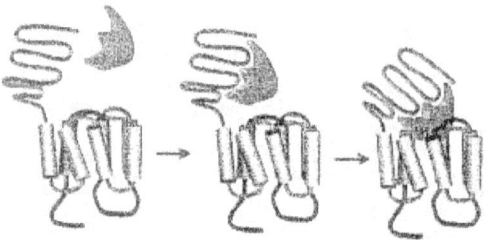

Fig.7 Schematic presentation of the receptor-hCG interaction.

hCG bind to the N-terminal segment of the receptor and the hCG-N-

terminal segment interacts with exo loops to generate a signal[150].

The initial high affinity interaction includes multiple contacts between

the exdomain and both subunits of the hormone[173][174].The precise

hormone contact sites in the exodomain are unclear. The most putative

contact sites are αC-terminal region, N-oligosaccharide at αAsn[52], and

unique αhelix in the α-subunit, as well as unusual loop (seat belt) in

the β -subunit and the peripheral β-hair pin loop of both subunits[175].

Between the initial interaction and the signal generation , hCG and

receptor undergo conformational changes. Studies including

photochemical crosslinking of hCG, mutational analysis of the receptor and serial truncation has been demonstrated a structural changes of hCG involving the intersubunit interaction[162][164][176-177].

1.5.2 The Role of hCC-R in Nongonadal Tissues and Tumor Tissues

It has long believed that the hCG-Rs were present only in gonads.

But the studies, using immunocytochemistry method and MAb for receptor or reverse transcription polymerase chain reaction technique, have demonstrated that various female as well as male nongonadal tissues (uterus, placenta, fetal membrane, deciduas, fallopian tubes, brain, breast, skin) contain low levels of hCG-R protein and hCG-R transcripts (cancer tissues are among these tissues)[178-187]. Moreover the direct action of ectopically synthesis hCG in regulating the growth of various cell types and its role in various cancers, implies the existence of the corresponding receptors in these tissues.

Studies on nonpregnant human uteri, demonstrated not only the presence but also different cellular distribution of hCG-R, where epithelial cells contain more receptors than that stromal cells of endometrial in turn, contain more than myometrial and vascular smooth muscle[178][188]. The hCG-R are increased from the proliferation to the secretary phase of the cycle. These differences suggest that other hormones regulate the receptor, which regulated

295

different functions. Evidences from in vitro studies supported these suggestion, for example , hCG was reported to have a relaxing effect on porcine myometrium[189] and can increase cAMP levels and progesterone synthesis in rat uterus[190]. The expression of receptor mRNA had been found higher in myometrial then in human endometrial blood vessels ,and there is possibility that hCG could an directly increase uterine blood flow [187].Human chorionic gonadotropin may regulate epithelial cell by increasing the local synthesis of steroid hormones[190]. In vitro , hCG can directly regulate proliferation of human myometrial smooth muscle cells causing hyperplasia as well as hypertrophy[188]. Increasing expression of receptor gene in human endometrial cancer has also been obtained [184].

Studies on human placenta , fetal membranes, decidua have been shown the presence of receptors as well as cellular localization differences and changes from mid to term pregnancy suggesting that hCG may regulate their function. In fact, there are data from in vitro studies support this possibility, in placenta, high hCG-R concentration have been shown to increase cAMP formation[191], glycogen breakdown[192], aromatization of androgens to estrogens[193], and interconversion of estron to estradiol[194]. In decidua, high hCG concentration have been shown to directly stimulate prolactin synthesis, which in turn, has been inhibited placental hCG synthsis.This finding indicates the presence of hCG- influenced short loop positive and negative regulatory mechanisms within the human fetoplacental unit[195][196]. Investigation for the presence of functional hCG-R in human breast, revealed that normal epithelial cell, benign lesion, and cancer biopsies content hCG-R[183][197]. The intensity of the immunolabeling of hCG-R varied in individual biopsies. The presence of receptor mRNA was also confirmed.In the breast, it has been proposed that hCG provokes differenentiation, which in turn renders the cells less susceptible to neoplastic transformation[198]. This mechanism would explain the decreased occurrence of breast cancer in women who had on early pregnancy. Studies on human breast cell lines showed the functional presence of hCG-R that can bind hCG to exert a direct antiproliferative effect on human breast epithelial cells through secretion of inhibin and decreasing estrogen receptor[199]. Indeed hCG has been shown to exert either stimulatory or inhibitory effects on the growth of various cancer in vitro. In bladder, lung and endometrial cancer as well as choriocarcinoma, hCG and/or its subunits promote the growth of these cancers while in breast and prostate cancers are growth inhibiting[115].

The Aim of the Work

The aim of this work includes the following :

1-Investigation the presence of intact hCG and free hCGβ in sera and tissues of patients with endometrial and epithelial ovarian cancers.

2-Development a quantitative radiorecptor assay for detection and analysis of membrane-associated hCG-Rs of human cancer tissues of endometrial and epithelial ovarian cancers.

3-Purification and characterization the hCG-Rs of epithelial ovarian cancer from detergent soluble membrane extracts .

4-Determination of the kinetic parameters of the binding reaction of hCG with it's receptor in epithelial ovarian cancer.

5-Investigation the CEA in the sera and tissues of endometrial and epithelial ovarian cancers patients.

6-Evaluation the levels of LDH, and ALP enzymes activities in sera of endometrial and epithelial ovarian cancers patients and analysis the different isoenzymes and forms of them.

7-Measuring the concentration of Copper, Zinc, and Calcium elements in sera of patients with endometrial and epithelial ovarian cancers.

Human Chorionic Gonadotropin in Sera and
Tissues of Patients with Gynecologic Cancers

Human chorionic gonadotropin is a clinically relevant marker of trophoblastic and nontrophoblastic cancers. Most studies have focused on serum determination of hCG, which have been reported to be elevated in a significant portion of patients with various nontrophoblastic cancers including gynecologic cancers [97-111]. The elevation of hCG reported vary considerably for similar cancer. This is possibly due to differences in patient selection and assay characteristic. Recently, the utilization of monoclonal antibodies, highly specific for intact hCG or its subunits have been re- evaluated the presence of hCG in the sera of nontrophoblastic tumors[102-111]. Several studies have shown that either hCG or its subunits may be localized to a variety of nontrophoblastic tissues and was extrac Table from malignant and normal human tissues[126-137]. Expression of membrane-associated hCG was found to be a phenotypic marker characteristic of all evaluated cultured human cancer cell lines, irrespective to their type or origin [114-125]. A stimulation of the growth of several tumor cells by hCG had also been reported[138-141]. In present work, a re-evaluation of presence of intact hCGand free hCGß in sera samples of patients with endometrial and epithelial ovarian cancer was carried out using a highly sensitive and specific radioimmunoassay (RIA) for these forms of hCG. Determination of intact hCG and free hCGß in these malignant tissues had been carried out to further definition of the role of hCG as tumor marker,

Materials and Methods:

2.4 Collection of Specimens and Preparation of Tissue Homogenates.

Serum: All blood samples were collected before treatment in all cases using venipuncture.Additional sample were obtained from 6 patients postoperatively while they were still in hospital. The samples were allowed to clot before separation by centrifugation at 1500xg for 15 min. The sera were subjected to RIA measurement.

Tissue: Tumor tissue specimens were obtained from patients during surgical operating. For comparison two term pregnancy placentas from spontaneous normal vaginal deliveries were used . The tissues were brought to the laboratory on crushed ice and washed extensively with ice–cold physiological saline to remove blood then stored frozen until analysis.The frozen tissues were weighted, minced finely then, homogenized in 50 mM Tris/HCL, pH 7.4 containing (0.25 M sucrose, 1mM $MgCL_2$, 5 mM EDTA, 1mM PMSF) with a ratio of 1:4 (w:v) by homogenizer at setting (2.5) using three 20s periods of homogenization . The homogenate was then filtered through a nylon mesh sieve in order to

301

eliminate fibers and cell debris then centrifuged at 600xg for

15min at 4^0c to remove the nuclei.The pellet was again homogenized and

centrifuged. The above supernatants were pooled and subjected to RIA

measurement and protein determination.

2.5 Quantitative Measurement of Intact hCG and Free hCGß

Intact hCG anf free hCGß of sera and tissues samples were

measured using highly sensitive and specific RIA Kit. The assay protocol

was described in Table (2.1)

Table (2.1) Assay protocol of intact hCG and free hCGß

	Total count (tracer)	hCG Blank (0mIU/ml)		hCG Standards (mIU/ml)	hCG Control (mIU/ml)	Patie nt sampl e
Tube number					302	

			5	10	25	50	100	200	90	X
	T_1, T_2	B_0 1,2	3,4	5,6	7,8	9,10	11,12	13,14	15,16	17,18
Standards, control, blank patients samples (µL)		←---------------------- 200 µL ---- ----------------------------------- ----------→								
^{125}I-hCGß red tracer (µL)	←-------------------------- ------ 100 µL --- ---------→									
^{125}I-hCGß blue antibody		←---------------------- 100 µL ------------------------------------- ----------→								
	1.vortex mixing, incubation for 1h at room temp.,total count set aside until counting in gamma counter									
Precipitating antiserum		←----------------------1ml--- ----→								
	1.Incubation for 5 min at room temp. 2.Centrifugation at 40^0C for 15 min at 1500xg 3.Decantation									

303

	4.Counting for radioactivity in a gamma counter for 1min

Calculation:

1. The standard curve was drawn by plotting the CPM bound for hCG standards versus their concentration(Fig 2.1)

2. The samples values of intact hCG and free hCGβ were read directly from the curve. Patients samples with assay values greater than 200 mIU/ml must be diluted.

Estimation of Protein Contents:

Protein was measured by the method of Lowry et.al.,[200] using bovine serum albumin as standard.

Statistical Analysis: Results were expressedas mean ± S.E.M.Student's t

- test

and one way analysis of variance were used for statistical comparisons and P values of less than 0.05 were considered statistically significant.

Results and Discussion:

Preoperative Data:

Results of hCG determination depend largely on the selection of antibody and the type of technique used. In present study, re-evaluation

of the presence of intact hCG and free hCGβ subunit immunoreactivity
in serum of patients with ovarian and endometrial cancer, using RIA
assay with the lower limit of sensitivity of (1.5 mIU/mI) and
monoclonal antibody recognize these forms of hCG,had been done.
Immunoreative intact hCG and free hCGß, was elevated (> 5mIU/ml)
in the sera of 11 out of 23 patients (48%) with gynecologic cancers (range
22.1 -166 mIU/ml)as shown in Table (2.2). Intact hCG and free hCGß
was found to be above normal range in the sera of 4 out of 9 patients
(44%) suffering from endometrial cancer range (22.1 -110.5 mIU/ml);
mean ± S.E.M (64.5± 41.8 mIU/ml) (Table 2.3). In patients with ovarian
cancer (n=14), elevated intact hCG and free hCGß serum values were
found in 7 of 14 (50%) , range (37.3 -166 mIU/ml).

Intact hCG and free hCGß production occurred exclusively in patients
with serous ovarian neoplasm (Table 2. 3).Analysis of the data indicated
no significant difference in the occurrence of hCG in patients with
endometrial and ovarian cancer (P> 0.05, NS). Furthermore, elevations of
intact hCG and free hCGß in the sera from patients with ovarian cancer
(100.55± 45.32) were significantly higher than in the sera from patients
with endometrial cancer (64.6±41.8).

The mean age of intact hCG and free hCGß positive group (61.5± 12.1)
was similar to that of intact hCG and free hCGß negative group (60±11.3)
of patients with endometrial and ovarian cancers (Table 2.2).

305

In benign condition positive findings were made in 7 of 59 cases (12%) including adenomyosis and myomas of the uterus, and various form of benign ovarian tumors (Table 2.3). The elevation level of intact hCG and free hCGß varied between (8.3-14.4) mIU/ml. The mean elevation (11.2± 2.2) mIU/ml was smaller than in the malignant group (87.6± 47.9)mIU/ml ($p<0.05$), the percentages of elevation intact hCG and free hCGß in benign and malignant conditions are shown in Fig 2.2. In the benign group hCG-positive patients were significantly older (60.6 ±5.8 years) than hCG- negative patients (44.2±8; $p<0.05$; Table 2.2). Human chorionic gonadotropin is one of the earliest embryonic gene products appearing in ontogeny. The finding of circulating hCG in association with cancers has been regarded generally as another expression of embryonic antigens in cancer. It's place in fetal survival and placental development has been related to its role in the control of "pseudo malignancy" because trophoblastic cell has angiogenic and invasive properties[201]. Trophoblasts express oncogenes and proto-oncogene[202] [203] and demonstrate cytokine expression[204] and resistance to immune rejection that we associate with malignancy. The percentage of elevated of intact hCG and free hCGβ was (48%) for patients with gynecologic cancer. This is comparable to that reported by Grossmann et.al.,[107] (37%) for gynecologic cancers based immunoradiometric design. Crawford et. al.,[111] demonstrated the usefulness of free hCGβ and hCG$_{βcf}$ in assessing prognosis of primary

cervical cancer. De-Bruijn et.al.,[109]studied the progressive vulvar

cancer(n=104) and found elevated free hCGβ in 50% of patients and

indicated that the synthesis of free hCGβ can be increased during

progression. Ind et.al.,[108] investigated the elevated free hCGβ and other

tumor markers in women with primary epithelial ovarian cancer. They

found a correlation between markers levels and cancer stage. Elevated

levels of intact hCG or free hCGβ were found also by other authors in

different nontrophoblastic tumors in addition to gynecologic cancers,such

as tumors of the head and neck, lung cancer ,gastrointestinal track tumors

and melanoma . Hoermann et.al.,[106] found elevated level of free hCGβ in

55% of patients with (breast, pancreas, colon, stomach, ovary, cervix,

bladder and hepatocellular cancer), whereas intact hCG was not elevated

in all serum malignant samples. Marcillac et.al.,[103] detected elevated free

hCGβ level in 47% of bladder, 32% of pancreatic and 30% of cervical

cancer, they also found low elevation level of intact hCG in the same

patients (1.3%). Alfthan et.al.,[104] observed elevated levels of serum free

hCGβ in 72% of pancreatic cancer and 86% of biliary cancer. Iles and

colleagues[105] demonstrated that the incidence of free hCGβ was

approximately 30% in serum of patients with bladder cancer and 15 out

of 36 patients with pancreatic adenocarcinoma had elevated plasma

hCGβ[110]. In all these studies, the hCG assay sensitivity was increased for

307

nontrophoblastic cancers by inclusion of free hCGβ subunit measurements.These studies indicated that most hCG-producing malignancies secret hCGβ in addition to the intact hCG molecule and free hCGβ subunit may even be the major form of hCG in nontrophoblatic cancers .This pattern of secretion contrasts with that observed in pregnant women who display a predominant secretion of intact hCG in large excess[79] .The result of an earlier studies based intact hCG determination confirm this observation where the values obtained are low. Donaldson et.al.,[99] in their assessment of markers of gynecologic cancers found low percentage (22%) of patients has total hCG serum level greater than 5 mIU/mI . Rutanen et. al.,[97]. also found an elevation of total serum hCG in only 18% of gynecologic cancers. In early studies[97-101], the overall incidence was in the range of 18-25% of all tumors studies. Serum intact hCG and free hCGβ levels were elevated in 44% of patients with adenocarcinoma of the uterus and in 64% of patients with serous epithelial ovarian cancers. On considering whether the histological type of tumor or cells give any clue of its ability to secrete hCG, it is obvious, by the spectrum of histological appearance of hCG-producing tumors , that the morphological features of neoplastic are not necessarily linked to hormone producing. Donaldson et.al.,[99] among their analysis of ovarian and cervical tumors found elevated levels of hCG in selected cases of epithelial ovarian cancer (serous 27%,

endometriod 100%, mucinous 0%, and Granulosa cell 0%) whereas
small-cell, keratinizing, and nonkeratinizing types of squamous
carcinomas had elevated levels in 13, 40 and 20% of cases respectively of
cervical cancer, while none of the cervical adenocarcinoma had elevated
levels of hCG. Mohabeer et.al.,[128] when examining ovarian epithelial
tumors, found no relationship between the hCGβ positive and the
histological type of tumors, or whether the tumor was of a benign, or
malignant type (with no trophoblatic proliferation), nor even the
histological grade of malignant tumors .Other authors such as Collins
et.al.,. [132] demonstrated that hCGβ positive was found in
adenocarcinoma of the uterine cervix in which the cells of tumor have
some histological resemblance to trophoblastic cells. Rutanen et.al.,[97].
did not find bias in the distribution of hCG in patients with poorly and
well–differentiated endometrial cancer, while Mc Manus et.al.,[100] have
commented that hCG positive was most frequent in poorly differentiated
anaplastic tumors. There are also nongestational and extragonadal tumors
which both produce hCG and bear a striking resemblance to trophoblastic
neoplasms such that many authors use the term "choriocarcinomatous" to
describe them. Cases have been reported with either poorly differentiated
transitional cell carcinoma of the bladder or adenocarcinoma of the
urothelial, stomach colon, and uterus[129-132].

Low elevated intact hCG and free hCGβ were found in 12% of patients with nonmalignant gynecologic tumors, and women with positive intact hCG and free hCGβ were older than women with negative intact hCG and free hCGβ, using cut off level 5mIU/ml. If we take an important consideration that hCG excreted in healthy subjects[80] and there are direct evidence for production of the intact hCG by the pituitary gland[62] and its expression is related to the age[81], then the elevated intact hCG and free hCGβ in benign group could be explained. It is highly likely that the low level of intact hCG and free hCGβ (11.2±2.2) found in the sera of nonmalignant gynecological patients originates from the pituitary gland and not from the tumor. This level is significantly low in comparison with malignant group (87.6±47.9).

Theories to explain the production of ectopic proteins in general involve the possibility of derepression of genes that are expressed in fetal life, or the recruitment of uncommitted cells, or the occurrence of random mutation[132]. These hypotheses assume that hCG are not a normal features of later life, but the presence of very low levels of hCG in both tissues and body fluids during normal metabolism and tissue turnover has been documented[136][137][81][80]. The source of such hCG in healthy subjects is postulated to be the normal stem cells of replicating tissues. If hCG is synthesized in many normal sites, then the neoplastic cells because of their increased number would produce larger quantities of stem cell proteins compared to the quantities produced by normal cells. Circulating intact hCG and free hCGß could be demonstrated in early as well as in advanced stage of the two kinds of gynecologic cancers (Table 2.4). Of the 9 patients with endometrial cancer, intact hCG and free hCGß elevated in 2 out of 6 and 2 out of 3 of the stage I and II, respectively . The highest intact hCG and free hCGß serum level (110 mIU/ml) was found in women with the stage II, however the analytical data indicated no significant differences in serum intact hCG and free hCGß concentration between two stages of endometrial cancer (p>0.05). In ovarian cancer, intact hCG and free hCGß was elevated in 2 out of 5 (40%) of stage I and 5 out of 9 (56%) of stages (II –III (Table 2.4). The highest level of intact hCG and free hCGß was found in patients with stage III (166 mIU/ml), but also no significant different in the serum intact hCG and free hCGß concentration found between different stages. It was found no correlation between the concentration of intact hCG and free hCGß and the spread of the tumor.

Although only a few cases could be examined, women with invasive endometrial and ovarian cancer as assessed by staging had the highest serum concentration of intact hCG and free hCGβ, but difference between stages was not statistically significant .These results confirm previous observation from other investigations, which characterize hCG as a key

311

factor defining the metastasis phenotype specifically of nontrophoblasic malignancies. Grossmann et.al.,[107] obtained that the advanced disease of cervical cancer was associated with elevated intact hCG and free hCGβ serum values (4/13 (31%) of stage II and 11/27(41%) of stages III-IV) , also obtained that women with more aggressive endometrial cancers had higher serum concentrations of intact hCG and free hCGβ. Sheth et.al.,[101] using RIA techniques, found elevated levels of serum hCG in 41% patients with squamous carcinomas of cervix FIGO stages II-IV with an increasing frequency in the higher clinical grades. Marcillic et.al.,[103] found that the production of free hCGβ was associated with tumors of high prognosis such as cancers of the lung, pancreas, and liver.

Walker[127] also noted a relation between the presence of hCG and metastases of breast cancer. Syrigos[110] and de-Bruijn[109] also indicated, that the patients with elevated serum hCGβ had a worse progressive tumor compared with the group of normal hCGβ in patients with vulvar and pancreatic cancer.

The sensitivity, specificity and predictive value of the intact hCG and free hCGß in the diagnosis of gynecologic cancers are shown in Table 2.5. When pre-treatment serum intact hCG and free hCGß levels were compared between patients with benign and those with malignant gynecologic tumors, they distinguished the malignant from benign tumor with a predictive value of (73% and 80%) in uterine corpus and ovarian tumor, respectively. In all healthy females sera, intact hCG and free hCGß activity was measurable. All females showed levels within the upper limit of normal range (5mIU/ml) (Table 2.2). In women older than 45 years the mean concentration (4.8 ± 0.5 mIU/ml) was significantly higher than that of the women younger than 45 year(3.8± 0.8 mIU/ml). It is noteworthy that hCG was present at low levels (<5 mIU/ml) in serum of many cancer patients as well as in healthy women's and patients with benign disease (Fig 2.3).

Postoperative Data:

Intact hCG and free hCGß levels were postoperatively measured in 6 hCG –positive cancer patients who had undergone radical surgery including hysterectomy and ovariectomy. The blood was obtained from them in the first postoperative week, while they were still in hospital. The data showed reversion of serum intact hCG and free hCGß levels in 4 patients , while 2 remained hCG–positive (Table2.6). On the basis of clinical examination no tumor was demonstrated in any of the 4 hCG negative patients, while the 2 hCG- positive patients had a metastasis (stage III). One of these 2 women, multiple serum specimens were obtained from her during the period of different weeks. intact hCG and free hCGß concentration paralleled the clinical course of this patient (Fig.2.4).

In several cases elevated intact hCG and free hCGβ levels returned to normal level after operation, and that indicate the hormone has been produced by the tumor itself, but in two ovarian cancer cases with metastasis, intact hCG and free hCGβ levels remained elevated after operation which give an example of usefulness of hCG in the following of patients with ovarian cancer. Crossmann et.al.,[107] reported the importance of intact hCG and free hCGβ in following the ovarian cancer cases and commented that for the optimal management of gynecologic cancer, multiple markers measuring could be helpful. Marcillac et.al.,[103] and Alfthan et.al.,[104] have also reported that free hCGβ is promising marker in diagnosis and following the bladder and pancreatic cancer. Donaldson et.al.,[99] obtained that measuring hCG with other markers could help to follow up patients with gynecologic cancers.

Malignant and Non Malignant Tissues:

Intact hCG and free hCGß immunoreactivity has been determined in tumor tissues of the patients with endometrial and ovarian cancer (n=23), and in tumor tissues of patients with the benign tumor (n=25). For comparison, placenta intact hCG and free hCGß content has also been determined in 2 term pregnancy women. In malignant tissues, intact hCG and free hCGß levels ranged between (14.5 -212 mIU/ml; Table 2.7). Statistical analysis of differences between blood serum and tumor tissue intact hCG and free hCGß content in patient with malignancies has been performed. The elevation of tissue intact hCG and free hCGß level appeared to be statistically significant than in the corresponding serum samples (P<0.05). Remarkably, of these 12 women, which showed normal serum values (<5mIU/ml) (Fig 2.5).

In 25 non-malignant tissues, intact hCG and free hCGß levels ranged from (5.3 -9.5 mIu/ml), mean 8.19 ± 1 mIU/ml which were significantly lower than in the specimen from women with ovarian and endometrial cancer (P<0.05) (Table 2.7). If the upper limit of normal range for tissue as 10 mIU/ml, then 23 out of 23 (100%) of the malignant tissue samples were considered pathological and 25 out of 25 (100%) of the benign were judged normal.Determination of hCG in placenta had been obtained for comparison. The term pregnancy placenta gives higher level of intact hCG and free hCGß, even more than cancer tissue (371 ± 11 mIU/ml) (Table 2.7).

Effort to improve the diagnosis efficiency in gynecologic tumors has been made by assessing intact hCG and free hCGß in tumor tissues. Malignant cells are assumed to be source of ectopic hormone production, however, the rate at which hCG is actually released into the circulation may vary considerably. Consequently, one might expect that measuring hCG in compartments within the neoplasm increases the sensitivity of marker detection. In our study, determining intact hCG and free hCGß in malignant tissue enhanced the sensitivity of this marker as compared to

315

serum. Concentrations of intact hCG and free hCGß were significantly higher in malignant tumor tissue than in the corresponding sera samples (p<0.05;(Table 2.6),and intact hCG and free hCGß was elevated even in patients with normal serum values (23/23) using 5mIU/ml as reference value (Fig 2.5). In benign tissues, the highest concentration of intact hCG and free hCGß measured in 25 specimens was (9.5 mIU/ml), using 10mIU/ml reference value as suggested by some studies, 23/23 (100%) of the malignant samples were considered pathological and 25/25 (100%) of the benign samples were judged normal.

These data are extended to other findings that intact hCG and free hCGß in tissue might be useful for the diagnosis of the malignancies and it expression in cancer, defines the metastic aggressiveness of the tumors in which it is found. There is several documentation of the localization of hCG, hCG like material, or free hCG subunits in a variety of nontrophoblastic tissues and was extrac Table from virtually all normal and malignant human tissues[126-137]. Using immunohistochemical technique, various investigators found hCG in adenocarcinoma of large bowel[134] and uterine cervix[132], breast cancer[127],hepatoblastoma[133] ,epithelial ovarian cancers[128] ,colorectal cancer[130], Urothelial carcinoma [129],and malignant gastric tumors[131]. Yoshimoto et.al.,[163] reported that extracts of cancer tissues from stomach, liver, colon, and lung contained hCG-like material higher than normal tissue. The work of Acevedo and other authors[114-124] has shown that free hCGß express in human fetal tissue and cancer cells of different histological types and origins. Bellet et.al.,[64] demonstrated that activation occurs with the gene cluster responsible for hCGβ in breast, bladder, prostate, and thyroid cancer and suggested that methylation play a role in maintaining the active/inactive status of the gene. The stimulation of growth of several cell lines by hCG has been reported[138-141] , also resolution of the three dimensional structure of hCG had shown this hormone to be a growth factor[76][72][77] , thus cancer cells are able to regulate independently its own growth. Indeed, hCG has been shown to exert inhibitory effects on the growth of breast and prostate cell lines[199]. In the breast, some patients have increasing hCG levels, and some breast cancer tissue and human breast cell lines contain native hCG.

Several hypotheses have been proposed to explain the origin of hCG producing cells and include the following:[132]

a. Displaced gonadal cell(extragonadol choriocarcinoma).

b. Metastasis from an intrauterine or gonadal lesion

c.An evaluation from a somatic cell that underwent a morphological and functional transformation into a cell functionally similar to the trophoblast.

Table 2.2: The Values of Intact hCG and Free hCGß Levels in Sera of Malignant and Benign Gynecologic Tumors (All details are explained in the text)

Clinical categories	No. of patients	Range of intact hCG and free hCGß (mIU/ml)	Range of age (year)
Malignancy			
Intact hCG and free hCGß positive*	11	22.1-166	40-80
	12	3.8-5	38-70
Intact hCG and free hCGß negative*	23	3.8-166	38-80

All patients			
Benign			
Intact hCG and free hCGß positive*	7	7.3-14.4	53-67
Intact hCG and free hCGß negative*	52	3.9-5	22-65
	59	3.9-14.4	22-67
All patients			
Normal	30	2.5-5	20-68

*positive:patients having levels of intact hCG and hCGß above 5mIU/ml

* negative:patients having levels of intact hCG and hCGß below

5mIU/ml

Table 2.3: Preoperative Elevated Serum Levels of Intact hCG and Free hCGß in Malignant and Benign Gynecologic Tumors

(All details are Explained in the text)

Diagnosis	*Elevated/Total	%	Range (mIU/ml)	Intact hCG and Free hCGß Conc.mIU/ml (mean±S.E.M.)
Malignancy	>5mIU/ml			
Endometrial				
Adenocarcinoma	4/9	44	22.1-110.5	64.6± 41.8
*Ovarian cancer				
Serous	7/11	64	37.3-166	100.55±45.32
Mucinous	0/3	Zero		
All patients	11/23	48	22.1-166	87.6±47.9
Benign				
Adenomyosis	1/4	25	11.2	11.2
Fibromyoma	3/20	15	8.3-13.1	10.2±2.5
Endometriosis	0/3	0		
Follicular cyst	1/10	14	12.3	12.3
Serous cyst	2/9	33	10.2-14.4	12.3±3.5
Musinous cyst	0/3	0		
Dermoid cyst	0/4	0		
Poly cystic	0/6	0		

All patients	7/59	12	8.3-14.4	11.2±2.2
Normal				
Female <45 year	0/15	0		
Female >45 year	0/15	0		

*Elevated /Total: Number of patients having levels of the intact hCG and

free hCGß above 5mIU/ml/total number of patients.

Table2.4: Elevated Serum Level of Intact hCG and Free hCGß in

Relation to Staging of Endometrial and Ovarian Cancers (All details

are explained in the text)

	Endometrial cancer			Ovarian cancer		
Clinical Stage*	**Elevated/total**	**%**	**hCG/ hCGß mean±S.E.M.**	**Elevated/total**	**%**	**Intact hCG and free hCGß mIU/ml**

							mean±S.E. M
I	2/6	33.3	62.9±36.34		2/5	40	95.4±82.17
II	2/3	66.7	66.3±62.5		1/3	33.3	66.1
III					4/6	67	112.1±44.4

*FIGO classification

NS:not significant

Elevated/Total: numbers of patients having levels of intact hCG and free hCGß above 5mIU/ml/ total number of patients.

Table 2.5 : Preoperative Serum Intact hCG and Free hCGß Levels: Diagnosis of Gynecologic cancers (All details are Explained in the text)

	Uterine corpus		Ovary	
	Benign	Malignant	Benign	Malignant
No. Of patients	4/24	4/9	3/35	7/14

*Positive/total				
Sensitivity	100%	100%	100%	100%
Specificity	83%	44%	91%	50%
Predictive value		73%		80%

* positive:intact hCG and free hCGß >5mIu/ml

Table 2.6: Pre and Postoperative Elevated Serum Intact hCG and Free hCGß in Gynecological Cancers (All details are explained in the text)

Time of study	No. of patient	Intact hCG and free hCGß(mIU/ml) mean±S.E.M.
Endometrial Pre-op*	4	64.6± 41.8
Pos-op*	2	4.7±0.14
ovarian Pre-op	7	87.4±59.6
Pos-op	2/4 negative	4.8±0.4
	2/4 positive	9±1.4

5

*pre-op. : preoperative

*pos-op. : postoperative

Table 2.7: Comparison of Levels of Intact hCG and Free hCGß in Sera and tissues of Benign and Malignant Gynecologic Cancers (All details are explained in the text)

Clinical categories	Intact hCG and free hCGß in blood		Intact hCG and free hCGß in tissue	
	No. of cases	mIu/ml mean±S.E.M.(range)	No. of cases	mIu/ml mean±S.E.M.(range)
Endometrial cancer	9	31.5±40.6 (3.8-110.5)	9	52.6±52.8(14.5-168)
Ovarian cancer	14	52.5±59.8(4.2-166)	14	79.7±74(15.2-212)
Benign tumor	25	6.3±3.2(3.9-14.4)	25	8.19±1(5.3-9.5)
Placenta	2		2	371±11(360-382)

Development of a Radioreceptor Assay for Detection and Analysis of hCG - Receptor in Benign and Malignant Gynecologic Tumors.

The hCG-R belongs to the family of glycoprotein hormone G protein –coupled receptors, which also comprise TSH-R and FSH-R[149].All three receptors are glycoprotiens containing a large extracllular leucin rich repeats (LRR), N-terminal domain with several N-linked glycosylation. A plasma membrane domain composed of seven hydrophobic α-helices ending with an intracellular C-terminus[154].These three receptors have been shown to transduce hormone binding via coupling to the heterotrimeric Gs protein which activates adenylyl cyclase, or other G proteins that activate phosphlipase C (as assessed by measuring inositol phosphates, diacylglycerol, and / or intracellular Ca^{+2}) [151].

The mechanism of the coupling in hCG-R is different from other G protein- coupled receptors whose ligands are much smaller and intercalate among the transmembrance helices[150].

The hCG-R, which is present on gonadal cells, plays a pivotal role in reproductive physiology. Until recently, it was believed that hCG-R were only present in gonadal cells, where they regulate steroidogenesis. However, it is now known that these receptors are also expressed in human and animal uteri[178] [188] [189], human pituitary[185], skin[186] fallopian tubes[179], human placenta, fetal membranes, decidua[178], human gestational trophoblastic neoplasms, human breast[197] and breast cancer[183], endometrial and myometrial blood vessels[187] and brain[182]. These studies have shown that hCG can directly regulate the functions of nongonodal tissues indicating that the receptor are functional in these tissues.

The evidence for hCG receptors has been obtained by ligand binding measurements or immunocytochemistry using receptor –specific antibodies or evaluation the presence of hCG receptor mRNA. The traditional hCG-R binding studies involved binding a radioactive form of either the hormone itself or a biologically active analog (agonist) to membrane preparations (particulate or solubilized)of target tissues, have been used to identify and characterize the hCG-R[154] [189] [205]. In most hCG-R binding studies,[125]I-labeled hCG prepared by radio iodination with chloramines or lactoperoxidase has been used. Tritium, has also been used in some studies for labeling.

The binding of LH or hCG to cell surface receptors was thought to be a reversible process, thus saturation binding experiments were performed under steady state conditions[206]. It has now become clear that the hCG-receptor interaction is much more complex and cannot be described as a simple bimolecular reaction[175]. The hormone-receptor complex is not only involved with the stimulation of adenylate cyclase, but also functions in the ligand-induced regulation of the receptors[154]. From different separation techniques of bound from free hormone, the choice was usually between centrifugation and precipitation of the hormone receptor complex[149].

9

The present investigation was undertaken to develop a radioreceptor assay for

hCG-R determination in benign and malignant ovarian and uterine tumors. The nature

of the binding was characterized by determination of the equilibrium dissociation

constant (k_d), Scatchard plots, inhibition studies, and rate constants.

Materials and Methods

3.1 Buffers and Reagents:

Buffers and reagents of chapter 2 (2.4) were used in the experiments of this

chapter. Other solutions used were indicated in each experiment.

3.2 Patients and Specimens:

The benign and malignant tissues of patients described in section (2.3) are

included in radio receptor experiments. The crude tissue homogenates were prepared

as described in section (2.4), but further centrifugation was carried out on the

supernatant at 9000xg for 30min. The pellet containing the receptor, was resuspended

in 50 mMTris/HcL, pH 7.4 containing 1mM PMSF and 5 mM EDTA,

20% glycerol,0.1% BSA in ratio of 1:4 (w:v) and then homogenized and subjected for

binding studies.

3.3 Binding Studies of ^{125}I-hCG with Its Receptor in Benign and Malignant

Ovarian and Uterine tumors

3.3.1 Preliminary Test of hCG-R Binding:

The binding of ^{125}I-hCG to the tissue homogenates was primarily checked. The

experiment was carried out in duplicate, 250µl of ovarian or uterine homogenates

(700 µg protein) were incubated with 80µl of I^{125}-hCG (1 µg/ml) and the volumes

were completed to 500µl with 50 mM Tris/HCL, pH 7.4 containing 0.1% BSA.

Incubation was carried out at 37°C for 1hr or at 4°C for 24h. This was followed by

centrifugation for 30 min at 1500xg and then decanted. The radioactivity of the bound

hCG(CPM) was counted in the pellet for each tube using gamma counter. Non

specific binding(NSB) was also determined by the same method in the presence of

200 fold excess of unlabelled hCG as competitor.

The specific binding (CPM) was calculated by subtraction of the radioactivity

(CPM) obtained in the presence of excess of unlabelled hCG (NSB) from total

binding (TB) .

SB (CPM) = TB (CPM) - NSB (CPM)

Percentage (%SB)= SB(CPM) / Total count (CPM) of the ^{125}I-hCG used in each tube

X100

3.3.2 The Effect of ^{125}I-hCG Concentration on the Binding:

Increasing concentration of ^{125}I -hCG ranging from (1-20 pM) were added to 250

μL (700 μg protein) of crude ovarian or uterine homogenates with a final volume of

500 μl (completed with 50 mM Tris/ HCL, pH 7.4 containing 0.1% BSA.

After incubation for 1hr at 37°C, the bound hCG was determined as described in

section (3.3.1). The specific binding (SB%) was calculated and plotted against the

concentration of ^{125}I-hCG.

3.3.3 The Effect of Receptor Concentration on the Binding:

Forty microlitres of ^{125}I –hCG (Iμg/mL) was added to 250 μl of increasing

amount (300,400,500,600,700,800μg) of crude ovarian homogenates in a final

volume of 500 μl (completed with Tris -0.1% BSA buffer pH7.4). After incubation

for 1hr at 37°C, the bound hCG was determined as described in section (3.3.1) The

same experiment was carried out using 250μl of increasing amount

(300,400,500,600,700,800,ug protein) of uterine homogenate added to a set of tubes

11

contained 20 μl of ^{125}I -hCG (1μg/ml) in a final volume of 500μl. The SB% was calculated and plotted against the concentration of receptor.

3.3.4 The Effect of pH on the Receptor Binding:

Two hundred fifty microliters of crude ovarian homogenates (500μg protein) were added to 40 μl (1μg/ml) of ^{125}I -hCG. The mixtures were then completed with buffers of different pH (5, 5.5, 6, 6.4, 6.8, 7, 7.2, 7.4, 7.6, 7.8, and 8.0) to 500μl. The experiment was repeated using 250 μl of crude uterine homogenates (700μg protein), added to 20 μl (1μg/mL) of ^{125}I -hCG and completed in the same manner. After incubation for 1hr at 37°C, the bound hCG was determined as mentioned in section (3.3.1).The SB% was calculated and plotted against pH .

3.3.5 Temperature Dependency of the Binding:

Fourty micro liters (1μg/ml) of ^{125}I -hCG and 250 μl (500μg protein) of crude ovarian homogenates were mixed in a final volume of 500μl (completed with Tris - 0.1% BSA buffer pH 7.2) .After incubation for 1hr at different temp. (4,25,37,45°C), the bound hCG was determined as described in section (3.3.1). The experiment was repeated using 250μL of crude uterine homogenates (700 μg protein) added to 20 μL of ^{125}I -hCG and completed in the same manner. The SB% was calculated and plotted vs. the temperature of incubation.

3.3.6 Time Course of Receptor Binding

Crude ovarian homogenate (500μg protein in 250μl) was added to 40 μl (1ug/ml) of ^{125}I -hCG in a final volume of 500 μl (completed with Tris -0.1% BSA buffer PH 7.2). The tubes were incubated at 4°C. At certain time intervals (0.5, 1, 2, 6, 8, 16,

24hr), two tubes were taken and the bound hCG was estimated as mentioned in section (3.3.1). The experiment was repeated at 25, 37°C. The same protocol was repeated for the uterine homogenate using 250µl (700µg protein) of this homogenate, added to 20µl (1ug/ml) of ^{125}I -hCG. The SB% was calculated and plotted vs. the time of incubation.

3.3.7 Stability of Receptor Homogenate and Hormone Receptor Complex :

In order to investigate the effect of temperature on receptor properties, the stability of receptor homogenate and receptor – hCG complex have been measured. For measuring receptor stability, 250 µL of crude ovarian homogenates were incubated at 25°C 37°C. At certain time intervals (1, 2, 3, 4hr), two tubes from each set were taken and mixed with 40ul of ^{125}I-hCG in a final volume 0f 500µL (completed with Tris-0.1% BSA buffer PH 7.2). After incubation for 1h at 37°C, the specific activity was determined as described in section (3.3.1) . In a control (with no preincubation) ovarian homogenate , the binding assay was performed and considered 100% binding .The relative binding was plotted against preincubation time,. The same protocol was repeated for the uterine homogenate using 250 µl (700µg protein) of this homogenate.

For measuring receptor-hCG complex stability , the experiment was performed as described in section 3.3.5 at 37°C. After the evaluation of the bound hCG, the receptor-hCG complex was reincubated at three temperatures (4, 25, 37°C). Between 0 and 8hr, the remaining binding of ^{125}I-hCG was measured and the relative binding was calculated and plotted against the time of incubation.

3.3.8 Determination of the Equilibrium Binding Constants of hCG-R

13

Ovarian homogenate (500µg protein in 250µL were added to 40µL of increasing

concentration (1-20pM) of [125] I -hCG with or without the addition of a 200 fold excess

of unlabelled hCG in a final volume of 500 µL (completed with Tris -0.1% BSA, PH

7.2). After incubation for 1hr at 37°C , the bound hCG was determined as described in

section 3.3.1. the same protocol was repeated for the uterine homogenate using 250µl

(700µg protein) of this homogenate added to 20µl of increasing concentration (10-

2000fM) of [125] I -hCG with or without the addition of a 200fold excess of unlabelled

hCG. The concentration of receptors and the association constant (K_a) were

determined according to Scatchard equation[205] .

$$B / F = B_{max} - B / K_d \text{ and } K_d = 1 / K_a$$

Where B= the concentration of bound hCG.

F= the concentration of free hCG.

B_{max}= the maximum number of binding sites (binding capacity).

K_d= equilibrium binding constant (dissociation constant).

K_a= equilibrium binding constant (association constant).

The bound and free hCG were calculated by multiplication of the ratios specific

bound (CPM) / total count (CPM) and free (CPM) / total count (CPM) with the

concentration of [125] I -hCG respectively. The B/F was plotted vs. B. The receptor

concentration and the association constant were calculated from the x-axis and the

slope of the straight line respectively.

3.3.9 Specificity of Binding and Determination of IC_{50} and K_i

Ovarian homogenates (500µg in 250µl) were added to 40µl (1µg/ml) of the [125] I -

hCG without or with the addition of increasing concentration (1-1000ng) of

unlabelled hCG in a final volume of 500µl. After incubation for 1hr at 37°C, the

bound hCG was determined as described in section (3.3.1). For the study of the competitive effect on the binding of uterine receptor, 250μl (700 μg protein) of this homogenate was added to 20 μl (1μg/ml) of [125]I -hCG without or with the increasing concentreation (5-500ng/ml) of unlabelled hCG in a final volume of 500μl. After incubation for 1h at 37°C, the bound hCG to uterine receptor was determined and the SB% was calculated as mentioned in section 3.3.1. The experiment was repeated with different competitors [FSH, LH,TSH , Serum from choriocarcinoma] . The relative binding of ^{125}I-hCG was calculated and plotted against competitors conc., competition curves were generated and the concentration of unlabeled ligand displacing 50% of specific radioligand binding (IC_{50}) was determined.The binding affinity constant of unlabeled ligand (k_i) were also determined according to the following equation:

$$k_i = \frac{^IC_{50}}{1+[L]/kd}$$

.   Where [L] :the concentration of radioligand

RESULTS AND DISCUSSION

Membrane Preparation

In a series of preliminary experiments, curde plasma membranes were prepared by centrifugation of ovarian and uterine homogenates at various centrifugal force from 3000 to 9000 xg. As expected, the recovery of the receptor increased with increased rotor speed, membranes were subsequently prepared by centrifugation at 9000xg in order to obtain maximal recovery of the receptor. The stability of the crude membrane receptor was markedly improved by supplementation of the buffer with glycerol; the hormone binding activity of the membrane extract was completely retained after storage at 4°C for at least 3 day. The proteolysis of the receptor (and/or nicking), by

15

endogenous protease, had been inhibited by the inclusion of an inhibitor cocktail containing PMSF, and EDTA in extraction buffer.

Previous reports describing the extraction of the hCG-Rs have been based on the use of either particulate membrane or soluble membrane extract from bovine[157][158] and rat[156][207][208] gonadal tissues. Other non gonadal tissues were also used such as rat kidney and liver[208] and porcine uterus[189]. The membrane fraction was prepared by centrifugation[207][149] at various centrifugal forces. While preparation of soluble hCG-R has been base almost exclusively on the use of triton X-100[157][158][149]. Emulphogene (anonionic detergent) has also been used[156]. Ligand-receptor binding experiments can be done on membrane preparation of tissues as particulate or solubilized, in contrast purification studies have been done only on solubilized receptors.

Human Chorionic Gonadotropin Receptors in Ovarian and Uterine Tumors: Initial studies were performed by ligand–receptor binding method; involve binding highly specific, purity, and biological active radiolabelled hCG (^{125}I-hCG) to particulate membrane preparations. The presence and binding activity of hCG-Rs in 48 cases of benign and malignant ovarian and uterine tumors were investigated (Table 3.1). The ^{125}I-hCG binding activity of the receptor after 24hr of incubation at 4°C was the same as at 37°C for 1hr, which indicates that the equilibrium of reaction was depended on the temperature. Table (3.1) shows that the malignant tumors of ovarian have a specific hCG-binding activity of 1.6±0.36 pmol/mg of protein, which is approximately 2 fold higher than that of benign tumors. In endometrial cancer, binding activity for hCG (0.2±0.15 pmol/mg of protein) is lower than that in malignant and benign ovarian tumors. Normally hCG-Rs are functional in gonad cells, where both LH and hCG regulate; through this receptor; the ovarian and testicular steroidogenesis[209] ,LH also increases ovarian blood flow in several species. Human chorionic gonadotropin and/or LH may also regulate glandular and Luminal epithelial cell functions in gonadal cells via cAMP mediation or by increasing the local synthesis of steroid hormones[210]. Crude homogenates prepared previously from ovarian of pseudo pregnant rats have a specific hCG-binding activity of 0.8-1.3 pmol/mg of protein (Bruch et.al.,[156], Shao K.[207], Segaloff et.al.,[149]) which is approximately 10 fold higher than that of homogenate prepared from porcine luteal tissue[149], rat testis[211], bovine luteal[157][158], or mouse leydig cell tumors[149].

The high specific hCG-binding activity (1.6 ± 0.36 pmol/mg) in ovarian tumor tissues seems to be compatible with the increasing the number of cell produced by malignant tumor. There was no obvious relation between the specific activity and staging of malignant ovarian tumor. Further studies in a greater number of patients will be necessary to determine whether the concentration of hCG-R also is correlated with aggressiveness of the tumor and the prognosis of the patients. In malignant tumor of uterus, it appeared important to detect a tumor containing hCG-Rs because most hormonal markers (including estrogen, progesterone), EGF receptors, and so-forth, are present in only a subset of the cancer[212]. Specific ^{125}I-hCG binding activity was observed for all uterine preparations (Table 3.1),revealing the presence of hCG-Rs in these tissues. Recent evidence shows that in addition to their classical endocrine effects, hCG and LH may also be ectopically synthesized and exert paracrine effects,regulating the growth of various cell types . This direct action implies the existence of the corresponding receptors in these tissues.

Reshef et.al.,[178] demonstrated for the first time the presence and cellular distribution of hCG-R in nonpregnant human uterus using specific immunostaining procedure. They obtained that the receptors are present in glandular and luminal

17

epithelial cells and stromal cells, of endometrial, and in circular and elongated

myometrial smooth muscle and in vascular smooth muscle of myometrium. Ziecik et.

al.,[189] reported that all of the porcine myometria and 30% of the endometria

examined contained hCG-Rs which increase from the proliferate to the secretary

phase of the cycle. The physiological significant of human uterine hCG-Rs is not

known, but the presence of receptors in different uterine cell types as well as

differences between them suggest that hCG may regulate different functions in

different cell type in the uterus. The presence of differences during the menstrual

cycle suggests that these receptors are regulated by other hormones and hCG was

reported to have a relaxing effect on porcine myometrium[189]. In vitro, hCG was

reported to increase cAMP levels and progesterone synthesis in rat uterus[190]. Lei.et.

al.,[187] found vascular hCG-Rs mRNA transcript and receptors protein in human

endometrial and myometrial, suggested that LH or hCG might directly regulate blood

flow in human uterus. Evidence already exists in support of such possibilities, for

example LH increases ovarian blood flow in several species[213][214]. Kornyel et.al.,[188]

considered human myometrium a direct target of gonadotropin regulation because of

the presence of hCG-R in this tissue. They demonstrate that hCG can directly regulate

myometrial smooth muscle cells, causing hyperplasia as well as hypertrophy.

Logically hCG and LH in uterine cells can make all their functions already exist in

gonadal cells[215][216]. The expression of hCG-R has been reported in human

endometrial carcinoma by immunocytochemistery[184]. The expression of receptor

varied among individual cancers. This receptor has also been reported in breast cancer

by two different monoclonal antibodies raised against human hCG-R, which allowed

Meduri and his coleagues[183] to detect this receptor in cancer and benign breast lesions. They also reported that the receptor was also present in epithelial cells of normal human and sow breast.

Factors Affecting the Binding of ^{125}I-HCG with Its Receptor

A binding saturation study could be performed at a steady state when criteria of radioligand purity, minimization of nonspecific binding have been satisfied. In addition, linearity of radioligand binding to the tissue must be demonstrated and the appropriate incubation time and temperature to reach a steady state must also be determined. Thus, the investigation of these effects is quite necessary to get reliable measuring for ligand binding in the tissue.

1 **The Effect of ^{125}I-hCG Concentration on the Binding**

Ligand receptor binding studies usually followed the kinetics of very similar to those of classic enzyme-substrate interactions[206]. For reversible ligand receptor interactions:

$$a[L] + b[R] \frac{K+1}{K \quad 1} c[RL]$$

Where: [L]=concentration of free ligand.

[R]= concentration of unoccupied receptor sites .

[LR]= concentration of ligand-receptor complex.

K_{+1}=association rate constant.

k_{-1}=dissociation rate constant.

$$\left(\frac{k \quad 1}{k+1}\right)$$
k_d=equilibrium binding constant

The classic law of mass action for enzyme-substrate interaction adapted to ligand-

$$\frac{B_{max}[L]}{[L]+Kd}$$ receptor interaction which is [LR]=

19

One of the property of ligand-receptor interactions is saturability, that is, only a finite number of specific receptor sites exist per unit of tissue, usually designated B_{max}. To fulfill this criterion, various concentrations of the ^{125}I-hCG with a fixed concentration of tissue have been incubated[217]. Saturation curves for specific binding of hCG to the receptor homogenates of malignant and benign tumors are shown in Fig. 3.1.

In ovarian tumors the hCG-Rs are saturated with ^{125}I-hCG at 17 pmol and 7.8 pmol for malignant and benign conditioned respectively, while in uterine tumors, the hCG-Rs saturated with ^{125}I-hCG at 4 pmol and 2 pmol for malignant and benign conditions respectively.

2 The Effect of Receptor Concentration on the Binding:

One of methodological problems apparent involves the choice of appropriate tissue (receptor) concentration to utilize in the binding experiment[218]. The receptor concentration influences the K_d value and the linearity of radioligand binding with tissue. In order to demonstrate that, increasing concentration of homogenate were incubated with fixed concentration of ^{125}I-hCG. As shown in Fig.(3.2) the percentage of ^{125}I-hCG bound was increased linearly with increasing of receptor concentration in benign and malignant conditions. This experiment shows the homogeneity of tissue preparation from ovaries and uterus with similar affinities of labeled ligand to these tissues. Jacobs and Cuatrecases[217] pointed out that non linearity may arise if both ligand and receptor preparation are heterogeneous. This situation also arises if the nonspecific binding (to tissue, to tube, etc) is not define or too high[218]. The correct definition of nonspecific (and thus specific) binding is very important.

3 The Effect of PH on The Receptor Binding

The effect of pH on the binding is shown in Fig. 3.3. The binding of ^{125}I-hCG to the human ovary and uterus homogenates exhibited pH optimum between 7.0-7.4. It was not determined whether the decreased binding at suboptimum pH values resulted from a decrease in binding affinity, binding rate, or inactivation of the receptors. It is known that these two homogenates incubated at pH 4.5 for 1h at 37°C loses irreversibly 75% of its binding capacity. Optimum pH binding has been reported for purified hCG-R by Pandian and Bahl[158] in bovine corpus luteal plasma membrane preparation to be (7.2-7.4). Bellisario et.al.,[208] observed that the optimum pH binding of rat testis hCG-Rs was between (6.3-7.3). The binding experiments of rat ovarian receptor in previous reports have been carried out almost exclusively at pH 7.4[156][207][149].

4 Temperature Dependency of The Binding

The temperature dependency of the association of ^{125}I-hCG with it receptor isolated from malignant and benign tumors of ovary and uterus was investigated. Fig.(3.4) shows that the binding of ^{125}I-hCG to the receptor was greater at 37°C than at 4, 25 and 45°C when incubation for 1hr. when binding was carried out for 1h at 37°C, 15-30% of the ^{125}I-hCG was bounded for different tissue preparations. It seems that the hCG has high binding affinity to the receptor and need only 1hr to reach equilibrium, also seems that the equilibrium of binding depend on temperature, at 4 and 25°C need more than 1hr to give maximum binding, while at 45°C thermal inactivation of the receptor may be occur. Thus, time course experiment is important to confirm these observations. In all previous reports, binding experiments have been done either at 37°C for 1hr or at 4°C for 24hr[154].

5 Time Course of Receptor Binding

21

Association characteristics of ^{125}I-hCG with human homogenates were examined at different temperatures (4, 25, 37°C). As illustrated by Fig.(3.5), maximum binding with both ovarian and uterine homogenates was greater at 37°C than 25°C.Furthermore, the maximum binding that occurred after 24hr of incubation at 4°C was nearly the same as at 37°C for 1hr. When binding was carried out at 25°C, the maximum binding of ^{125}I-hCG was at (6-10hr). As shown in Fig.(3.5) incubation of ^{125}I-hCG with ovarian and uterine homogenates for time periods longer than that required for maximum binding resulted in decreased binding, the loss of binding was more rapid at 37°C than at 25°C. This inactivation process could result from inactivation of ^{125}I-hCG or the human receptor during the binding assay. The results (as shown later) from stability experiment confirmed a time-dependent loss of binding activity of receptor at various temperature. Bellisario et.al.,[208] observed partial degradation of ^{125}I-hCG occurs during the binding assay in addition to the loss of rat testis receptors activity depending on temperature and time incubation. The results from previous reports are in agreement with our results. Bruch et.al.,[156] observed that the maximum binding of ^{125}I-hCG to the rat ovarian receptor at 4°C, was after 24hr of incubation. Pandian et.al.,[158] found that the binding of ^{125}I-hCG to the bovine corpus Luteal receptor was greater at 37°C than at 4 and 25°C and the equilibrium reached in 2 to 10hr depending on the temperature. Huhtaniemi an Catt[211] observed in their work on testicular receptor that the maximum binding with ^{125}I-hCG was at 24°C for 16h.

6 Stability of Receptor Homogenate and Hormone Receptor Complex

To prove the receptor inactivation at various temperatures at time course experiment, preincubation of the ovarian and uterine homogenates at 25°C and

37°C were performed. Time-dependent loss of binding activity was shown in Fig. (3.6) for hCG-Rs at these two temperatures.

The loss of receptor activity was greater at 37°C than at 25°C and was irreversible. Preincubation of the receptor homogenates in benign and malignant conditions at 37°C and 25°C for 2hr resulted in a loss of (45-50) and (9-10) of the initial binding activity respectively. In this regard, the stability was similar to the stability observed previously with ovarian and testicular receptor[156][208].

For further investigation, the effect of temperature on receptor properties, the ^{125}I-hCG-receptor complex was reincubated at three temperature (4, 25, 37°C) and the relative binding was estimated. As shown in Fig.(3.7), hCG-receptor complex were readily dissociated at the higher temperature. Approximately, 80% of dissociation was observed at 37°C after 8hr. This result was consistent with the apparent thermal sensitivity of the crude native receptor homogenate at 37°C when incubated in the absence of hCG. The hCG binding characteristic of the receptor at 4°C was stable, while (40-45%) of performed complex were dissociated at the 25°C after 8hr Thermal sensitivity of the hCG-receptor complex has been previously observed by Bruch et.al.,[156] when they studied the dissociation of hCG receptor complex at different temperature (4, 22, 37°C). Approximately 60% of preformed complex were dissociated at 22°C while complete dissociation was observed at 37°C after 24hr.

7- Determination of the Equilibrium Binding Constants and Maximum Binding Capacity

Ligand - receptor interaction usually follow a reversible binding reactions, thus they require to be performed under steady state or equilibrium conditions. At equilibrium or steady state the rate of the forward reaction equals the rate of the reverse reaction. The equilibrium binding constant may then be defined either as an association binding constant (K_a) or as dissociation binding constant (K_d). Knowing the concentrations of ligand bound (B) and free (F) at equilibrium allow to determine of both the equilibrium binding constant (K_d) and the maximum number of binding sites (B_{max}) by Scatchard equation[206]

$$\frac{B}{F} = \frac{B_{max}}{Kd} \quad B$$

the Scatchard equation allows a linear transformation of binding data so that K_d and B_{max} may readily be determined from radioligand saturation experiments, by incubating the concentrations of the radioligand with a fixed concentration of tissue receptor. A binding saturation study can then be performed over a range of radioligand concentration, from 10-20% of the estimated K_d to four to five time this value[217].

Scatchard analysis of saturation curves in our study (Fig. 3.8) indicated a single class of binding sites for hCG-R in benign and malignant tissues and, also indicated high affinity and low capacity for receptor in uterus tissue. The values of K_a of malignant and benign ovarian and uterine receptor did not alter significantly and were of the order of 10^{10} M^{-1} (Table 3.2). This result was consistent with the previous results of the determination of K_a . Bruch et.al.,[156] demonstrated that the value of K_a of the crude receptor from rat ovarian was 6.88($\pm$0.33) x 10^{10} M^{-1}. Pandian and Bahl[158] reported the value of K_a of the receptor in bovine corpus Luteal membrane, which was 4.9x10^{10} M^{-1}, while Dattatreyamurty et.al.,[157] pointed out that the value of K_a of the crude receptor did not alter from that of purified. Dufau et.al.,[219] showed the presence of a single order of binding sites with high affinity (10^{10} M^{-1}) for hCG of gonadotropin receptor of the rat testis, Bellisorio and Bahl[208] confirmed this result in their study. Keutmann[229] indicated that there was only modest increase in the association constant of the purified receptor over that was determined in crude receptor from bovine corpora lutea homogenate. ($3.28(\pm0.21) \times 10^{10}$ M^{-1}, $8.88(\pm 1.08) \times 10^{10}$ M^{-1}, respectively). Huhtaniemi and Catt[211] in their study found a differential binding affinities of rat testis hCG-R for hLH and hCG obtained that the value of K_a for hCG was 6.5×10^{10} M^{-1} where for LH was 2.25×10^{10} M^{-1}.

8 Specificity of Binding

The specificity of hCG binding was evaluated in competition experiments with unlabeled glycoprotein hormones[218]. A fixed concentration of ^{125}I-hCG was incubated with increasing concentration of unlabeled hormone, competition curves were then generated, and the concentration of unlabeled hormone displacing 50% of specific ^{125}I-hCG (IC$_{50}$), and affinity constant of unlabeled ligand (K_i) were determined.

The ^{125}I-hCG binding to the receptor was inhibited in a dose-dependent manner by the hCG (native and from serum of choriocarcinoma (chCG)) and LH (Fig.3.9). as shown in the Figure, the binding of ^{125}I-hCG by homogenates is specifically displaced by low concentration of hCG,unlabeled hCG, and LH. The curves of hCG and LH yield similar slopes.

The doses of hCG and LH that resulted in 50% displacement of the ^{125}I-hCG (IC$_{50}$) were shown in (Table 3.3). The ChCG was about (1.5-2.5) times more effective in competition for binding than native hCG. Other glycoprotein hormones such as FSH, TSH are inactive in competition for binding, with relative potency 0.014, 0.008, respectively. The binding inhibition observed with TSH and FSH may result from low level contamination with LH in these preparations. The results of

25

competition experiments revealed a high affinity receptor sites for hCG and LH in malignant and benign homogenates, but hCG was more effective in competing with ^{125}I-hCG for binding sites than LH, this results was expected for hCG receptor, where hCG is higher affinity for these receptor as compared to LH[149]. The same binding affinities for the hCG, LH have been previously observed[156][208][158]. In addition, hCG from serum of choriocarcinoma was more effective in competing with ^{125}I-hCG than native hCG (Fig. 3.9),this may results from asialo hCG produced by malignant cells[221] . Choriocarcinoma produce tumor-specific glycosylation variant of hCG. Numerous studies have demonstrated that asilo hCG exhibited greater binding to the hCG-R than native hCG. Bellisario and Bahl[158], in their study, demonstrated that asialo hCG exhibited greater binding to the rat testis and liver homogenates than native hCG, they indicated to the presence of additional binding sites for the asialo, hormone. Bruch et.al.,[156] also obtained that asialo hCG had higher binding affinities than intact hCG to ovarian homogenate. Keutmann et.al.,[222] in their characterization of deglycosylated hCG obtained a high affinity of asialo hCG to receptor than native hCG. However, it has been believed that hCG by its carbohydrate chains bind to a lectin-like membrane component to give the biological response and remove of the terminal sialic acid enhance binding to these lectine component by decreased electrostatic repulsion[19][223].

Table 3.1 Binding activity of ^{125}I-hCG with hCG-R in particulate membrane

preparations of benign and malignant ovarian and uterine tumors

(All details are explained in the text)

Crude membrane preparation		protien mg	^{125}I-hCG Binding activity pmol($\pm$S.E.M)	specific activity pmol/mg protein
ovary	Malignant	0.7	1.1$\pm$0.25	1.6$\pm$0.36
	Benign	0.7	0.55$\pm$0.28	0.8$\pm$0.4
uterus	Malignant	0.7	0.2$\pm$0.15	0.3$\pm$0.2
	Benign	0.7	0.08$\pm$0.014	0.11$\pm$0.2

27

	Ovarian	homogenates	Uterine	homogenates
	Benign	Malignant	Benign	Malignant
$K_d x 10^{-10}$ (M^{-1})	0.15 (±0.06)	0.13 (±0.09)	0.13 (±0.02)	0.12 (±0.07)
$K_a x 10^{10}$ (M^{-1})	6.6 (±1.2)	7.7 (±1.7)	7.7 (±1.0)	8.3 (±1.5)
B_{max} (pM/mg)	3.2 (±0.49)	3.6 (±0.28)	0.93 (±0.33)	1.3 (±0.3)

Table 3.2 Scatchard analysis of saturation binding curves for hCG-R in

ovarian and uterine homogenate.

(All details are explained in the text)

Effectors	IC_{50} (ng)	Relative potency	$K_i x 10^{-12}$ M^{-1}
With ovarian homogenate			
hCG	2.4	1	0.78
LH	4.0	0.6	1.3
chCG	1.0	2.4	0.32
FSH	900	0.0026	290
TSH	1000	0.0024	322
With uterine homogenate			
hCG	0.95	1	0.31
LH	1.8	0.53	0.6
chCG	0.8	1.2	0.26
FSH	-	-	-
TSH	-	-	-

Table 3.3 Specificity hCG binding to the receptor.

(All details are explained in the text)

Evaluation of Some Biochemical Constituents in

Gynecologic Cancers

5.1 CEA,LDH, and AIP Kits

1- Carcinoemryonic antigen (CEA) IRMA Kit was provided by (OCPA.France) and contains one vial of ^{125}I-rabbit-antiCEA antibody, one hundred test tubes coated with anti CEA antibodies, seven vials of human CEA standard with concentrations ranging of (0-200 ng/ml), two vials of control serum, one vial of assay buffer, and tube of wash reagent.

2- Lactate dehydrogenase (LDH) Kit for colorimetric determination was provided by (Randox, England) and contains one vial of 0.8 mmol/l sodium pyruvate in phosphate buffer PH 7.45, 10 Vial of NADH (1mg/ml)(each vial content reconstituted with 10ml of buffer before used), and one vial of color reagent (1mmol/L 2,4-dinitrophenydrazine in hydrochloric acid).

3- Alkaline phosphates Kit for colorimetric determination was provided by (bio Merieux-Frane) and contains substrate buffer vial (5mmol/l Dinatriumphenylphosphate in 50 mmol/l carbonate bicarbonate buffer pH 10), standard phenol reagent equal to 20 Kind and King U, inhibitor reagent (60mmol/l amino -4antipyrine with 75 g/l sodium arsenate), color reagent (150mmol/l potassium ferricyanide).

5.2 Apparatus

The apparatus, mentioned in section 2.2 were used in the

experiments of this chapter.

5.3 Patients and Specimens

The study group consisted of benign and malignant patients, and

control group described in section 2.3. The sera of these groups were

collected as described in section 2.4.and tissues homogenates and were

prepared as described in section 2.4.

5.4 CEA Quantitative Measurement

The level of CEA was measured in the sera and tissues of patients by the

immunoradiometric assay (IRMA). The assay protocol was described in

Table 5.1., according to manufacturer instructions.

5.5 Determination of LDH Activity

Colorimetric method was used to determine LDH activity. The

method is based on the reduction of pyruvate to lactate in the presence of

NADH by the action of lactate dehydrogenase.

LDH

$$\longrightarrow \text{Pyruvate} + NADH + H^+$$

The pyruvate that remains unchanged reacts with 2,4-dinitrophenylhydrazine to give the corresponding phenylhydrazone which is determined calorimetrically in alkaline medium at 520 nm. The assay protocol was described in Table 5.2, according to manufacture instructions

Table (5.1): Assay protocol of CEA

Tube number	CEA standards ng/ml							Control serum	Samples
	0	2.3	4.8	9.6	19.6	60.0	210.0		
	1,2	3,4	5,6	7,8	9,10	11,12	13,14	15,16	17,18
Standard Control Patient samples (μL)	←-------------------------------- 100uL ----------------- -------------→								
Assay buffer (μL)	------------------------------- 100 μL -------------- ←--- -------------→								
	Shaking for 2h at 25 ℃								
Wash buffer	←---------------------------1 ml ----------------------------								

(ml)	------------→
	Aspirate, wash once with wash buffer
^{125}I-anti CEA(µL)	←----------------------------100uL --------------------- ---------→
	Shaking for 1h at 25°C
Wash buffer (ml)	←--------------------------1 ml -------------------------- -------------→
	Aspirate,wash once with wash buffer, measurment of the radioactivity bound in gamma counter

Calculation

1- The radioactivity of all standards measured in (CPM) bound was

plotted vs. their concentration (Fig 5.1).

2- The samples and control values of CEA were read from standard

curve.

Table 5.2 : Assay protocol of LDH

Tube number	Sodium pyruvate with NADH(U/L)						Serum sample
	0	111.4	223.1	334.9	390.6	446.3	

	1,2	3,4	5,6	7,8	9,10	11,12	13,14
Sodium pyruvate with NADH(ml)	0.9	0.7	0.5	0.3	0.2	0.1	0.9
Distilled water(ml)	0.1	0.3	0.5	0.7	0.8	0.9	
Serum sample(ml)							0.1
	Mixing, incubation in a water bath at 37^{0}C for exactly 30 min						
Color reagent	←--------------------------------1 ml --------------------------- ----------------→						
	Mixing, let stand at room temperature for 20 min						
1.6% NaoH(ml)	←-----------------------------10 ml --------------------------------- ----------------→						
	Mixing, let stand at room temperature for 10 min. Reading absorbance of sample or standards against distilled water at 520 nm						

Calculations:

1-The absorbance of samples (1-12) are plotted vs. the corresponding

values in U/L (Fig 5.2).

2-The serum LDH activity was determined from calibration curve.

5.6 Analysis of LDH by Electrophoresis

LDH isoenzyme was separated by poly acrylamide gel electrophoresis as described in section (4.6.2). The enzyme activity bands were

LDH developed according to following reactions[272]:

Lactate+NAD$^+$ Pyryvate+NADH+H

NADH+Phenazain methosulfate NAD$^+$ +Phenazin methosulfate

Phenaz methosulfate (PMS) +nitroblue tetrazolium (MBT)

Nitroblue tetrazolium formazan

(Violt

ppt)+phenazain methosulfate

After electrophoresis , the working solution was added on the gel, then incubation for 60 min at 37^{0}C, The violet bands appeared and the gel was placed in fixing solution for 10 min to fix the bands.

Solutions:

Working solution : was prepared by mixing 1ml of 2 mol/l sodium lactate, 3ml of

1mg/ml NBT, 0.3ml of 1mg/ml/PMS and 1ml of

0.056 mol/l Tris

buffer pH 7.4 then 15 mg of NAD$^+$ was added .

Fixing solution: was prepared by mixing methanol, distilled water, glacial acetic acid in ratio of 5:4:1

5.7 Determination of Alkaline Phosphates Activity

Colorimetric method was used to determine AIP activity according to

the following reaction

Alkaline phosphatase, pH10

Phenylphosphate   phenol +phosphate

The liberated phenol was measured in the presence of amino 4-

antipyrine and potassium ferricyanide. The presence of sodium arsenate

in the reagent stops the enzymatic reaction. The assay protocol was

described in Table 5.3: according to manufacturer instructions.

Table 5.3 Assay protocol of ALP

	Serum	Serum blank	Standard	Reagent

Tube number	sample			
	1,2	3,4	5,6	7,8
Substrate buffer (ml)	←-------------------------------2 ml ---→			
	Incubation for 5 min at 37^{0}C			
Serum sample (µL)				←--50 µl ---→
Standard (µL)				←--50 µl ---→
	Incubation exactly 15 min at 37^{0}C			
Inhibitor	←-----------------------------0.5 ml ---→			
	Mixing			
Color reagent	←-----------------------------0.5 ml ---→			
Serum sample				←--50 µl ---→
Distilled water				←--50 µl ---→
Mixing, let stand for 10 min in the dark. Reading absorbance at 510 nm against reagent blank				

Calculation

$$A_{\text{serum sample}} - A_{\text{serum blank}} / A_{\text{standard}} \ X \ 142$$

Kind and king U/L=Enzyme activity unit=One kind and king unit is that

an mount of enzyme which in the given conditions liberates 1mg of

phenol in 15 min at 37^0C

4.8 Determination of Heat Stable Alkaline Phosphatase Activity

(HSAP):

Heat stable alkaline phosphatase (HSAP) activity was measured after

the complete inactivation of all AIP isoenzymes by heating the sample for

15 min at 55^0C in a water bath[50]. Fifty microliter of serum sample was

incubated for 15 min at 55^0C in a water bath. Immediately after

incubation the inactivated serum was cooled at ice temperature. The

remaining activity was measured by the same methods of AIP (section

5.7)

4.9 Determination of the Elements (Cu^{++}, Zn^{++}, Ca^{++}) Concentrations

in the Sera of Tumor Patients

Copper, zinc,Ca were determined by flame atomic absorption

spector- photometry[73].Serum trace element levels were measured using

serum diluted (1:2) with deionized distilled water, while Ca^{++} level was

measured using serum diluted (1:10) with deionized distills water. The

concentrations of the elements were determined by comparing the signal

from diluted serum with that from appropriate aqueous calibration

39

standards, which were prepared. Patients with metastases were excluded

when calcium was determined.

Results and Discussion

Biochemical Constituents in Ovarian and Endometrial Cancer

Patients

The levels of the biochemical constituents in the sera of patients

studies were as summarized in Tables 5.4, 5.5, and 5.6. As can be seen

from the Tables, all the biochemical constituents had higher mean values

in patients as compared to the controls.

CEA levels of sera of ovarian and endometrial cancer patients were

slightly elevated and most modestly elevated in endometrial cancer. CEA

was elevated in 43% of ovarian cancer and 33% of endometrial cancer

patients as compared to 7% in the control population Table (5.4). The

incidence of antigen elevation in patients with invasive cancer was 25%

higher than that in patients with stage I cancer. The higher levels of CEA

were found in patients with mucinous ovarian neoplasms. CEA

immunoreactivity also has been determined in the patient's tissues. The

elevation of tissue CEA levels appeared to be statistically significant than

in the corresponding sera samples ($p < 0.05$) in ovarian malignant

condition (Fig 5.3), while the difference was not significant in

endometrial cancer. The results of determination of the CEA in the sera and tissues of gynecologic tumor patients indicated that CEA was not tumor specific and was found in some benign conditions. These results confirms previous observation from other investigator, where CEA activity in tissues can be demonstrated in most gynecological cancers while serum levels are often too modestly elevated to be useful for diagnosis or for monitoring. Stall et.al.,[255] showed slightly elevated plasma CEA level in approximately 50% of ovarian cancer patients , and mucinous tumors tend to have highest levels. Tuxen et.al., [26] also found elevated serum CEA levels in patients with mucinous histotypes ovarian cancer.Bast et.al., [39], and Tuxen et.al., [26][254] obtained that the combination of CEA and CA125 would have a higher sensitivity and specificity than CA125 alone, in monitoring human ovarian cancer. In the uterus, adenocarcinoma that arise in the endocervix express a greater amount of CEA than adenocarcinomas of the endometriums [251-253]. It is reflected in the reported frequency of elevated plasma CEA level:68% in cervical adenocarcinoma and 34% in endometrial adenocarcinoma, therefore, have therapeutic consequences when doubt exists as to the origin of a uterine tumor[40]. Squamous cell carcinoma of cervical cancers also express CEA and high levels indicated in advanced disease[41]. In immunohistochemical studies, CEA was detected in 60-63% of cervical squamous cell carcinoma , and in 77% of cases of cervical adenocarcinoma [256-258].Generally, in gynecologic cancers a high

41

pretreatment values of serum CEA indicate awide spread of tumor[99] and

poor prognosis[251-253]. CEA have also been demonstrated in a large

variety of malignancies included, cancers of the colon and pancreas and

elevated concentration, varies with the tumor type and the stage of

disease [249][250]. CEA also elevated in several non cancerous condition,

such as smoking or hepatic dysfunction.

It is evident from the Table 5.5 that the mean levels of LDH

activity were higher in cancer patients then those of healthy individuals

but the differences were not statistically significant. The highest elevation

of LDH activity was observed the invasive stage of ovarian cancer (stage

I FIGO.133±24.343 U/L, and satageII+III FIGO.185.6±47.54U/L). The

electrophoresis pattern of serum LDH isoenzyme in ovarian cancers (Fig

5.4) showed an additional band (extra band). This extra isoenzyme moved

faster than LDH_1 which means that its charge is more negative than

LDH_1.LDH, is elevated in the sera of patients with a variety of

cancers[259]. Evaluation of serum levels of this enzyme was documented

to be significantly advantageous in diagnosis and treatment monitoring of

patients with gynecological cancers[43-47], and its level reflect tumor

burden as well as tumor growth or regression .However LDH as single

marker has not proved sufficient to meet the full requirements of clinical

application. Increased serum LDH value in malignancies is

multifunctional and no single explanation can be put forward of account for whole spectrum of malignancies. LDH is often elevated in epithelial

ovarian cancer[259], cervical cancer[47] and many solid

malignancies[17],making it a non-specific tumor marker. This isoenzyme

provide marginal specificity for organ involvement[44]. The elevation of

LDH_5 was associated with liver metastases and central nervous system

metastases[17]. In dysgerminom, the two fast fraction(s)(LDH_1 and LDH_2)

were increased and their activity appeared to parallel the response to

therapy[45],LDH_3 was found to be elevated in multiple myeloma. Add

ional band has been found in hepato cellular cancer patients[17].

The results of total AIP determination indicated that the mean

values in cancer patients were higher than control and significantly

different (Table 5.6). Different stages of ovarian and endometrial cancers

appeared different levels of total AIP. The results of HSAP estimation

showed that mean value in patients with ovarian and endometrial cancers

were significantly increase compared to the control group (Table 5.6).

The HSAP levels did not correlate with tumor stage. This

isoenzyme has been found to be more useful as tumor marker in

gynecologic cancers than total AIP because the differences between

cancer and control groups were clear. It has been reported that HSAP

43

appeared in 21-22% of cases of cervical cancer and in 25% of cases of endometrial cancer[260][261]. Elevated serum HSAP has been found in 64% of ovarian cancer patients[49], but by using a radioimmunoassay and a polyclonal antibody for placental AIP determination, only 18% of cases showed elevated levels .HSAP has previously been reported to be useful in combination with lipid bound sialic acid (LSA), in diagnosis, and treatment monitoring for cancer patients [50][274]. The changes in the HSAP level were also reported in benign tumor of ovary[49][261].

Copper, Zinc, Calcium in the Sera of Ovarian and Endometrial Cancer Patients

The results of determination copper, zinc, and calcium ions concentration are illustrated in Table (5-7). These results showed that sera zinc levels were significantly higher ($p < 0.05$) in ovarian and endometrial cancers groups than in the control group. In benign group, zinc levels remained without alteration .Serum copper levels were not significantly higher in the two cancer groups when compared with those of controls, although the mean values were higher in cancers groups. No alteration in the level of copper ion was observed in the sera of benign tumor as compared to healthy individual. The patients with ovarian and endometrial cancers showed no significant difference in their sera calcium levels from those of the control group. However, two patients of ovarian cancer and one of endometrial cancers were hypercalcemic (10.5, 11.1 and 10.6 mg/dl respectively).

High levels of zinc in the ovarian and endometrial cancer are in agreement with studies that indicate, the zinc level was increased in different cancer patients[275][265][261]. It has been suggested that the zinc might play a possible role in tumor growth promotion.

The copper in serum exists largely in the form of ceruloplasmin (more than 90%) a metalloprotein of Mwt (132 kDa) contain 6 atoms of copper/ molecule[275].

The copper levels of cancer sera in our study did not significantly change but some studies reported elevation in ceruloplasmin level in some cancer such as breast and lung cancers[256]. It is known that copper plays some role in angiogenesis, where it is required for development of new tissue as well as tumor growth possibly through the mediation of copper –dependent amine oxidases. The increase of zinc to copper ratio in the sera of cancer patients reflects the implication of the zinc and copper in the cancerous process of the tissue, so it may be useful as a tumor marker for the evaluation of the status of gynecologic cancers.

Although the mean values in the present study for ovarian and endometrial cancers patients showed no significant difference in their sera calcium levels, from those of the control group, but some cancer patients were hypercalcaemic. Hypercalcemia is a common complication of cancer and usually associated with bone metastasis[270]. Calcium is present in serum in three distinct fractions, free or ionized calcium account for about 50% of total calcium, about 5% complexed with variety of anions particularly phosphate and citrate, and the remaining 45% of Ca is bound to plasma protein especially to albumin[276].Calcium homeostasis involves three major organs, the small intestine, the kidney and the skeleton. Hypercalcemia has been reported in breast, lung, kidney cancers without the presence of bone metastases[268].PTH like peptides were found in about 49% of patients with malignant hypercalcaemia and 16% of patients with malignant normocalcaemic state. It have also been reported that cancer tissue in the human being was capable of direct osteolysis(277). Rieke et.al.,(269) reported a hypercalcemic state (with the absence of bone destruction) in Hodgkins disease. They suggested elevated levels of 1,25 dihydroxy Vit D3. Hypercalcamia on malignancy was thought to be due to progression of the tumor tissue[277]. Hypercalcacmia has also referred to osteoclast activating factors which are released locally by tumor. These include prostaglandin E2[278], interlukin I, tumor necrosis factor[279] such as Beta lymphotoxin, epidermal growth factor [280], and transforming growth factor beta[281].

Table 5.4 The values of CEA levels in sera of patients with

gynecologic tumors

(All details are explained in the text)

Tumor	Group	%of elevated CEA >5ng/ml *(Elevated /total)	Mean ± S.E.M of all patients ng/ml	Statistical *significant
Ovarian	*C	7(2/30)	3.96±1.25	
	*B	11(4/35)	4.11±1.79	*NS
	*M	43(6/14)	12.25±12.8	P<0.05
Uterine	C	7(2/30)	3.96±1.25	
	B	13(3/24)	3.97±1.76	NS
	M	33(3/9)	6.33±3.64	P<0.05

*C: control

*B: benign

47

*M: malignant

NS: not significant

Elevated/Total:numberof patients with CEA above 5mg/ml/number of

patients with CEA below 5mg/ml.

Table 5.5 Lactate dehydrogenase (LDH) activity in sera of patients

with gynecologic tumors (All details are explained in the text)

Tumor	Group	*N	mean±S.E.M(U/ml)	Statistical significance
Ovarian	*C	30	144.78±32.5	
	*B	35	145.6±24.7	NS
	*M	14	156.57±28.8	NS
Uterine	C	30	144.78±30.5	
	B	24	143.93±26.5	NS
	M	9	146.51±67.34	NS

C:control

B:benign

M:malignant

NS:not significant

N:number of patients.

Table 5.6 AIP activity and HSAP activity in sera of patients with

gynecologic tumors (All details are explained in the text)

T tumor	Group	*N	mean ±S.E.M of AIP U/L	Statistical significance	mean ±S.E.M. of HSAP U/L	Statistical significance
Ovarian	C	30	58.5±19.4		2.3±0.3	
	B	35	60.3±12.3	NS	2.2±0.6	NS
	M	14	81.5±26.5	P<0.05	5.5±0.4	P<0.05
Uterine	C	30	58.5±19.4		2.3±0.3	
	B	24	65.9±14.6	NS	2.4±0.9	NS
	M	9	78.5±32.3	P<0.05	4.6±0.5	P<0.05

*M: Malignant

*B: Benign

* C control

*N: Number of patients

*NS: Not Significant

Table 5.7 Copper (Cu^{++}), Zinc (Zn^{++}) and Calcium (Ca^{++})

concentration in the sera of ovarian and endometrial cancers patients

Tumor	No. of patients	Copper mean±S.E.M	Zinc mean±	Zn^{++}/Cu^{++}	Calcium men±S.E.mg/100ml

		μmol/l	μmol/l		
Ovarian					
*M	8	17.3±1.5	13.3±3.2	0.75	10.1±1.2
*B	10	16.6±1.6	7.4±1.1	0.44	9.5±0.08
*C	25	16.7± 0.71	7.1 ± 0.45	0.42	9.7 ± 0.7
Uterine	9	17.4±1.8	10.7 ± 2.15	0.61	9.9±0.3
*M	10	17.1± 0.85		0.4	9.6±0.16
*B			6.8 ± 1.9		
*C	25	16.7± 0.71	7.1 ± 0.45	0.42	9.7±0.7

*M: Malignant

*B: Benign

*C: Control

most important tumor marker for early detection, staging and monitoring men **with prostate cancer** [5].

Further analysis with this molecule revealed that it is identical to both the protein ==

1.1 Introduction

Prostate specific antigen (PSA) is a 33-34 KD, single- chain glycoprotein of 240 amino acid residues with four glucidic side chains .The molecular features   7-10% carbohydrate contents, 3.1 S sedimentation coefficient and isoelectric point at pH 6.8-7.5[1,2]. It is secreted by the epithelial cells lining the acini and ducts of the prostate gland [3], and found exclusively in the tissue of normal, benign hyperplastic, and cancerous prostate gland as well as in seminal plasma and prostatic fluid [1].

This antigen which was first identified in 1978[4], is a member of the human *kallikrein* family, and nowadays is widely used as the eminal fluid by *Hara et al* in 1974, and the *protein p30*, also isolated from plasma seminal fluid by *Sensabaugh et al* in 1978 [6].

Prostate specific antigen is known to be a serine protease enzyme with chymotrypsin and trypsin like activity [7]. Its physiological role is believed to be liquefaction of the seminal coagulum forming after ejaculation [8].

A percent of 60-80% of the PSA secreted in the seminal plasma have chymotrypsin and trypsin like activity, while the remaining 20-40% are enzymatically inactive, presumably due to an internal bond cleavage between two lysine residues [7]. But when PSA is released in the blood, 70-90% of its total amount (t-PSA) is inactivated by the major extracellular serine protease inhibitors: α_1 - *antichymotrypsin* (α_1ACT), α_2-*macroglobulin* (α_2M), and other acute phase proteins. In addition, about 10-30% of it may exist in a free uncomplexed form   (f-PSA) [9-10].

Total PSA, (i.e.: all of the immunologically detectable forms), consisting primarily of (PSA-ACT) and (f-PSA), has served as an excellent indicator of prostate disease when the concentration exceeds 4.0 ng/ml in serum [11]. While the portion of PSA in the blood inactivated by (α_2M) is non–immunoreactive because it is probably engulfed in the (α_2M) structure [3]. The serum concentration is also increased with the prostate volume and the stage of the prostate cancer [12].

Lilja et al and *Stenman et al* demonstrated that the proportion of (PSA-ACT) complex increases as a function of (t-PSA) concentration, they also showed that this proportion in BPH is somewhat less than that of PCA [13]. Accordingly many studies have suggested that the ratio of (f-PSA/t-PSA), (f-PSA%) allows a better discrimination between BPH and PCA [14].

Although previously thought to be produced exclusively by the epithelial cells of the prostate, PSA at present is considered a wide spread biochemical marker present in many non–prostatic tissues and fluids [15]. Many studies indicate that the PSA expression in both physiological and pathological conditions, is not organ or sex – specific, but rather a steroid hormone mediated response [16].

1.2 The Prostate [17-20]

The prostate gland, figure (1-1), is the largest accessory sex organ in males. It consists with the *Cowper's glands* and the seminal vesicles a system of exocrine glands whose secretions constitutes the bulk of seminal fluids in which sperm are conveyed. It starts to develop at the twelfth week of fetal life under the influence of androgenic hormones from the fetal testes.

The prostate is situated immedialty below the internal urethral orifice surrounding the neck of the bladder and urethra. The normal prostate in an adult weighs about 20 grams and it has the shape of a blunted cone. Anteriorly and laterally, a capsule composed of fibrous and smooth muscle tissue surrounds the prostate.

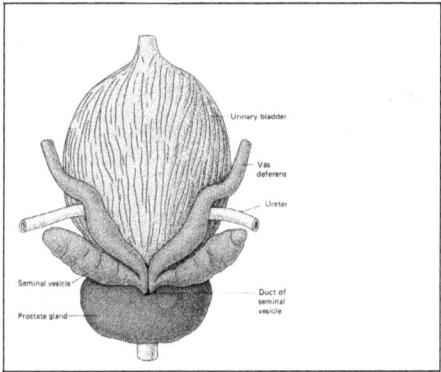

Figure (1-1): A posterior view of the bladder, seminal vesicle, and prostate gland [19].

1.2.1 Histology [17,21]

The prostate is a complex organ consisting of acinar, stromal, and muscular elements. In the early 1970's **Mc Neal** proposed a concept of zonal anatomy, figure (1-2), based on histology and anatomy that is currently used as the basis for describing the location and perhaps the origin of neoplastic processes within the prostate. According to this concept, the glandular portion of the prostate is composed of a large peripheral zone and a small central zone, which together constitute about 95% of the gland. The transition zone forms the other 5%. This zone is located just outside the urethra at the verumontanum and is composed of the periurethral glands, which presumably are responsible for all of the BPH. Sixty to seventy percent of prostatic cancer occurs in the peripheral zone, 10-20% in the transition zone, and 5-10% in the central zone.

Based on embryologic, ultrastructural and arterial injection studies, the prostate is now regarded as essentially two separate organs; figure (1-3):

1- The periurethral, female portion, which is sensitive to androgens and estrogens, and this represents the inner group of glands, commonly referred to as the female prostate. It gives rise to benign nodular hyperplasia. For this reason benign enlargement mainly produces urinary symptoms.

2- Subcapsular true male prostate, which is sensitive to androgens, this represents the outer group of glands which forms a horseshoelike sheath around the female prostate.

Figure (1-2): **A**- Schematic lateral view of the prostate. **B**- Cut section of the same. **C**-Transverse view of area shown in **A** [21].

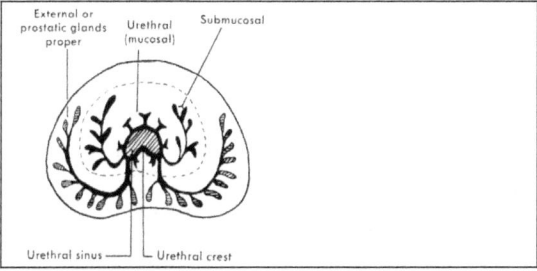

Figure (1-3):   Distribution of normal prostatic glands slightly modified. Urethral

(mucosal) and submucosal glands together form inner group, which is

separated from outer gland group by an inconstant capsule [17].

1.3 Pathological Conditions of the Prostate [17]

The pathological conditions of the prostate may be classified as:

1-*Non – tumours conditions:* these include

- acute prostatitis.
- chronic prostatitis.
- granulomatous prostatitis.
- parasitic infection.
- corpora amylasea and calculi.
- thrombosis and infarction.

2-*Tumours conditions:* these are subdivided into:

- **tumorlike lesions:** such as prostatic cysts, amyloid deposits and prostatic hyperplasia.
- **benign tumors**.
- **malignant tumors :** which includes various types of prostatic carcinoma .

1.3.1 Benign Prostatic Hypertrophy (BPH)

1.3.1.1 Incidence [17,22]

Non–neoplastic nodular enlargement of the prostate –*nodular hyperplasia*– is the most common symptomatic tumorlike condition in humans. It seldom occurs before the age of 50, but the incidence increases with age, and it can be found in 75% to 80% of men over age of 80. It appears a decade earlier in **Blacks** than in **Whites** and it is rare in **Orientals**.

The normal prostate in an adult weighs about 20g while the enlarged one can be two to four times larger, but seldom weighs more than 200g. However, one weighing 2,410 g has been reported two year ago [22] .

1.3.1.2 Theories of Causation of BPH [23]

- *The Hormonic Theory:* As age advances the male hormone diminishes while the quantity of the estrogenic hormone is not decreased equally. According to this theory the prostate enlarges due to disturbance of the ratio and quality of the circulating androgens and estrogens.
- *The Neoplastic Theory:* Postulates that the enlargement is a benign neoplasm. As the prostate is composed essentially of fibrous tissue, muscle tissue and glandular tissue, the neoplasm is *fibro-myo-adenoma*.

1.3.1.3 Clinical Stages in BPH [24,17]

The anatomic location of the prostate readily explains the symptoms of hyperplasia. Clinical features are variable depend upon the lobs effected:

Stage 1: Frequency, nocturia, and delayed initiation of voiding.

Stage 2: Benign decompensation, residual urine. Increasing frequency and pollakiuria.

Stage 3: Detrusor decompensation, over flow incontinence, constant dribbling, upper tract obstruction and kidney damage.

1.3.1.4 Diagnosis [24-26]

The diagnosis of the different stages can be made on the basis of the typical history. Rectal examination and measuring residual urine by sonography is used to diagnose the first and second stages, while in acute or chronic retention a catheter is diagnostically and therapeutically indicated. Latest methods recommend the use of digital rectal examination, serum PSA, urianalysis, serum creatinine and the AUA (American Urological Association) symptom score for the initial evaluation of BPH.

1.3.1.5 Treatment

Indications for treating patients with BPH may be absolute, in that treatment is urgently needed due to serious complications, or they may be relative depending on the degree to which the symptoms disrupt the patient's quality of life [27]. On a review of current treatment, an increasing number of options now exist, these include:

1- ***Operative Treatment*** [28-31]**:** Surgery is the gold standard in treatment of BPH. Trans urethral resection of the prostate (TURP) is the most frequently performed procedure, despite the continuing debate over its relative benefits and risks vs. open surgery. Instrumental techniques such as ***balloon dilation, stetnting*** and ***hyperthermia*** are still under investigation.

2- ***Laser Treatment of the prostate*** [32]**:** The use of laser technology in the ablation of prostatic tissue (***Laser prostatectomy***), is one of the new thermotherapies which has rapidly become a widely used procedure, primarily because of its ease to use, the minimal bleeding and the impressive safety profile in comparison to TURP. The tissue removal can be done by two different ways:

a- indirectly by heating the tissue to a maximum of 100°C, thus causing the coagulated tissue to slough after the procedure.

b- instantaneously by vaporizing the tissue while the temperature rise over 300°C; this modality causes the tissue to convert into vapors of water and hydrocarbons, thus creating immediate cavitations.

3- ***Pharmacologic Treatment*** [27]**:**

a- **α-Adrenergic Receptor Blockers:** Medical treatment of BPH is presently dominated by α-adrenergic blockers, they increase urinary flow and improve symptoms. The use of α-adrenergic blockers is based on a sound principle, since α-adrenergic receptors are wide spread in the prostate and bladder neck, where they increase smooth muscle tone. α-Blockers reduce muscle tone, there by reducing the dynamic component of prostatic obstruction.

b- **Plant Extracts** [27]**:** plant extracts are used extensively in a number of countries. The active ingredients are often not known. Some of these extracts are claimed to exert α-adrenergic blockers effects or *5α-reductase* inhibiting effects.

c- **Hormonal Therapy:** There are several options in this type of treatment :

- *Androgen Deprivation Therapy:* Androgens are essential to the growth of the prostate, notably the glandular epithelium. Androgen deprivation provides a mean of shrinking the prostate, thereby relieving obstruction and improving quality of life. This can be achieved by medical castration, using drugs with antiandrogenic activity [27,33,34], or drugs that act on the *hypophyseal teticular axis* such as *gonadotropin releasing hormone GnRH* analogue [35].

- *Aromatase Inhibitors* [27]*:* Aromatase, the enzyme that converts androgens to estrogens in peripheral tissue is responsible for producing a major part of circulating estrogens in men. Estrogens are believed to act synergistically with androgens in controlling prostate growth and predominantly on the stroma. Therefore aromatase inhibitors should diminish and improve symptoms.

- *5α-Reductase Inhibitors:* Such as *Finesteride,* which promotes stabilization of testosterone and *dihydroxy testosterone (DHT)* [36].

1.3.2 Prostate Cancer

1.3.2.1 Incidence

Prostate cancer is a malignancy of older age groups. The incidence increases between 60 and 80 years of age [37]. It is less common in the *Japanese*, while it is higher and its behavior is more aggressive in *Negros* compared with *Caucasian* population [23].

Carcinoma of the prostate usually originates in the external group of glands, this location is distant from the urethra, and the growth is therefore initially assymptomatic [24].

1.3.2.2 Etiology [17]

Although the cause of carcinoma of the prostate is unknown, androgens have been suspect. Testosterone accelerates the activity of carcinoma cells, whereas orchiectomy or estrogen therapy causes regression of tumor. These observations have led to the theory that androgens are responsible for carcinoma of the prostate. But prolonged administration of androgens has not produced any tumors, and cancer of the prostate occurs at the time of life when the level of androgens is low. The most prevalent hypothesis is that carcinoma of the prostate may begin at the stage of life when androgen levels are high and decline with advancing age.

1.3.2.3 Types of Prostate Carcinoma [17]

- *Latent carcinoma:* This type is found in autopsies of men dying of other causes.
- *Incidental carcinoma:* In 6-20% of tissue removed surgically for clinically BPH, histologic examination shows carcinoma of the prostate.
- *Occult carcinoma:* It is found in a number of patients who have no symptoms of prostatic carcinoma and show evidence of metastases on clinical examination.

- *Clinical carcinoma:* This includes all cases in which rectal examination has aroused suspicion of carcinoma and the diagnosis is confirmed by pathologic examination of the tissue removed from the prostate.

1.3.2.4 Signs and Symptoms [17, 21]

The only sign of prostate carcinoma may be an abnormal digital rectal examination (DRE), therefore any irregular, firm, or hard nodule, palpable on rectal examination should be biopsied.

In early carcinoma of the prostate, there are no distinct symptoms, and when present, they are indistinguishable from those of BPH. Late cancers usually manifest themselves through back pain, and anemia, which indicate bone metastasis.

1.3.2.5 Diagnosis [21,38,39]

The standard technique to delineate the local extent of disease is digital rectal examination (DRE) followed by CT* or MRI* to delineate lymph node involvement. In the last few years, transrectal ultrasonography (TRUS) with biopsy has been introduced to assess both volume of cancer within the prostate as well as extracapular extension of prostate cancer. Bone scintigraphy is still the preferred method to rule out metastatic involvement, acid phosphatase is being used less commonly, while cancer diagnosis has been aided greatly by the availability of PSA.

1.3.2.6 Treatment

The following alternative treatment options exists:

1- *Radical Prostatectomy (RP):* In the early stages the radical prostatectomy may be curative, i.e.: it is indicated only if the tumor is confined to the gland and no metastases detected [24].

2- *Orchiectomy:* The basic treatment for advanced prostate cancer is the bilateral orchiectomy (total or subcapsular) [24].

---

* See list of abbreviations

3- *Radiation Therapy*: The indication for *curative radiation* is given if the tumor is confined to the prostate and no metastatic spread is found while *palliative radiation* is used in advanced stages [24].

4- *Hormonal Treatment* [24,37,40]: The goal of the hormonal treatment is the suppression of androgen action. This can be achieved by interfering with *hypothalamus pituitary-axis* (extraprostatic) or by blocking the hormonal effect in the prostate (introprostatic), figure (1-4):

a- **Bilateral Orchiectomy**.

b- **Estrogen Treatment**: the estrogens administration suppress the *pituitary gonadotrophic hormone* (GnRH) production and inhibits *Leydig cell* activity.

c- **LHRH Analogues (medical castration):** these drugs cause a down regulation in pituitary (LHRH) receptors, thus suppressing the release of androgen from the testes.

d- **Antiandrogens:** antiandrogens acts by competitively blocking the binding of testosterone and its metabolite dihydroxy testosterone (DHT) to the nuclear androgen receptors in prostate cancer cells.

e- **Combined androgen blockade (CAB):** although castration, (medical or surgical), causes a reduction of about 90% in serum testosterone concentration, the androgen biosynthesis in the adrenal which contributes 8-10% of the total amount of androgens is not effected. This illustrates the extra benefit of (CAB) by the addition of antiandrogens to castration (medical or surgical), to create a completely free milieu.

5- *Chemotherapy*: due to sever side effects of chemotherapy, this treatment modality is only considered if all other treatment modalities have failed. Chymotherapeutic agents such as *estramustin phosphate*, *5- flouruuracil*, and *cyclophosphamide* have been tested with some success [24].

Figure (1-4): The goal of hormonal treatment for prostate cancer is the suppression of androgen action. This can be achieved by interfering with the hypothalamus-pituitary axis (extraprostatic) or by blocking the hormonal effect in the prostate (intraprostatic).

1.4 Tumor Markers

A tumor marker is a substance present in or produced by a tumor or by the tumor's host in response to the tumor's presence, that can be used to differentiate a tumor from normal tissue or to determine the presence of a tumor based on measurement in the blood or secretions [41]. It can be measured qualitatively or quantitatively by chemical, immunological, molecular biological methods to determine the presence of cancer [41].

A tumor marker can either be *specific* (unique to single tumor type) or *non- specific* (present in a variety of tumor types) [42]. Most tumor markers are present in normal, benign, and cancer tissues and are not specific enough to be used for screening cancer [43]. In fact the clinical utility of a tumor marker becomes almost totally dependent on its specificity and sensitivity. When a tumor marker assay said to be 100% sensitive, this means the assay can detect all patients with that particular type of cancer whereas, a 100% specific assay means the assay will identify only the patients with the specific type of a tumor and not those with benign or non-neoplastic disease [44].

Tumor markers are useful in screening, in determining therapy, in providing prognostic information, in monitoring the response to therapy and in detecting the relapse [45].

Table (1-1) lists different tumor markers classified according to their biochemical and biological characteristics, and their associated malignancies [45].

Table (1-1): Tumor markers, classified according to biological or biochemical characteristics, and their associated malignancies [45].

Marker type	Example		Associated Malignancy
Oncofetal antigens	Alpha-fetoprotein		Germ cell tumor, hepatoma
	Carcinoembryonic antigen		Colorectal, breast, stomach, lung
Tumor-associated antigens (carbohydrate antigens)	Carbohydrate determinant, e.g.CA 19-9		Gastrointestinal, pancreas
	Epithelial mucins, e.g. cancer-associated tumor antigen		Ovary, colorectal
	Glycoproteins	CA-125	Ovary, colorectal, breast, lung
		Prostatic-specific antigen	Prostate
Hormonal peptides	Beta-human chorionic gonadotrophin		Germ cell tumor, chorionic carcinoma
	Adrenocorticotrophic hormone		Pituitary, small-cell lung
Neuromediators	Catecholmines (24-hour urine)		Neuroblastoma
	5-hydroxyindoleacetic acid (24-hour urine)		Carcinoid
Proteins	Thyroglobulin		Thyroid
	Immunoglobulins		Myeloma, lymphomas
Enzymes	Neuron-specific enolase		Neuroblastoma, small-cell lung, medullary carcinoma of the thyroid
	Prostatic acid phosphatase (labile tartarate)		Prostate
	Lactate dehydrogenase		Most malignancies
	Placental alkaline phosphatase		Seminoma, dysgerminoma of breast, ovary
Oncogenes	c-*erb* B-2		Breast, stomach
Cytogenetic markers	Philadelphia chromosome		Chronic myeloid leukemia

1.5 Tumor Markers in Prostate Cancer

The incidence of prostate malignancy led to the search of markers to use for its detection. These are:

1.5.1 Prostatic Acid Phosphatase

Prostatic acid phosphates (orthophosphoric monoester phosphohydrolase EC.3.1.3.2) or PAP, is synthesized by the prostate gland and is one of the many acid phosphatase isoenzymes found in different human tissues and cells including liver, spleen, kidney, erythrocytes, platelets, osteoclasts, and hairy cell leukemias [46-50].

In 1938, **Gutman and Gutman** reported elevated serum acid phosphates activity in prostatic cancer patients, especially those with bone metastasis. This increased enzyme activity was subsequently shown to be of prostatic origin[51].

Normal levels of serum PAP have been reported in patients with BPH [52-54]. A transient increase of serum PAP Levels has been reported to occur after manipulation of the prostate gland [55]. Because other tissues may cause elevation in the enzyme activity, many efforts have been made to distinguish the prostatic isoenzyme from the isoenzymes of other origin. These efforts have been based on the different effect of various substrates and inhibitors on enzymes from these sources [44]. One of the most common inhibitors used is **L-tartarate**, which was shown to be useful as a specific inhibitor of PAP [56].

Development of immunoassay techniques that utilize the immunological reactivity of PAP rather than its enzymatic activity has resulted in greater specificity for the prostatic isoenzyme and greater sensitivity than the earlier enzyme   assays [55,18]. However, the specificity and sensitivity of PAP are low in diagnosing, staging and following patients with prostate cancer [57].

Presently PSA is superior to PAP for diagnosing, screening and monitoring prostate cancer. PAP may have an adjuvant value in the management of prostate cancer, because a combination of PSA and PAP testing has revealed a high sensitivity and specificity in detecting prostate cancer [57].

1.5.2 Prostrate Specific Antigen

This antigen was first discovered *by Albin and coworkers* in prostatic tissue in 1970 [58], and in seminal plasma in 1971 by *Hara et colleagues* [59]. They called it *gamma semino protein*.

In 1978 *Senabough* characterized this glycoprotein with isoelectric points from 6.5-8 in seminal plasma. They called it *p30* and regarded as a semen marker for use in forensic science [60]. In 1979, *Wang et al* were the first to isolate and purify PSA from prostatic tissue after injecting crude extracts of human prostatic tissue into rabbits. They discovered its importance as a prostate tumor marker and they were the first to name it PSA [2].

Few years later, several investigators proved that *gamma semino protein*, *p30*, and *PSA* are very similar biochemically [61,62].

Currently, PSA represents the best serum marker for prostate carcinoma, and it has the highest validity of any circulating marker for cancer today [63].

1.5.2.1 Nature

Prostate specific antigen is a 33-34 KD single chain glycoprotein, that is a 7-10% carbohydrate contents, 3.1S sedimentation coefficient and isoelectric point at pH 6.8-7.5[1,2], with a molecular weight 26,079 for the peptide moiety [6]. It has 240 amino acid residues with four carbohydrate side chains with linkages at amino acids 45 (asparagine), 69 (serine), 70 (alanine), and 71 (serine). The N-terminal amino acid is isoleucine, while the C-terminal residue is proline [43]. At least five PSA isoforms based on differences in isoelectric point have been described [64]. *Halbeek et al* [65], suggested that these isoenzymes may differ in their structure by their carbohydrate composition, ranging from non-glycosylated to fully glycosylated [66].

Prostate specific antigen is encoded from a (6 kb) gene in the *human glandular kallikrein* gene locus on chromosome (19) [67,68], which harbors the gene for the *pancreatic/renal tissue kallikrein (hk1)*, and the genes for *human glandular kallikrein-1 (hk2)* and *PSA* or *(hk3)*. The expression of *hk2* and PSA is restricted to the prostatic epithelium under androgen control, although low levels of PSA are also expressed in other tissues [69,70]. The coding region of PSA and *hk2* genes is 85% identical and 91% of their promoter region are the same. This high homology between the two genes could cause cross reactivity between PSA and *hk2* as antigens because of their extensive similarities [71], *hk2* has 78% sequence identity with PSA [72]. Recent studies indicate that *hk2* is a new potential marker that may be useful as an adjunct to PSA in the diagnosis and monitoring prostate cancer [72,73].

1.5.2.2 Activity and Functional Role

Functionally, PSA is a serine protease with trypsin like and chymotrypsin-like activity. It is produced almost exclusively in the cytoplasm of normal and neoplastic epithelial cells, and secreted into the lumina of the prostatic duct during the formation of seminal plasma [74,75]. The proteolytic activity of PSA is mainly directed against the major gel-forming proteins in freshly ejaculated semen. It cleaves these biological substrates including *semenogelin I, II* and *fibronectin* into small peptides. This results in liquefaction of semen coagulum and increasing sperm motility [76,77].

About 70% of PSA in seminal fluid is present in the active single-chain form, where as a minor part (~30%) is devoid of enzyme activity. This is mainly due to an internal lys-lys cleavage, resulting in an inactive two-chain form of PSA [78]. Up to 5% PSA in seminal fluid is devoid of protease activity due to complex formation with *protein C inhibitor*, a 55 KD extracellular protease inhibitor [79].

By a mechanism yet unknown, small quantities of PSA are released from the prostate into the circulation [80]. Its enzymatic activity in blood posses mitogenic activity may be involved in growth regulation and high concentrations might favor growth of cells, especially the formation of metastasis [81,82].

In serum, the proteolytic activity of PSA is inhibited by forming complexes with α_1-anti-chymotrypsin (α_1ACT, Mwt: ~70 KD), and α_2-macroglobulin (α_2M, Mwt: ~800KD), two major hepatocellular derived extracellular protease inhibitors occurring at 10^4 to10^5 fold molar excess to that of PSA in serum [69,83], figure (1-5).

Complex formation with α_1ACT results in exposure of limited number of epitops of PSA, where complex formation with α_2M encapsulates the antigenic determinants [84], rendering the PSA-α_2M complex undetectable by current immunoassays [3]. This results in an incorrect calculation of the level of PSA when released from prostate into the blood [85].

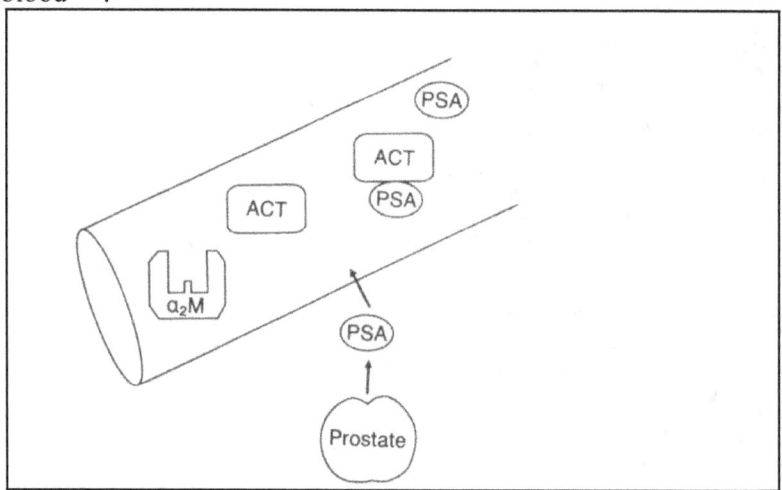

Figure (1-5): Schematic representation of two major protease inhibitors in serum, α_2-macroglobulin and α_1-antichymotrypsin [4].

The Major form of PSA in serum (about 80%), forms a 1:1 molar ratio complex with α_1-antichymotrypsin (PSA- α_1ACT: ~ 90 KD) in an irreversible reaction that splits the reactive center in (α_1ACT) between Lue $_{360}$ and Ser $_{361}$ [69]. This Position is identical to that reported from the reaction between ACT and chymotrypsin [84].

Smaller quantities of PSA are bound to α_2M [4]. The binding is initiated by the cleavage of the peptide bond between the amino acids Tyr $_{686}$and Glu $_{687}$

of the bait region indicating a chymotrypsin–like activity of the PSA. Kinetic analysis revealed faster binding of PSA to α_2 M than to ACT [85].

A minor fraction is free (f-PSA: ~30 KD) non-complexed with proteinase inhibitors despite the large excess of α_1ACT and α_2M in blood. This suggests that this form in serum lacks enzymatic activity [84,86]. This inactive form could represent the PSA zymogen or an internally cleaved inactive form that is similar but not identical to that in seminal plasma [66,84,87]. The low molecular mass of (f-PSA) suggests it to have a high turnover rate in blood, thus it may be eliminated rapidly from the circulation by renal clearance (half life in serum ~1.5h), while the ~90 KD size of serum PSA-ACT complex may well prevent renal clearance [88].

For a reason yet unknown, patients with prostate cancer have a lower proportion of (f-PSA) than patients with BPH have [89-91]. The molecular basis is unclear, but this may reflect the high incidence of prostate tumor cells, producing both PSA and ACT, This in contrast to the lack of ACT production in BPH epithelium [7,86,92,93].

1.5.2.3   Physiological Properties

The metabolic clearance rate of PSA follows first order elimination kinetics and has a half life of 2-3 days, because of this relatively long half life, 2-3 weeks may be necessary for the serum PSA to return to base levels after certain procedures[43], including TRUS*, DRE*, TURP* RP* or any kind of biopsy [97,43,81]. This is why the collection of blood for PSA assay is not recommended after such manipulation [4,98,99].

Other conditions such as prostatitis, acute urinary retention, and renal failure can also elevate the PSA level [100]. In addition, serum PSA concentration does not present diurnal rhythm [101]. *Tuan et al* reported a daily biological variation of (7-12)% [102]. *Stamey et al* found that serum PSA concentration decreases by a mean of 18% 24 h. after hospitalization [99]. Multiple authors have referenced the variation in out patients and inpatients

---

* See list of abbreviations

values [103]. Even the influence of ejaculation on PSA concentrations is not clear [104,105].

1.5.2.4   Non – Prostatic Sources of PSA

Improved highly sensitive methods for measuring PSA have shown that PSA is present in many non-prostatic tissues and fluids [106,107].

Recently, PSA was found in 30-40% of breast tumors and at a lower percentage in other tumors including lung, colon, skin, ovary, liver, kidney, salivary gland, adrenal and parotid tumors [108].

PSA was also found in normal endometerium, in normal breast [108], in milk of lactating women [109], and many biological fluids such as amniotic fluid [110] nipple aspirate fluid from the female breast [111], CSF* [112], pleural fluid [113], ascitic   fluid [114] and female serum [15]. The physiological role of PSA in these sources is unknown and currently is under investigation [108].

The gene expression and protein production of PSA in these sources are under the regulation of steroid hormone via their receptors [115,116]. Androgens, glucocorticoids, and progestins up-regulate the PSA gene expression, resulting in an increase of protein production. Estrogen by it self seems to have no effect on PSA regulation but it can impair PSA production induced by androgens [115].

In non-prostatic tissues PSA exists mainly in its free molecular form, but PSA-ACT complex is also present in most of the fluids that contain PSA. It remains unknown whether PSA is enzymatically active in these sources [115].

In urine, many investigators concluded that urine is free of PSA in the upper urinary tract [117,181], and that the presence of PSA is detectable following passage in the prostatic urethra, even in men having had radical prostactomies, most likely due to the   *priurethral glands* [119-121].

1.5.2.5 Measurement

1- Methods used for measuring total serum PSA concentration [43,122]:

---

* See list of abbreviations

Several immunoassays are commercially available including RIA and immunoradiometric assays using radioactive, enzyme, or fluorescent label.

The t-PSA immunoassays available today recognize the immunoreactive forms: f-PSA and PSA-ACT complex, but not PSA-α_2 M which is non-immuno- reactive. Their results for t-PSA refers to the sum of free and ACT bound forms as measured by the immunoassay.

Total-PSA assays differ from one another in an important respect: they do not recognize free and ACT bound species equivalently. *"Equimolar response assays"* measure equal molar concentrations of f-PSA and PSA-ACT equivalently; *"Skewed response assays"* measure these PSA forms differently. The following are some of these assays [43] :

a- **Pros Check Assay :** Many earliest studies of PSA used this assay which uses the traditional RIA approach. Rabbit polyclonal antibody against PSA is used to bind radioactively labeled PSA and the PSA in the patient sample. After overnight incubation, a second goat antirabbit antibodies precipitates the primary antibody-PSA complex. The detection limit of this assay is reported to be 0.2 μg/L.

b- **Tandem-R or Tandem-E Assay:** The Tandem assay is a solid phase two site immunometric assay (IRMA) that uses two monoclonal antibodies directed against different epitops on the PSA molecule. Tandem-R uses radioactive label whereas Tandem-E uses alkaline phosphates label. PSA's detection limit is 0.1μg/L and a high dose hook effect is observed at approximately 5000 μg/L.

c- **IMX Assay :**The automated IMX analyzer uses microparticles coated monoclonal antibodies against PSA on the solid phase to capture PSA . Alkaline phosphatase linked polyclonal (goat) antibodies bound to other sites to from a sandwich. The particle bound reactants are separated from the other reagents by a microfilter. The substrate 4-methylumbelliferyl phosphate is converted to the florescent product 4-methylumbellifron [123]. The detection limit is 0.1μg/L. No high dose hook effect was seen at 50.000 μg/L.

2 - Methods used for measuring serum PSA isoforms:

In order to increase PSA sensitivity and specificity for diagnosing prostate cancer, assay procedures have been developed to measure different PSA immunoreactive isoforms (i.e., f-PSA and PSA-ACT) [91,124].

Figure (1-6) describes three different non-competitive assays designed by **Christensson et al** [87]. One of these assays measures t-PSA by detecting f-PSA and PSA-ACT forms. The second assay measures PSA-ACT complex whereas the third one detects f-PSA form.

In a recent study, **Esapana et al** have developed an immunoassay for quantifying the non-immunoreactive form of PSA: (PSA-α_2 M) too [3] .

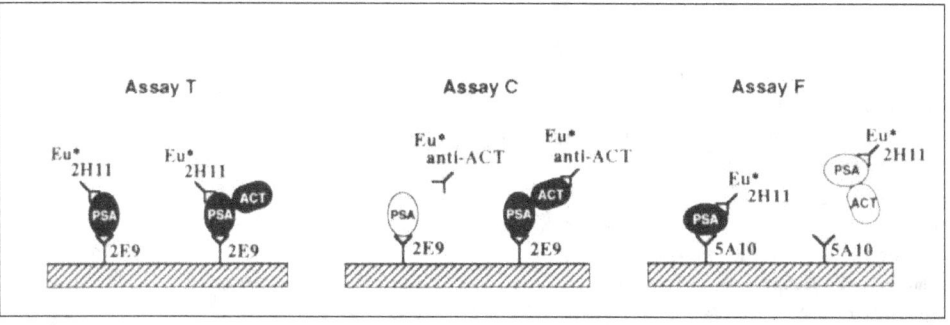

Figure (1-6): Schematic representation of three PSA assays. Assay T (total PSA), with 2E9 anti -PSA monoclonal antibody as capture antibody and Europium *(Eu*)*-labeled 2H11 anti-PSA monoclonal antibody as detection antibody, detects epitops available on noncomplexed PSA and PSA complexed to α_1-antichymotrypsin (ACT). Assay C (complexed PSA), using same catching antibody as assay T and polyclonal tracing antibody against α_1-antichymotrypsin, solely measures PSA complexed to α_1-antichymotrypsin. Assay F (free PSA), with same detection antibody as assay T but with 5A10 anti-PSA monoclonal antibody as capture antibody, detects noncomplexed PSA [87].

3- Ultrasensetive methods:

During the last few years, investigators and commercial concerns have made efforts to produce PSA assays with improved detection limit (below 0.1µg/L) [87,125]. The rational behind the development of these assays is that the relapse of prostate cancer or tumor doubling time after radical prostactomy, can be detected much earlier when patients are monitored with them [126].

An ultrasensitive PSA assay is characterized by its lowest limit of detection (LLD), which by definition is the least amount of analyte that can be detected with a predetermined confidence, usually 95% or 99% [125].

An example of these methods is the modified tandem-E assay by *Liedtke et al* which has a detection limit of 0.009 µg/L [127].

1.5.2.6 Methods for Improving the Clinical Usefulness of PSA

The substational overlap in serum PSA between men with BPH and those with PCA, coupled with the lack of specificity and sensitivity of serum PSA for alone detecting PCA has led to the development of better methods of using PSA as a marker for PCA [4]. These methods are:

1. **PSA Density or Index:** PSA density *(PSAD)* which was first introduced by *Benson et al* [128], is identified as the ratio of serum PSA and transrectal ultra- sound detected prostate volume. Although initial studies have claimed an enhancement in the ability of predicting PCA when serum PSA level where between 4 and 10 ng/ml by using *(PSAD)*. However, this was not supported by the following studies, which suggested that *(PSAD)* did not enhance the ability of PSA in predicting PCA [129].

2. **PSA Velocity or Slope:** PSA velocity is the rate of change of PSA over time. This measure is based on the fact that serum PSA increases more rapidly with PCA than with BPH [130]. *Carter et al,* first introduced this concept and determined that a PSA velocity of 0.75 ng/ml per year or greater was indicative of PCA [131].

3. **Age Specific Reference Ranges:** A third concept proposed, is the use of age referenced serum cutoffs. The rational for this method is that, because the prevalence of BPH increases with age, serum PSA concentrations are higher in older men [130,132].

4. **f-PSA/t-PSA or (f-PSA%) Ratio:** Many studies [84,133,134], confirmed that the proportion of f-PSA is significantly lower in patients with PCA than in

patients with BPH. Thus, the mean *(f/t)* ratio or *(f%)* in PCA is lower than that in BPH and may be helpful to distinguish PCA from BPH especially in the gray zone (4.0-10.0) ng/ml [84,133,134].

5- **Serum–to–Urinary PSA Ratio:** *Irani et al* showed that BPH for a yet unknown reason is associated with high urinary PSA levels while PCA and prostatitis are not [135]. They suggested that the serum to urinary PSA ratio might be useful in distinguishing PCA from BPH particularly in the gray zone (4.0-10.0) ng/ml [136].

1.5.2.7 Clinical Role

1- **Early detection of PCA:** PSA testing by it self is not effective in the screening or early detection of PCA because PSA is specific for prostatic tissue but not for prostatic cancer [43]. However, if combined with DRE* and/or TRUS* it may become a vital part of any early detection program [137].

   Attempts to improve PSA ability in early detection of PCA [43,138], are mentioned in section (1.5.2.6).

2- **Staging of PCA:** several studies have shown that serum PSA correlates with clinical stage, tumor volume, and pathological stage [99,139,140]. Higher PSA levels as well as higher percentages of patients with elevated PSA concentrations are associated with advanced stages. However, PSA testing is not sufficiently reliable to determine stages on an individual basis [43].

3- **Monitoring treatment:** the greatest clinical use of PSA is in the monitoring of definitive treatment of PCA:

   a- *PSA following radical Prostatectomy:* after radical prostactomy any detectable serum PSA signals tumor recurrence [141].

   b- *Radiation therapy:* numerous reports have attempted to establish a reference range of post-radio therapy PSA that is associated with cure , or long term control. Most agree that achievement of a *Nadir* PSA less than 1-1.5 ng /ml is essential [141].

---

* See list of abbreviations

c- *Androgen deprivation therapy (ADT):* treatment of BPH and PCA
with *ADT* usually decreases the serum PSA concentration . Hence,
PSA is a valuable tumor marker for prognosticating the response to
ADT and portending progression [142].

1.5.3 Prostrate Specific Membrane Antigen [143,144]

Prostatic specific membrane antigen *(PSMA)*, is a membrane bound
antigen that is highly specific for normal, benign, and malignant prostate
epithelial cells. It is elevated in prostate cancers especially in poorly
differentiated, metastatic and hormone refractory carcinomas. It has been
measured in serum with immuno-competitive and Western blot analysis,
and its levels have been found to be correlated with the prediction of
treatment failure and disease prognosis. Another current application of
PSMA is in immunotherapy of PCA.

References

1. Disaia, P.J., and Creasman, W.T. (1989) In Breast Diseases and Colorectal Cancer in Clinical Gynecologic Oncology. Third ed., pp. 1-5, The C.V. Mosby Company, Toronto.

2. Parkin, D.M, Idara F., and Muir, C.S. (1988) Int. Cancer **41**, 184-97.

3. Coleman, M.P., Esteve, J., Damiecki, P., Arston, A., and Renard, H. (1993) Trends in cancer incidence and mortality, Lynos: International Agency for Research on Cancer (IARC. Scientific Publication No. 121).

4. Steven, A., Schroeder, Marcus, A., Krupp, Lawrence, M., Tierney, and Stephen, J. Mcphee (1989) In Current Medical Diagnosis & Treatment, pp 429-435.

5. Wooster, K., Neunausen, S.L., Mangion, J. et al (1994) Science **265**, 2088-2090.

6. Nowak, R. (1994) Science **265**, 1796-1799.

7. McPherson, K., Steel, C.M., and Dixon, J.M. (1994) BMJ **309**, 1003-1007.

8. Wealheral, Ledinglaic, and Warrel (1984) Oxford Text Book of Medicine, Oxford University press.

9. Anderson, D.E., and Badzioch, M.D. (1985) Cancer **56**, 383.

10. Gilbertsen, V.A. (1975) Semin. Oncol. **1**, 87-90.

11. Canellos, G.P., Hellman, S., and Veronesi, U. (1982) N. Engl. J. Med. **306**, 1430.

12. Calson, H.E. (1980) N. Engl. J. Med. **303**, 795-799.

13. Trialists Collaborative Group (1992) In: Early Breast Cancer Lancet 339, 1-15, 71-85.

14. Singleton, W.V., and Mecarty, K.S. (1987) Gyncol. Oncol. **26,** 271-275.

15. Gelber, R.D., and Goldhirsch, A. (1986) J. Clin. Oncol. **4,** 1696.

16. Donegan, W.L., and Spratt, J.S. (1979) In Cancer of the breast, W.B. Saunders, Philadelphia.

17. Horris, J.R, Leven, M.B., and Helman, S. (1987) Semin Oncol. **5,** 403.

18. Butta, A., Maclennan, K., Flanders, K.C., and et al. (1992) Cancer Res. **52**, 4261.

19. Slevin, M.L., Stubbs, L., Plant, H.J., and et al. (1990) Br. Med. J. **300,** 1458.

20. Wilson, J.D., Aiman, J., and MacDonald, P.C. (1980) Adv. Inter. Med. **25**,1.

21. Bailey & Love's, In Short Practice of Surgery, 21st edition (1991) pp. 806-810.

22. Helman, S. (1983) In Controversies in Breast Cancer, Conference Sponsored by the MD Aderson Hospital and Tumor Institute, Chicago, Year Book, Medical Publishers, Inc.

23. Chetty, U. (1979) Br. J. Surg. **67**, 789.

24. Humphrey, U. et al (1983) Contemp Surg. **23,** 97.

25. Cole, P., Elwood, J.M., and Kaplan, S.D. (1978) AM. J. Epidemiol. **108**, 112.

26. Oluwole, S.F., and Freeman, H.P. (1979) AM. J. Surg **37**, 786.

27. Rao, B.R.(1981) Cancer **47**, 2016.

28. Devitt, J.E. (1972) Surg. Gynecol Obstet. **134**, 803.

29. Yamamota, K. (1985) Ann. Rev. Genet. **19**, 209-252.

30. Reddik, K, and Holland, J.F. (1976) Proc. Natl. Acad. Sci. USA, **73**, 2308.

31. Wood, C.H., Varela, V., and Palmquist, M. et al (1977) J. Surg. Oncol. **5**, 251.

32. Secreto, G., Recchione, C., and Caralleri, A., et al (1983) Br. J. Cancer, **47**, 269.

33. Sharon, P. (1984) Scientific American **6**, 86-95.

34. Handas, S., and Nakamura, K. (1984) J. Biol. Chem. **95**, 1323-9.

35. Magdelenal, I.I. (1992) J. Immunol Meth. **150**, 133-143.

36. Suresh, M.R.(1944): Cancer markers In: The immunoassay handbook (Wild, D. ed.) pp. 441-460 NY. Stockton Press.

37. Suresh, M.R., Noujam, A.A., and Longeneeker, B.M. (1991): Recent developments in monoclonal antibodies In: biotechnology Current Progress, Vol. **1**, (Cheremisinoff, P.N., and Ferrante, L.M. eds), pp. 83-101, USA Technomic Publ.

38. Sano, T, Smith, L.S., and Cantor, C.R. (1992) Conjugates Science **258**, 120-122.

39. Suresh, M.R. (1996) Anticancer Research **16**, 2273-2278.

40. Suresh, M.R. (1991): Immunoassay for cancer-associated carbohydrate antigens In, Seminars in cancer Biol., Vol. **2,** pp. 367-377, London W.D. Saunders Publ.

41. American Society of Clinical Oncology (1996) J. Clin. Oncol. **14,** 2843-2877.

42. Greene, G.L., Sobel, N.B., and King, W.J. et al (1984) J. Steroid Biochem. **20**, 51-56.

43. Green, S., Gronemeyer, H., and Chambon, P. (1987) In Structure and function of steroid hormone receptors in Sluyser M. ed.: Growth Factors and Oncogenes in Breast Cancer, England, Mlis pp. 728, Horwood.

44. Walter, P., Green, S., and Green, G. et al. (1985) Proc. Nail. Acad. Sci. U.S.A. **82**, 7889-7893.

45. Orti, E., Bodwell, J.I., and Munck, A. (1992) Endocr. Rev. **13**, 105-128.

46. Ruh, T.S., Ruh, M.F., and Singh R.K. (1988) In Nuclear acceptor Sites: Interaction with estrogen-versus antiestrogen-receptor complexes, in Moudgil V.K. ed.: Steroid Receptors in Health and Disease, pp. 233-250, New York, N.Y. Plenum.

47. Bauer, K.D., Bagwell, C.B., and Giaretti, W. et al. (1993) Cytometry **4**, 486-491.

48. Tandon, A.K., Clark, G.M., and Chamness, G.C. et al. (1990) N. Engl. J. Med. **322**, 297-302.

49. Reid, P.E., Culling, C.F.A., and Dunn, W.L. (1978) J. Histochem. Cytochem. **26**, 187-192.

50. Culling, C.F.A., and Reid, P.E. (1979) J. Histochem. Cytochem. **27**, 1177-1179.

51. Bouchier, I.A.D., and Clamp, J.R. (1971) Clin. Chim. Acta., **35**, 219-224.

79

52. Horowitz M.I.(1977), "Gastrointestinal glycoproteins' In: "The glycoconjugates" eds., Horowitz M.I. and Pigman W., 1st ed. Vol. **1**, pp. 189-213 Academic Press.

53. Tuppy, H., and Gottschalk, A. (1972) "The structure of sialic acids and their quantitation" In: "Glycoproteins" ed. Gottschelk A., 2nd ed., pp. 403-449 Amsterdam.

54. Schauer, R. (1982) Adv. Carbohydr. Chem. Biochem., Vol. **40**, in press.

55. Schauer, R. (1978) Methods Enzymol. **50C**, 64-89.

56. Buscher, H.P., Casals-Stenzel, J., and Schauner, R. (1974) Eur. J. Biochem. **50**, 71-82.

57. Reuter, G., Vielgenthart, J.F.G., Wember, M., Schauer, R. and Howard, R.J. (1980) Biochem. Biophys. Res. Commun. **94**, 567-572.

58. Sheshadri, N. (1994) Annals. of Clinical and Laboratory Science, Vol. **24** No. 4, 376-384.

59. Warren, L. (1959) J. Biol. Chem. **234**, 1971-5.

60. Shukla, A.K., and Schauer, R. (1981) Physiol. Chem. **362**, 236-7.

61. Shamberger, R.J. (1986) Anticancer Res. **6**, 717-20.

62. Hara, S., Takemori, Y., Yamaguchi, M., Nakamura, M., and Ohkura, Y. (1987) Anal. Biochem. **164**, 138-45.

63. Pigman W., (1977): Blood group glycoproteins" In: "The glycoconjugates" eds. Horowitz M.I. and Pigman W., 1st ed., Vol. **1**, pp. 181-188 Academic press.

64. Schwick, H.G., Heide, K., and Haupt, H. (1977) "Plasma" In: "The glycoconjugates" eds., Horowitz M.I. and Pigman W., 1st ed., Vol. **1**, pp. 261-321 Academic press.

65. Patel, V. (1978) "Degradation of glycoprotein" In: "the glycoconjugates" eds., Horowitz M.I. and Pigman W., 1st ed., Vol. **2**, pp. 185-229 Academic press.

66. Baumann, H. and Doyle, D. (1984) "Determination of carbohydrate structures in glycoproteins and glycolipids", Molecular and chemical characterization of membrane receptors, pp. 125-160.

67. Horowitz M.I., (1978) "Immunological aspect and lectins" In: "The glycoconjugates" eds., Horowitz M.I. and Pigman W., 1st ed., Vol. 2, pp. 387-425 Academic press.

68. Yogeeswaran, G., and Salk, P. (1981) Science 212, 1514-6.

69. Bahl, O.P., and Shah, R.H. (1977) "Glycoenzymes and glycohormons" In: "The glycoconjugate" eds., Horowitz M.I. and Pigman W., 1st ed., Vol. 2, pp. 385-422 Academic press.

70. Schauer, R. (1985) Trends Biochem. Sci. 10: 357-60.

71. Reid, P.E., Culling, C.F.A., Dunn, W.L., and Clay M.G. (1978) J. Histochem. Cytochem. 26, 1033-1041.

72. AL-Suhail, A., Reid, P.E., Yeung, M., Corret, S., Frolich, J., and Brooks, D.E. (1981) "Serum level of sialic acid: Effect of age, smoking and heart disease". C.S.C.C. 25th annual convention No. 5.

73. McNeil, C., Berrett, C.R., Lucia, Y.S.U., Trentelman, E.F., and Helmick, W.M. (1965) Am. J. Cli. Path. 43, 130-133.

74. Carter, A., and Martin, N.H. (1962) J. Clin. Path. 15: 69-72.

75. Erbil, K.M., Jones, J.D., and Klee, G.G. (1986) Cancer 57, 1889.

76. Khanderia, V., and Keller, J. (1983) J. Surg. Oncol 23, 163-166.

77. Stefnelli, N., Klotz, H., Engel, A., and Bauer, P. (1985) J. Cancer Res. Clin. Oncol. 109, 55-59.

78. Shamberger, R.J. (1984) J. Clin. Chem. Clin. Biochem. 22, 647-651.

79. Silver, H.K.B., Rangel, D.M, and Morton, D.L. (1978) Cancer 41, 1497-1499.

80. Brozmanova, E., and Skrovina, B. (1972) Neoplasma 19, 115-123.

81. Silver, H.K.B., karim, K.A., Archibald, E.A., and Salinas, F.A. (1979) Cancer Res. 39, 5036-5042.

82. Moss, A.J., Bissada, N.K., Bayed, C.M., and Hunter, W.C. (1979) Urology **13**, 182-184.

83. Silver, H.K.B., Karim, K.A., Salinas, F.A., and Swenterton, K.D. (1981) Surg. Gynecol. Obstect. **153**, 203-213.

84. Harvey, H.A., Lipton, A., White, D., and Davidson, E. (1981) Cancer, **47**, 324-327.

85. Bradely, W.P., Blasco, A.P., Weiss, J.F., Alxander, J.C., Silverman, N.A., and Chretien, P.B. (1977) Cancer, **40**, 2264-2272.

86. Culling, C.F.A., Reid, P.E., Burton, J.D., and Dunn, W.L. (1975) J. Clin. Pathol. **28**, 650-656.

87. Culling, C.F.A., Reid, P.E., Worth, A.J., and Dunn, W.L. (1977) J. Clin. Pathol. , **30**, 1056.

88. Corfield, A.P., Michalski, J.C., and Schauer, R. (1981) "In perspective in inherited metabolic diseases", (Tettamanti G., Durand P. and Di Donato S., eds.), Vol. **4**, pp. 3-70, Edi Ermes Publ., Milano.

89. Varki, A., and Kornfeld, S. (1980) J. Exp. Med. **152**, 532-544.

90. Culling, C.F.A., Reid, P.E., Clay, M.G., and Dunn, W.L. (1973) J. Histochem. Cytochem. **22**, 826-831.

91. Casals-Stenzel, J., Buscher, H.P., and Schauer, R. (1975) Anal. Biochem. **65**, 501-507.

92. Erbil, K.M., Jones, J.D., and klee, G.G. (1985) Cancer **55**, 404-409.

93. Silver, H.K.B., Rangel, D.M., and Morton, D.L. (1978) Cancer **41**, 1497-1499.

94. Fukushima, K., Hirota, M., and Terasaki, P.I., et al. (1984) Cancer Res. **44**, 5279-5285.

95. Kessel, D., and Allen, J. (1975) Cancer Res. **35**: 670-672.

96. Berg, E.L., Robinson, M.K., and Mansson, O., et al. (1991) J. Biol. Chem. **266**, 14869-14872.

97. Lundblad, A. (1980) Scand. J. Clin. Lab. Invest. **40**, 3-11.

98. Reintgein, D.S., Cruse, C.W., Wells, K.E., Saba, H.I., and Fabri, P.J. (1992) Ann. Plast. Surg. **28**, 55-9.

99. Patel, P.S., Adhvaryn, S.G, and Baxi, R.B. (1991) Int. J. Biol. Markers **6**, 177-82.

100. Xing, R.D., Chen, R.M., Wang, Z.S., and Zhang, Y.Z. (1991) J. Oral Maxillofac. Surg. **49**, 843-7.

101. Horowitz, M.I., and Pigman, W. (1977) "The glycoconjugate" eds., Horowitz, M.I., and Pigman, W, 1st ed., Vol. **1**, pp. 1-10, Academic Press.

102. Martin, D.W. Jr. (1985) "Glycoproteins, proteoglycons, and glycosaminoglycans" In.: "Harper's review of biochemistry" eds., Martin, D.W.Jr., Mayer, P.A., Rodwell V.W., and Granner, D.K. 20th ed., pp. 464-479, Lange Medical Publications.

103. Filipe, M.I., and Fengar, C. (1979) Histochem. J. **11**, 277-287.

104. Shehan, D.G., and Jervis, H.R. 1(1976) Am. J. Anta. **146**, 103-132.

105. La Mont, J.T., Smith, B.F., and Moore, J.R.L. (1984) Hepatology **4**, 515-565.

106. Zinn, A.B., Plantner, J.J., and Carlson, D.M. (1977) "Nature of linkages between protein core and oligosaccharides": In "The glycoconjugates" eds., Horowitz, M.I., and Pigman, W. 1st ed., Vol. **1**, pp. 69-85, Academic Press.

107. Lenten, L.V., and Ashwell, G. (1970) J. Biol. Chem. **246**, 1889-1894.

108. Glick, M.C., and Flowers, H. (1978) "Surface membrane" In: "The glycoconjugates" eds., Horowitz, M.I., and Pigman, W. 1st ed., Vol. **2**, pp. 337-384, Academic Press.

109.   Hoskins, L.C. (1978) "Degradation of mucus glycoproteins in the gastrointestinal tract" In: "The glycoconjugates" eds., Horowitz, M.I., and Pigman, W. 1st ed., Vol. **2**, pp. 235-253, Academic Press.

110.   Holden, K.G., and Griggs, L. (1987) "Respiratory tract" In: "The glycoconjugates" eds., Horowitz, M.I., and Pigman, W. 1st ed., Vol. **1**, pp. 215-237, Academic Press.

111.   Ferguson, R.N., Edelhoch, H., and Saroff, H.A. (1975) Biochem. **14**, 282-289.

112.   Wasserman, R.L., and Capra, J.D. (1977) "Immunoglobulins" In: "The glycoconjugates" eds., Horowitz, M.I., and Pigman, W. 1st ed., Vol. **1**, pp. 323-348, Academic Press.

113.   Glandemans, C.P.J. (1975) Adv. Carbohydr. Chem. Biochem. **31**, 313-346.

114.   Pazur, J.H., and Forsberg, L.S. (1978) Carbohydr. Res. **60**, 167-178.

115.   Stern, P.L., Willison, K.R., Lennox, E., Calfre, G., Milstein, C., Secher, D., Ziegler, A., and Springer, T. (1978) Cell **14**, 775-785.

116.   Granner, D.K. (1985) "Hormone action" In: "Harper's review of biochemistry" eds., Martin, D.W., Mayes, P.A., Rodwell, V.W., and Granner, D.K. 20th ed., pp. 505-515, Lange Medical Publications.

117.   Macbeth, R.A.L., and Bekesi, J.G. (1962) Cancer Res. **22**, 1170-1175.

118.   Seibert, F.B., Seibert, M.V., Atno, A.J., and Campbell, H.W. (1974) J. Clin. Invest. **26**, 90-102.

119.   Nigelson, G.L., and Postle, G. (1976) N. Engl. J. Med. **295**, 253-258.

120.   Cunietti, E., Vaiani, G., Gandini, M, Monti, M, Locatelli, E., Gandini, R., and Reggiani, A. (1985) Cancer Detec. Prev. **8**, 222-232.

121.   Schachter, H. (1978) "Glycoprotein biosynthesis" In: "The glycoconjugates" eds., Horowitz, M.I., and Pigman, W. 1st ed., Vol. **2**, pp. 87-181, Academic Press.

122.   Both, S.N., King, J.P.G., Leonard, J.C., and Dykes, P.W. (1973) Gut **14**, 794-799.

123.   Barondes, S.H., (1981) Annual Review of Biochemistry **50**, 207-231.

124.   Toyoshima, S., Osawa, T., and Tonomura, A. (1970) Biochem. Biophys. Acta, **221**, 514-521.

125.   Kornfeld, S., and Kornfeld, R. (1978) "Use of lectins in the study of mammalian glycoproteins" In: "The glycoconjugates" eds., Horowitz, M.I., and Pigman, W. 1st ed., Vol. **2**, pp. 437-449, Academic Press.

126.   Powell, J. (1980) Biochem. J. **187**, 123.

127.   Sammel, H. (1984) Science **223**, 4639.

128.   Springer, G., and Desai, P. (1971) Biochemistry **10**, 3749.

129.   Lis, H., and Sharon, N. (1981) Ann. Rev. Biochem. **50**, 207-31.

130.   Miller, J.B., Hsu, R., Heinrikson, R., and Yachnin, S. (1975) Proc. Natl. Acad. Sci. USA, **72**, 1388-91.

131.   Ceri, H., Kobiler, D., and Barondes, S.H. (1981) J. Biol. Chem. **256**, 390-94.

132.   Pereira, M.E.A., and Kabat, E.A. (1979) Crit. Rev. Immunol. **1**, 1-73.

133.   Barondes, S. (1981) Annu. Rev. Bioche. **50**, 207.

85

134.   Boldt, D.H., et al. (1975) J. Immunol. **114**, 1532-1536.

135.   Scott, R.E., and Rosenthal, A.S. (1977) J. Immunol. **119**, 143-148.

136.   Alhadeff, J.A. (1989) Crit. Rev. Oncol. Hematol. **9**, 37-47.

137.   Taner, O., Nursen, E., and Limrin, A. (1990) Clin. Chem. **36**, 393-397.

138.   Shamberger, R.J. (1984) J. Clin. Chem. Clin. Biochem. **22**, 647-651.

139.   Vegh, Zs., Kremmer, T., Boldizsar, M., Gesztes, K.A., and Szajani, B. (1991) Clin. Chim. Acta **203**, 259-268.

140.   Raynes, J.G. (1983) Biomed. Pharmacother. **37**, 136-138.

141.   Lipton, A., Harvey, H.A., and De Long, S. et al. (1979) Cancer **43**, 1766-1771.

142.   Dnistria, A.M., Schwartz, M.K., and Katopodis, N. (1982) Cancer **50**, 9.

143.   Katopodis, N., Hirshaut, Y., and Geller, N.L. (1982) Cancer Res. **42**, 5270-5.

144.   Rothenberg, R.E., La Ruja, R.D., Mueller, O.T., and Pryce, E.H. (1994) Breast Dis. **7**, 3, 197-202.

145.   Lowry, O.H., Rosebrough, N.J., Farr, A.L., and Randall, R.J. (1951) J. Biol. Chem. **193**, 265-75.

146.   Wilkinson, L. SYSTAT. (1990) The system for Statistics Evanston, II: SYSTAT Inc.

147.   Crook, M. (1993) Clin. Biochem. **26**, 31-38.

148.   Cohen, S.L., Lincoln, S.T., and Rosen, S.T. (1986) Cancer Invest. **4**, 305-327.

149.   Patel, P.S., Baxi, B.R., Desal, S.S., and Balar, D.B. (1990) Ind. J. Pathol. Microbiol. **33**, 124-128.

150.　　　Fukushima, K. (1991) J. Exp. Med. **163**, 17-30.

151.　　　Itai, S., Arii, S., Tobe, R., Kitahara, A., and Kim, Y.C. et al. (1988) Cancer **61**, 775-87.

152.　　　Hakomori, S. (1985) Cancer Res. **45**, 2405-14.

153.　　　Warren, L., Fuhrer, J.P., and Buck, C.A. (1972) Proc. Natl. Acad. Sci. **69**, 1838-42.

154.　　　Schutter, E.M.J., Vissr, J.J., and Van kamp, G.J. et al. (1992) Tumor Biol. **13**, 121-32.

155.　　　Kakari, S., Stirngou, E., Toumbis, M., Ferderigos, As., and Poulaki, I. et al. (1991) Anticancer Res. **11**, 2107-10.

156.　　　Dnistrian, A.M., and Schwartz, M.K. (1981) Clin. Chem. **27(10)**, 1737-1739.

157.　　　Mannello, F., Bocchiotti, G., Troccoli, R., and Gazzanelli, G. (1993) Breast Cancer Res. Treat. **24**, 167-170.

158.　　　Patel, P.S., Baxi, B.R., Adhvaryu, S.G., and Balar, D.B. (1990) Cancer Lett. **51**, 203-208.

159.　　　Haq, M., Haq, S., Tutt, P., and Crook, M. (1993) Ann. Clin. Biochem. **30**, 383-386.

160.　　　Hansen, H.J., Snyder, J.J., Miller, E., Vandevoorde, J.P., Miller, O.N., Hines, L.R., and Burns, J.J. (1974) Hum. Pathol. **5**, 139-147.

161.　　　Harshman, S., Reynolds, V.H., Neumaster, T., Patikas, T., and Worrall, T. (1974) Cancer **34**, 291.

162.　　　Barlow, J.J., and Dillard, P.H. (1972) Obstet. Gynecol. **39**, 727.

163.　　　Aronson. N.N., and De Duve. C. (1978) J. Biol. Chem. **243**, 4564.

164.　　　Robert, A. (1962) Cancer Res. **22**, 1170.

165.   Lawrence, M., Gerald, B., and Zoltan, A. (1977) Clin. Chem. **23**, 2055.

166.   Yogeswarar, G. (1983) Advance Cancer Res. **38**, 289.

167.   Weimer, and Mashin, J. (1965) Clin. Chem. Principle and Techniques.

168.   Waalkes, P.T., Mrochek, J.E., Dinsmore, S.R., and Tormey, D.C. (1978) J. Natl. Cancer Inst. **6**, 703.

169.   Bradley, W.P., Blasco, A.P., and Weiss, J.F. (1977) Cancer **40**, 2264-2272.

170.   Bhuvarahamurthy, V., Balasubramanian, N., Subramanian, S., and Govindasamy, S. (1992) Bichem. Int. **28**, 105.

171.   Scambia, G., Panici, B., Perrone, L., Sonsini, C., Giannelli, S., and Gallo, A. et al. (1990) Br. J. Cancer **62**, 147.

172.   Sherblow, A.P., Buck, R.L., and Carraway, K.L. (1980) J. Biol. Chem. **255**, 783.

173.   Yogeeswaran, G., and Salk, P.L. (1981) Science **212**, 1514.

174.   Yamamooto, K. (1984) Eur. J. Biochem. **143**, 133.

175.   Bolmer, S., and Davidson, E. (1981) Biochemistry **20**, 1047.

176.   Yaskhiko T., Wataru I. and Mitsunon Y., Am. J. Nephrol 1988; **2**: 21.

177.   McCord, J.M., and Fridovich, I. (1969) J. Biol. Chem. **244**: 6049-6055.

178.   Fridovich, I. (1972) Acc. Chem. Res. **5**, 321-326.

179.   Wever, R., Oudega, B., and Van, Gelder, B.F. (1972) Biochem. Biophys. Acta, **302**, 475-478.

180.   Batalie, R., Klein, B., Durie, B., and Sany, J. (1989) Clin. Exp. Rheumatol. **7**, 319-28.

181.   Sigureirsson, B., Lindelof, B., Edhag, O., and Allander, E. (1992) N. Engl. J. Med. **326**, 363-7.

182.   Polivakova, J., Vosmikova, K., and Horak, L. (1992) Neoplasma **39(4)**, 233-6.

183.   Borrello, S., De Leo, M.E., Wohirab, H., and Galeoti, T. (1992) FEBS Lett. **310**, 249-54.

184.   Van Balgooy, J.N.A, and Roberts, E. (1979) Comp. biochem. Physiol. **62B**, 263-8.

185.   Winterbourn, C.C., Hawkins, R.E., Brian, M., and Carrell, R.W. (1975) J. Lab. Clin. Med. **85(2)**, 337-341.

186.   Knee, J.K., Mitidieri, E., and Affonso, O.R.b (1991) Cancer Lett **57**, 199-202.

187.   Bolzan, A.D., Bianchi, M.S., and Bianchi, N.O. (1993) Cancer Res. **6**, 142-6.

188.   Yoshimitsu, K., Kobayashi, Y., and Usui, T. (1984) Acta Paediatr. Scand., **73**, 92-6.

189.   Abella, A., Clerc, D., Chalas, J., Baret, A., Leluc, R., and Lindenbaum, A. (1987) Ann. Biol. Clin. **45**, 152-5.

190.   Tsurn, S., Nomoto, K., Aiso, S., Ogata, T., and Zinnaka, Y. (1983) Int. Arch. Allergy appl. Immunol. **71(1)**, 88-92.

191.   Galeotti, T., Masotti, L., Borrello, S., and Casali, E. (1991) Xenobiotica **21(8)**, 1041-51.

192.   Oberley, L., and Oberley, T.D. (1988) Mol. Cell Biochem. **84**, 147-53.

193.   Wong, Y.F., Wong, W.S.H., and Fung, Y.H., et al. (1993) Med. Sci. Res. **21**, 397-8.

194.   Mizuno, K., and Kozutsumi, T. (1981) J. Biol. Chem. **256**, 4247.

195.   Briles, E., and Gregory, W. (1979) J. Cell Biol. **81**, 528.

196.   Bishayee, S., and Dorai, D. (1980) Biochem. Biophys. Acta **623**, 89.

197.   Bohlool, B.B., Schmidt, E.L. (1976) J. Bacteriol. **125**, 1188-94.

198.   Burger, M., and Goldberg, A. (1967) Proc. Nat. Acad. Sci. USA **57**, 359.

199.   Kaplan, R., Li, S., and Kehoe, J. (1977) Biochemistry **16**, 4297.

200.   Hans J., Attila, B., Sigrun, G., and Michael, K. (1989) Biochem. Biophys. Res. Commun. **163**, 506.

201.   Ronald, L., James, F., and Wayne, W. (1982) J. Biol. Chem. **257**, 7574.

202.   Liener, I. (1955) Arch. Biochem. Biophys. **54**, 223.

203.   Lis, H., and Sharon, N. (1972) Methods Enzymol. **28**, 360.

204.   Gabius, H., Bandlow, G., Schirramacher, V., and Vehmeyer, K. (1987) Int. J. Cancer **39**, 634.

205.   Kaplan, A. (1998) Clinical Chemistry Theory, Analysis and Correlation, 2nd edition pp. 180.

206.   Ahmed, H., Chatterjee, B.P., Klem, S., and Schauer, R. (1986) Biol. Chem. Hoppeseyler **367**, 501-506.

207.   Basu, S., Sarkar, M., and Mondal, C. (1986) Mol. Cell biochem. **71**, 149-157.

208.   Varki, A., and Kornfeld, S. (1980) J. Exp. Med. **152**, 532-544.

209.   Schauer, R., Shukla, A.K., Schroder, G., and Muller, E. (1984) Pure and Appl. Chem. **57**, 907-921.

210.   Shukla, A.K., and Schauer, R. (1982) Hoppe-Seyler's and Physiol. Chem. **363**, 255-262.

211. Ravindranath, M.H., Higa, H.H., Copper, E.L., and Paulson, J.C. (1985) J. Biol. Chem. **260**, 8850-8856.

212. Elvin, A., and Manfred, M. (1967) Experimental Immuno Chemistry, Second edition, Illinois, USA.

213. Gottschalk, A. (1960) In: The chemistry and biology of sialic acids and related substances, Cambridge University Press, London.

214. Bakhtear, M. (1992) Ph.D. thesis, College of Science, Baghdad University.

215. Wild, J., Robinson, D., and Winchester, B. (1983) Biochem. J. **21**, 167.

216. Dolichos, R. (1983) Biochemistry **22**, 2741.

217. Finstand, C., Good, R., and Litman, C. (1974) Ann. N. Y. Acad. Sci. **234**, 170.

218. Dipti, G., Fred, C., and Brewer, J. (1994) Biochemistry **33**, 5526-5530.

219. Pemberton, R. (1970) Vax Song. **18**, 74.

220. Goldstein, I., and Hays, C. (1978) Adv. Carbohydr. Chem. Biochem. **35**, 127.

221. Goebel, W., et al. (1934) J. Exper. Med. **60**, 599.

222. Nassir M. (1995) Ph.D. thesis, College of Science, Baghdad University.

223. Nowak, T., and Barondes, S.(1975) Biochimica et Biophys. Acta **393**, 15.

224. Finstad, C., Litman, G., Finstand, J., and Good, R. (1972) J. Immunol. **108**, 1704.

225. Oppenheim, J., Nachbar, M., Salton, M., and Aull, F. (1974) Res. Commun. **58**, 1127.

226. Peters, B.P. et al. (1979) Biochemistry **18**, 5505-5511.

227. Roche, A.C. et al. (1975) FEBS Lett. **57**, 245-249.

228.   Mohan et al. (1982) Biochem. J. **203**, 253-261.

229.   Miller, R.L. (1982) J. Invertebr. Pathol. **39**, 210-214.

230.   Babal, P. (1994) Biochem. J. **229(2)**, 341.

231.   Kawagishi, H. (1994) FEBS Lett. **340**, 56.

232.   Scopes, R. (1982) Protein purification principles and practice, Springer Verlag, pp. 162, New York Heidelber Berlin.

233.   Pharmacies fine chemical: Gel filtration calibration kit instruction mannual for protein molecular weight determination.

234.   Csizman, L. (1960) Proc. Soc. Exp. Biol. N. Y. **103**, 157.

235.   Laemmli, U.K. (1970) Nature **227**, 680.

236.   Hans, F. (1977) Application note 306 LKB-Produkter AB., pp. 1-15, Bromma, Sweden.

237.   Huda, H. (1998) M.Sc. thesis, College of Science, Baghdad University.

238.   Isamu, M., Heruko, K., Naoko, I., and Yukiko, S. (1986) Carb. Res. **151**, 261.

239.   Goldstein, I.J., Hughes, R.C., Monsigny, M., Osawa, T., and Sharon, N. (1980) Nature **285**, 66.

240.   Czech, M.P., Lynn, W.S. (1973) Biochem. Biophys. Acta **297**, 368-377.

241.   Scatchard, G. (1949) Ann. N. Y. Acad. Sci. **51**, 660.

242.   Emil, L. (1985) In: Principles of biochemistry, seven edition, pp. 289, International Student Edition.

243.   Rae-Venter, B., and Dao, T. (1982) Biochem. Biophys. Res. Commun. **107**, 624.

244.   Hussain, M. (1990) M.Sc. thesis, College of Science, Baghdad University.

245.   Waelbroeck, M., Van Obeerghen, E., and Demeyts, P. (1979) J. Biol. Chem. **254**, 7736.

246.   Blumenthar, D.K., and Stul, J.T. (1982) Biochemistry

        Laport, D.C., Wierman, E.M., and Storm, D.I. (1

Curriculum Vitae of Prof.
Sami Al-mudhaffar

Prof. Al-Mudhaffar was born on 14 March 1940 in Basra, Iraq.

He received early education at Basra High School, and obtained a BSc Hons Degree from the University of Baghdad, Iraq (1959-1960). In 1962 he moved to the University of Virginia Tech., USA, for advanced studies under a merit assistantship awarded by that university, culminating in a PhD (1967). He returned to Iraq and began teaching and research as a Lecturer in the College of Science of the University of Basra. He became Assistant Professor (1971), and full Professor of Biochemistry (1979) at the University of Baghdad, Iraq.

He is one of the most senior Biochemists of Iraq, and has played an important role in promoting in that country Biochemistry, Molecular Biotechnology research and related subjects. He is primarily responsible for the initiation and establishment of many scientific and bilateral educational programmes with scientific organizations and laboratories in the advanced world and become active member of Iraqi academy of science (almajma alilmi) in 1996.

Prof. Al-Mudhaffar has been teaching undergraduate and postgraduate students in various branches of Biochemistry at the Universities of Basra and Baghdad for over 35 years (1968-2003). He has supervised 50 PhDs and 100 MSc students in related fields, and published more than 250 scientific papers. He also has 50 inventions to his credit.His guidance and active participation in the promotion of scientific activities has resulted in the formation of a sound base for the growth of the scientific culture in the country.He was awarded several prizes and medals for his activities in both science and culture.

Prof. Al-Mudhaffar was elected as a Fellow of the IAS in 2000 and vice chairman of Iraqi national academy of science in 2004and also 93 was democratically elected president of Baghdad university in 2003.

Sami A.Al-Mudhaffar is one of the senior chemist (Biochemist) of Iraq. He is presently the member of Academy of science An organization employing the largest No. of scientists in Iraq and well known for its scientific excellence. He is also member of national of Iraqi Academy of science and Islamic Academy of science. Dr. Sami has also played an important role in promoting research in Iraq. In spite of enormous difficulties and numerous problems he has been largely successful in his endeavours to develop scientific tradition in the country and bringing the research level in certain areas at par with many of the advanced countries. His guidance and active participation in the promotion of scientific activities has resulted in the formation of a sound base for the growth of the scientific culture in the country. He established several specialized fields, such as clinical enzymology, hormones receptors, Tumor Markers, and has published over 250 research papers.

In sept. 1962, he proceeded to USA (University of Virginia Tech.) for advanced studies under merit assistantship awarded by this University. Dr. Al-Mudhaffar returned to Iraq in Sept. 1967 after obtaining the Ph.D. Degree. On return from abroad, he was posted in the University of Basrah on teaching and research assignment as a lecturer in college of science. In 1971, Dr. Sami was promoted as assistant Prof. And in 1979 as a Professor of Biochemistry in Baghdad University.

Dr. Sami A. Al-Mudhaffar is has played an important role in promoting Biochemistry and related subjects such as Molecular Biotechnology research in Iraq. He worked with complete dedication in research in Biochemical science. Dr.Al-Mudhaffar is mainly responsible for initiating and establishing many scientific and educational bilateral programmes with scientific organizations and laboratory of the advanced world.

From 1968 till 2004 Prof. Dr. Sami Al-Mudhaffar was lecturing to undergraduate and postgraduate students at the college of science, U. of Basrah and U. of Baghdad. He was a scientific supervisor of 150 Ph.D's and Msc. students in the field of Biochemistry and related subjects. He published more than 50 inventions and 250 scientific papers. He had so far over 44 years of teaching experience in different branches of Biochemistry to undergraduate and postgraduate students.

www.ingramcontent.com/pod-product-compliance
Lightning Source LLC
Chambersburg PA
CBHW081714220526
45468CB00008B/1839